Traditional Medicine

Traditional Medicine

A global perspective

Edited by

Steven B Kayne BSc, PhD, MBA, LLM, MSc, DAgVetPharm, FRPharmS, FCPP, FIPharmM, FFHom, MPS(NZ), FNZCP

Honorary Consultant Pharmacist, Glasgow Homeopathic Hospital;
Honorary Lecturer, University of Strathclyde School of Pharmacy, Glasgow, UK

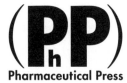

London • Chicago   **Pharmaceutical Press**

Published by the Pharmaceutical Press
An imprint of RPS Publishing

1 Lambeth High Street, London SE1 7JN, UK
100 South Atkinson Road, Suite 200, Grayslake, IL 60030–7820, USA

© Pharmaceutical Press 2010

(**PP**) is a trade mark of RPS Publishing
RPS Publishing is the publishing organisation of the Royal Pharmaceutical Society
of Great Britain

First published 2010

Typeset by New Leaf Design, Scarborough, North Yorkshire
Printed in Great Britain by TJ International, Padstow, Cornwall

ISBN 978 0 85369 833 3

Contents

Preface

My good friend, Dr Gill Scott, and I were sitting in the gardens of the Mount Nelson Hotel (affectionately known as 'The Nellie') in Cape Town discussing Traditional African Medicine. We both thought that it would be good to bring descriptions of a representative number of traditional medical systems together in one text, aimed at academics, students and interested members of the public. I was delighted when Gill immediately agreed to contribute a chapter.

Over one-third of the population in developing countries lack access to essential medicines. Countries in Africa, Asia and Latin America use traditional medicine to help meet some of their primary health care needs. In Africa, up to 80% of the population uses traditional medicine for primary health care. The provision of safe and effective Traditional Medicine Therapies could become a critical tool to increase access to health care. Migration, both within countries and across continents, means that host communities, in particular health care providers working in multicultural environments, may well come into contact with unfamiliar practices. A compact yet wide ranging source of knowledge such as that provided in this book will help them understand the basics of medical systems that are being used by patients, often concurrently with western medicine. However, health care providers need more than just knowledge, for it is necessary to understand and effectively interact with people across cultures. In short, there is a need to develop cultural competence. With this in mind a method by which orthodox health care providers can approach patients using their traditional practices in a sympathetic manner is introduced in Chapter 3. Although it specifically refers to North American aboriginal medicine it can be adapted to other health care environments.

This book covers medical systems practised on five continents, chosen to offer readers an awareness of different approaches to health care around the world. For example, Traditional Chinese Medicine and Ayurvedic medicine, two complete health systems that form the basis of almost all Asian medicine, are covered in detail, using material derived from both observation and published literature. Medicine from the Amazonian region of Colombia is presented through a series of fascinating interviews with local healers that emphasises the importance of ritualistic practice. In the African chapter the importance of using indigenous plants as remedies and the involvement of WHO are highlighted. Chapters on Japanese, Korean and Traditional Medicine in the Pacific provide an insight into the way other cultures have contributed to the development of their health care practices. Two chapters on folk medicine are also included: one covers the history and practice of secular and ecclesiastical practices with their origins across the continent of Europe, while the other seeks to demonstrate the wide ranging influence that a global religion can have on the health care of its believers.

I am grateful to my colleagues around the world for their generous support.

Steven Kayne
Glasgow
September 2009
steven.kayne@nhs.net

About the editor

Steven Kayne practised as a Community Pharmacist in Glasgow for more than 30 years before retiring from active practice in 1999. He is currently Honorary Consultant Pharmacist at Glasgow Homeopathic Hospital and Honorary Lecturer in CAM at the University of Strathclyde School of Pharmacy.

Dr Kayne was a member of the UK Advisory Board on the Registration of Homeopathic Products from its formation in 1994 until he retired in 2008, and currently serves on two other UK Government Expert Advisory Bodies: the Herbal Medicines Advisory Committee and the Veterinary Products Committee. He has also acted as an advisor to the WHO Collaborating Centre for Traditional Medicine.

As well as authoring, editing and contributing chapters to many books, Dr Kayne has written numerous papers and journal articles on a variety of topics associated with health care and has presented at conferences as an invited speaker on four continents. He is a member of the editorial advisory board of several journals, lectures to undergraduate and postgraduate students and acts as an Examiner, in the UK and overseas.

Contributors

Rosemary Beresford ONZM, BPharm, MSc, PhD

Rosemary Beresford began her career as a High School teacher, subsequently joining what is now the School of Pharmacy at Otago in 1982. She served as convenor of the University's distance learning programme, Associate Dean of Graduate Studies in Health Sciences, and finally Associate Dean of pharmacy admissions and undergraduate programmes before retiring in 2008. Dr Beresford's many academic and other contributions to the pharmacy profession in New Zealand were recognised by her appointment as an honorary member of the Pharmaceutical Society of New Zealand in 2004 and acceptance into the International Academy of History of Pharmacy in 2005. She was created an Officer of the New Zealand Order of Merit 'for services to medicine', in 2007. Dr Beresford currently holds honorary appointments as Associate Professor at the Universities of Hong Kong and Auckland.

Tony Booker MRSC, MRCHM, MBAC

Tony Booker has been practising Chinese medicine since 1994. He works as a practitioner in several clinics in Kent and maintains his own Chinese herbal dispensary integrated within an allopathic pharmacy. He has a particular interest in the treatment of debilitating conditions such as multiple sclerosis and rheumatoid arthritis. He is President of the Register of Chinese Herbal Medicine and, since 2005, has sat on the Herbal Medicines Advisory Committee.

Il-Moo Chang BSc, MSc, PhD

Il-Moo Chang is currently Director of the WHO Collaborating Center of Traditional Medicine, Chairman of the Technical Committee of Quality Assurance and Information, Forum on Harmonization of Herbal Medicines (FHH), and Director of the Korean Natural and Traditional Medicines Research Center. Professor Chang has written more than 120 research papers, 22 book chapters and monographs, including *Treatise on Asian Herbal Medicines* (9 volumes, 8804 pages).

Kenneth Collins MPhil, PhD, FRCGP

Kenneth Collins is a general practitioner with a special interest in medical history. He is a Research Fellow at the Centre for the History of Medicine at the University of Glasgow and has written widely on medical ethics, the medical aspects of Jewish immigration, and the medical practice of the great mediaeval physician and philosopher Rabbi Moses Maimonides.

Blanca Margarita Vargas de Corredor

Blanca Margarita Vargas de Corredor has spent over 30 years working on traditional medicine and conservation projects with different indigenous groups such as Uitotos, Muinanes, Andokes, Yukuna-Matapi, Tikuna, Cocama in the Caquetá medio region of the Colombian Amazon rain forest. Professor Vargas continues to co-direct the project 'Sabedores–sabedoras (wisemen/wisewomen) of the tropical rainforest' and is an associate researcher at the Centre for the Study of Religion and Politics (CSRP), University of St Andrews. She is cofounder of the Colombian 'Asociación para la Investigación Científica, Sociocultural y Ecológica (AICSE)'.

John K Crellin MSc, LRCP, MRCS, PhD

John Crellin's career spans three countries: the Wellcome Institute for the History of Medicine in the UK, Southern Illinois and Duke Universities in the USA, and Memorial University of Newfoundland, Canada, where he was John Clinch Professor of Medical History from 1988 until 2002. He currently teaches complementary and alternative medicine at the Faculty of Medicine, Memorial University of Newfoundland. His papers and books span a variety of topics, but with a sustained interest in the history of therapy from the eighteenth century onward, both conventional and complementary/alternative.

Owen Davies PhD

Owen Davies is Professor of Social History and Associate Head of School (Research) at the University of Hertfordshire, England. Much of his research has concerned the belief in the supernatural in the early modern and modern periods, which has led to work on popular medicine and interdisciplinary research applying anthropological and biomedical knowledge to historical topics. He has written chapters in several books and his latest book, published by Oxford University Press, is *Grimoires: A history of magic books*. His teaching specialisms include popular religion in Reformation Europe, crime and society in early modern England, landscape history and the history of European witchcraft, and custom and community in nineteenth-century England.

Bong Hyun Kim BSc, MSc, PhD

BH Kim received his degrees from Daegoo Hanny University, Daegoo, Korea, where, after internship and training at Seoul Hana Oriental Medicine Hospital, he became an instructor at the College of Oriental Medicine. Since 2004 he has been a Research Associate at Professor Il-Moo Chang's laboratory, Natural Products Research Institute, Seoul National University. Dr Kim is a specialist in acupuncture therapy.

Seon-Ho Kim OMD, PhD

From 1990 Seon-Ho Kim was based at the College of Oriental Medicine of Kyung-Hee University, Seoul, Korea. He is currently Adjunct Associate Professor at the Department of SMC of the College of Oriental Medicine, Kyung-Hee University, Director of Computer and Information, the Korean Society of SCM and Director of Oriental Medical Clinic, Suwon, Korea. He is Research Associate at Professor Il-Moo Chang's laboratory, Seoul National University and is an expert on Sasang Oriental Medicine, which is a unique theory of traditional medicine.

Ann Mitchell (Simpson) BSc, PhD, MRPharmS

Since 1987 Ann Mitchell has worked on traditional medicine and conservation projects with the anthropologist Blanca de Corredor with different indigenous groups such as Uitotos, Muinanes, Andokes, Yukuna-Matapí, Tikuna and Cocama in the Caquetá medio region of the Colombian Amazon rain forest. Ann is currently a teaching fellow at the Strathclyde Institute of Pharmacy and Biomedical Sciences, and a research fellow at St Mary's College, coordinating the Scottish–Colombia project at the Centre for the Study of Religion and Politics (CSRP), University of St Andrews. She is cofounder of the Colombian Asociación para la Investigación Científica, Sociocultural y Ecológica (AICSE)' and 'Fundación Biofuturo, Ecuador', which strives to work with communities on recuperation and preservation of the environment and recuperation of indigenous identity.

Gillian Scott BSc, PhD

Gillian Scott has an interest in plant species used as traditional medicines by indigenous South African peoples, particularly the Khoi-khoi and San. While employed at the then South African National Botanical Institute at Kirstenbosch, she was instrumental in the establishment of TRAMED (a traditional medicines programme for South Africa). She has worked since 1995 as a consultant in the field of African traditional medicines conservation, industrial development and application in formal healthcare. As an honorary research associate in the Department of Botany, University of Cape Town, she publishes regularly on aspects of traditional medicine research.

Haruki Yamada PhD

Haruki Yamada is the Director and a Professor at the Kitasato Institute for Life Sciences, and the Dean of the Graduate School of Infection Control Science, Kitasato University in Japan. He is also the Director of the research division of the Oriental Medicine Research Center at Kitasato University, and involved with the Scientific Advisory Board of Drugs for Neglected Diseases initiative (NDD*i*). He was former director of WHO Collaborating Center for Traditional Medicine at the Kitasato Institute. Professor Yamada received the Li-Fu Academic Award for Chinese Medicine in 1999 and an Academic Award of Medical and Pharmaceutical Society for WAKAN-YAKU (Traditional Medicine) in 2004. He is well known in the field of the scientific elucidation of Kampo medicines, and the bioactive polysaccharides from medicinal herbs.

1

Introduction to traditional medicine

Steven Kayne

Foolish the doctor who despises the knowledge acquired by the ancients.
Hippocrates

Almost 20 years ago the World Health Organization (WHO) estimated that 'In many countries, 80% or more of the population living in rural areas are cared for by traditional practitioners and birth attendants'.[1] It has since revised its view, adopting a rather safer position, now stating: 'most of the population of most developing countries regularly use traditional medicine.'[2] Whereas most people use traditional medicine in developing countries, only a minority have regular access to reliable modern medical services:[3]

- In China, traditional herbal preparations account for 30–50% of the total medicinal consumption.
- In Mexico the government is building regional health centres staffed by traditional healers who also receive training in how to detect diseases. The practitioners include traditional midwives (*parteras*), herbalists (*herbalistos*), bone-setters (*hueseros*) and spiritual healers (*curanderos* or *prayers*).
- In Ghana, Mali, Nigeria and Zambia, the first line of treatment for 60% of children with high fever resulting from malaria is the use of herbal medicines at home.
- In South Africa an estimated 250 000 traditional healers supply healthcare to around 80% of the black population using knowledge that dates back as far as 1000 BC.[4]
- In several African countries traditional birth attendants assist in most births according to WHO estimates.

- In industrialised nations some traditional therapies, in particular traditional Chinese medicine, and ayurveda, have become popular, diffusing out from immigrants into the host community.

Countries in Africa, Asia and Latin America use traditional medicine to help meet some of their primary healthcare needs. In Africa, up to 80% of the population use traditional medicine for primary healthcare. Over one-third of the population in developing countries lack access to essential medicines. Figure 1.1 shows the global distribution of traditional medicine, indicating which countries have specific policies as to its practice.

The provision of safe and effective traditional medicine therapies could become a critical tool to increase access to healthcare. In 2004 the South African Health Minister, Manto Tshabalala-Msimang, suggested that the use of African traditional medicines may eventually replace antiretrovirals in the treatment of HIV and AIDS.

In a number of industrialised countries many people regularly use some form of traditional complementary and alternative medicine (TCAM) with Germany (75%),[5] Canada (70%)[6] and England (47%)[7] being examples.

Definition

The WHO defines TCAM as referring to health practices, approaches, knowledge and beliefs incorporating plant-, animal- and mineral-based

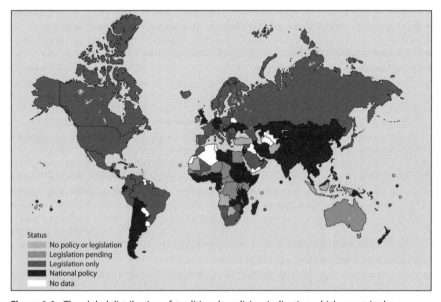

Figure 1.1 The global distribution of traditional medicine, indicating which countries have specific policies as to its practice. (Adapted from WHO *Global Atlas of Traditional, Complementary and Alternative Medicine*, Map Volume. Kobe, Japan: WHO Centre for Health Development, 2005: 49.)

medicines, spiritual therapies, manual techniques and exercises, applied singularly or in combination to treat, diagnose and prevent illnesses or maintain well-being.[2]

This definition makes no mention of the fact that the term 'traditional medicine' differs from other types of complementary and alternative medicine in that it is usually considered to be associated with discrete populations or geographical locations.

In this book the term 'traditional medicine' is used to describe:

> Health traditions originating in a particular geographic area or ethnic group and which may also have been adopted and/or modified by communities elsewhere.

Disciplines such as aromatherapy, medical herbalism, homoeopathy and others, usually known collectively as complementary and alternative medicine, are described in detail in a companion volume.[8]

The major traditional healing systems that have survived the impact of modern biomedicine driven by germ theory are traditional Chinese medicine and its associated therapies (see Chapter 6), Indian systems of medicine (see Chapter 7) and traditional African medicine (see Chapter 5).[9] The last differs from the two Asian systems in that it is largely an oral tradition with no written records whereas the Asian systems have written philosophies and pharmacopoeias.

The distinction between traditional medicine and what is known as folk medicine is not clear cut and the terms are often used interchangeably. Folk medicine may be defined as 'treatment of ailments outside clinical medicine by remedies and simple measures based on experience and knowledge handed down from generation to generation'. Another simpler definition is 'the use of home remedies and procedures as handed down by tradition'. In traditional medicine there is usually a formal consultation with a practitioner or healer and such practices may be integrated into a country's healthcare system, while in folk medicine advice is passed on more informally by a knowledgeable family member or friend and there is generally no such integration. Thus, acupuncture may be considered as being traditional medicine while the use of chicken soup – 'Jewish penicillin' – to manage poor health is folk medicine (see Chapter 11).

The role of medicines in traditional communities

The study of traditional medicines and their manufacture has much to offer to sociocultural studies of many medical systems. Medicines constitute a meeting point of almost any imaginable human interest: material, social, political and emotional.[10] They also play their many roles at different levels of social and political organisation: in international policy and funding, in national politics, and as vehicles of ideology and identity construction.[11] Ultimately medicines affect the private lives of individual patients, e.g. in the context of a consultation with the healthcare provider they are the conduit through which ill-health is transformed to good health. In the context of the family, buying a medicine for a relative can emit a message of love and care. Within a religious context medicines may be seen as gifts to the ailing community from holy leaders.

WHO activities in traditional medicine

The driving force for traditional medicine is provided by the people who use it. However, the ability of governments in the developing world to implement the opportunities offered by traditional medicine is, in many instances, beyond their capability. WHO initiatives are crucial in stimulating traditional healthcare.

The International Conference on Primary Health Care, meeting in Alma-Ata on 12 September 1978, declared a need for urgent action by all governments, all health and development workers, and the world community to protect and promote the health of all the people of the world.[12] The goal of the Alma-Ata Declaration was health for all by the year 2000 through promotion and strengthening of systems based on primary healthcare. The Alma-Ata Declaration was especially significant for traditional medicine. Although traditional medicine has been used for thousands of years and the associated practitioners have made great contributions to human health, it was not until the Alma-Ata Declaration that countries and governments were called upon to include traditional medicine in their primary health systems for the first time, and to recognise the associated practitioners of traditional medicine as a part of the healthcare team, particularly for primary healthcare at the community level. It was at this time that the WHO's Traditional Medicine Programme was established.

The main objectives of the WHO programme are:

- to facilitate integration of traditional medicine into the national healthcare system by assisting Member States to develop their own national policies on traditional medicine
- to promote the proper use of traditional medicine by developing and providing international standards, technical guidelines and methodologies
- to act as a clearing house to facilitate information exchange in the field of traditional medicine.

Many Member States and many of WHO's partners in traditional medicine (UN agencies, international organisations, nongovernmental organisations [NGOs], and global and national professional associations) contributed to a Strategy for the WHO and expressed their willingness to participate in its implementation. The Strategy was reviewed by the WHO Cabinet in July 2001 and, after Cabinet comments, was revised before being printed in January 2002. In 2003, the 56th World Health Assembly called on countries to adopt and implement the Strategy.[13] The Strategy advocates national policies and regulations, drug-safety monitoring systems, measures to protect knowledge of traditional medicine and plant resources and, where appropriate, the intellectual property rights of traditional practitioners.

Traditional medicine in practice

The following two examples will serve to illustrate studies on the practice of traditional medicine. The first study aimed to highlight the new or lesser known medicinal uses of plant bioresources along with validation of traditional knowledge that is widely used by the tribal communities to cure four common ailments in the Lahaul-Spiti region of western Himalaya.[5] The study area inhabited by Lahaulas and Bodhs (also called Bhotias) is situated in the cold arid zone of the state of Himachal Pradesh (HP), India. During the ethnobotanical explorations (2002–6), observations on the most common ailments, such as rheumatism, stomach problems, liver and sexual disorders, among the natives of Lahaul-Spiti were recorded. Due to strong belief in the traditional system of medicine, people still prefer to use herbal medicines prescribed by local healers. A total of 58 plant species belonging to 45 genera and 24 families, have been reported from the study area to cure these diseases. Maximum use of plants is reported to cure stomach disorders (29), followed by rheumatism (18), liver problems (15) and sexual ailments (9). Among the plant parts used, leaves were found most widely in herbal preparations (20), followed by flowers (12) and roots (11), respectively. Most of these formulations were prescribed in powder form, although juice and decoction forms were also used. Plants with more than one therapeutic use were represented by 24 species; however, 34 species have been reported to be used against a single specific ailment. Validation of observations revealed 38 lesser known or new herbal preparations from 34 plant species, where 15 species were used to cure stomach disorders, 7 for rheumatism, 10 for liver disorders and 6 for sexual problems. Mode of preparation, administration and dosage are discussed along with the family and local names of plants and plant parts used.

The second study investigated the use of traditional herbal medicine by AIDS patients in Kabarole District, western Uganda.[14] Using systematic sampling, 137 AIDS patients were selected from outpatient departments of 3 hospitals and interviewed via questionnaire. The questions related to such areas as type and frequency of herbal medicine intake, concomitant herb–pharmaceutical drug use (including herb–antiretroviral drug cotherapy) and the perceived effectiveness of herbal medicine. Overall, 63.5% of AIDS patients had used herbal medicine after HIV diagnosis. Same-day herbal medicine and pharmaceutical drug use was reported by 32.8% of AIDS patients. Patterns of traditional herbal medicine use were quite similar between those on antiretroviral therapy and those who received supportive therapy only. The primary conclusion is that AIDS outpatients commonly use herbal medicine for the treatment of HIV/AIDS.

When many people from developing countries of the world emigrate, they continue to seek medical advice from traditional practitioners working in their own communities, even in countries where all citizens have free access to good-quality western medicine.[15] They have difficulties adjusting to a new lifestyle, let alone to a new system of medicine. It is not surprising that they turn to their own healers, who emigrated before them and practise healthcare much the same as they did in their home countries. Although the main reasons for this are probably cultural and linguistic, the role of mistrust and fear should also be acknowledged. However, the situation is complex. Despite gaining skills that help immigrants improve their socio-economic status and overcome barriers to the mainstream host healthcare system, their health status may still decline as acculturation increases. Waldheim suggests that migration need not always lead to disease.[16] Working with Mexican immigrants in the USA she concluded that the maintenance of a Mexican culture that is distinct from the rest of American society helps ensure that traditional medical knowledge is not lost, whereas the social networks that link Mexicans to each other and to their homeland help minimise threats to health, which are usually associated with migration. Thus, increased access to professional medical care may not improve the health of migrants if it comes with the loss of traditional medical knowledge.

The ethnic medical systems embrace philosophies very different to those of the west. They are derived from a sensitive awareness of the laws of nature and the order of the universe. Practised according to traditional methods, their aim is to maintain health as well as to restore it. The ideas are complex and require much study to grasp their significance and the nuances of practice.

Traditional medical systems are challenging because their theories and practices strike many conventionally trained physicians and researchers as incomprehensible. Should modern medicine dismiss them as unscientific, view them as sources of alternatives hidden in a matrix of superstition or regard them as complementary sciences of medicine?[17]

National policies for traditional medicine

There has been intense debate on public health issues associated with traditional medicine in many parts of the world. The focus is to determine the most appropriate official policy towards traditional medicines. Some countries have policies that discourage traditional medicines, whereas others have supportive policies. Most countries do not have official policies and have simply left traditional medicines to individuals to decide.[18] For indigenous peoples, the existence of traditional medicine policies is crucial. The ability to use and control their own, culturally defined, traditional health system is the most fundamental right of self-determination of 'fourth world' peoples.

Figure 1.2 shows those countries of the world that have policies and legislation covering the practice of traditional medicine.

Asia

In Asia medical pluralism – the use of multiple forms of healthcare – is widespread. Consumers practise integrated healthcare irrespective of whether integration is officially present. In Taiwan, 60% of the public use multiple healing systems, including modern western medicine, Chinese medicine and religious healing. A survey in two village health clinics in China's Zheijang province showed that children with upper respiratory tract infections were being prescribed an average of four separate drugs, always in a combination of western and Chinese medicine.[19] The challenge of integrated healthcare is to generate evidence on which illnesses are best treated through which approach. The Zheijang study found that simultaneous use of both types of treatment was so commonplace that their individual contributions were difficult to assess.

Asia has seen much progress in incorporating its traditional health systems into national policy. Most of this began 30–40 years ago and has accelerated in the past 10 years. In some countries, such as China, the development has been a response to mobilising all healthcare resources to meet national objectives for primary healthcare. In other countries, such as India and South Korea, change has come through politicisation of the traditional health sector and a resultant change in national policy.

Two basic policy models have been followed: an integrated approach, where modern and traditional medicine are integrated through medical education and practice (e.g. China), and a parallel approach, where modern and traditional medicine are separate within the national health system (e.g. India).

Africa

In Africa the heads of state and government of the then Organization of African Unity (OAU) recognised that about 85% of the African population resort to it for their health delivery needs.[20] In 2001, the OAU declared a

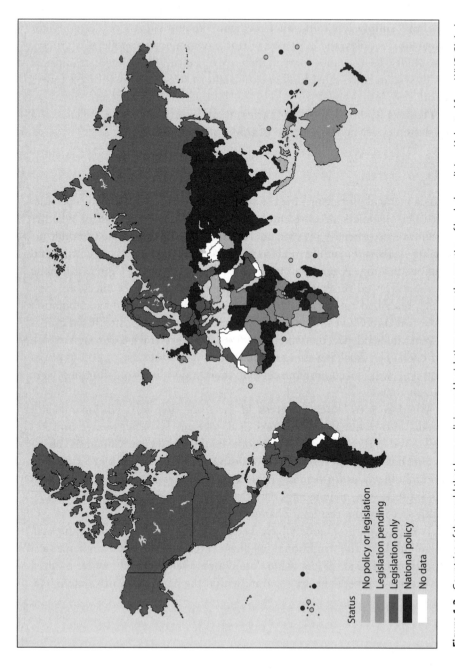

Figure 1.2 Countries of the world that have policies and legislation covering the practice of herbal medicine. (Adapted from WHO *Global Atlas of Traditional, Complementary and Alternative Medicine, Map Volume.* Kobe, Japan: WHO Centre for Health Development, 2005: 12.)

Decade of Traditional Medicine. After this landmark commitment by African leaders, the First AU Session of the Conference of African Ministers of Health (CAMH1), held in April 2003 in Tripoli, Libya, adopted the Plan of Action and implementation mechanism that was endorsed by the AU summit heads of state and government in Maputo in 2003. The main objective of the Plan of Action is the recognition, acceptance, development and integration/institutionalisation of traditional medicine by all Member States into the public healthcare system in the region by 2010. Moreover, the Maputo Declaration on Malaria, HIV/AIDS and Other Related Infectious Diseases (ORID) of July 2003 further resolved to continue supporting the implementation of the Plan of Action for the AU Decade of African Traditional Medicine (2001–10), especially research in the area of treatment for HIV/AIDS, tuberculosis (TB), malaria and ORID. In July of the same year, the Lusaka Summit declared the period 2001–10 as the OAU Decade for African Traditional Medicine. The 11 priority areas, which have been developed as strategic activities, are:

- Sensitisation of the society to traditional medicine
- Legislation of traditional medicine
- Institutional arrangements
- Information, education and communication
- Resource mobilisation
- Research and training
- Cultivation and conservation of medicinal plants
- Protection of traditional medical knowledge
- Local production of standardised African traditional medicines (SATMs)
- Partnerships
- Evaluation, monitoring and reporting mechanisms.

Since 2001, AU Member States have been implementing the plan of action of the AU Decade of African Traditional Medicine and the priority interventions of the WHO regional strategy, namely policy formulation, capacity building, research promotion, development of local production including cultivation of medicinal plants and protection of traditional medical knowledge and intellectual property rights.

Commonwealth

Key policy issues in integration have been outlined by Commonwealth health ministers.[15] Ministers established the Commonwealth Working Group on Traditional and Complementary Health Systems to promote and integrate traditional health systems and complementary medicine into national healthcare.

Europe

Unfortunately, at the present time it is generally recognised that regulation of traditional systems of medicine, the products used in traditional systems and the practitioners of these systems is very weak in most countries.[21] Despite being made up of 27 European Member States in which a significant proportion (at least 33%) of the population use non-orthodox medicine (including traditional medicine) as part of their healthcare provision, the EU currently has hardly any policies that specifically refer to traditional therapies. In 1997 the European Parliament adopted a resolution that called for steps to regulate and promote research in 'non-conventional medicine', including Chinese herbal medicine and shiatsu.[22] The report's rapporteur, Paul Lanoye MEP, was so disappointed in the way that the report had been weakened by negative amendments that he abandoned it at the last minute and forced the Parliament's Chairman at the time, Mr Collins, to add his name to it to enable it to be adopted.

One of the main reasons for this is that the EU Treaties are worded so as to protect the area of healthcare delivery as the responsibility of individual member states.

The lack of regulation leads to misuse of the medicines by unqualified practitioners and loss of credibility of the system. In traditional medicine, practitioners and manufacturers (particularly the small ones) usually oppose any steps to strengthen regulation by the health administration. Their fears are that regulation such as applies to allopathic medicine is not suitable for traditional medicine. The World Health Organization has initiated an effort in this direction and may be the appropriate body to help countries not only to develop a regulatory system but to take steps to meet the obligations under the Trade-related Intellectual Property Rights Agreement, when this became applicable in developing countries in 2005. It means that traditional healers (*hakkims*) who have come to the UK may practise within a culture that is oblivious to the highly regulated status of western medicine. Healthcare providers should be vigilant to ensure that any risks to patients are minimised.

All the foregoing may seem to indicate that integrating traditional and western medicine is at best difficult and at worst impossible. Most of the remarks in this chapter are directed at Chinese and Asian medicine, these two systems being the two traditional disciplines that health care providers are most likely to meet in the UK. It should be noted that traditional medicines in other cultures also flourish and many are integrated into local healthcare. In their own countries Australian Aboriginals,[23] New Zealand Maoris,[24] North American Indians,[25,26] Africans,[27,28] Pacific Islanders[29] and the peoples of Latin America[30] continue to make important contributions to their national cultures and fulfilling healthcare needs.

Each culture has its own range of remedies, although some elements are common to all. One notable success to cross the cultural divide is an essential oil obtained from the Tea tree (*Melaleuca alternifolia*) native to Australia. The oil is claimed to be anti-fungal, and antibiotic, and is used topically. It has become a popular and effective remedy in Europe.

Traditional healers may be called shamans. They practise a method of healing that is supplemented by rituals and explanatory systems appropriate to their particular culture and environment. The healing often includes meditation, prayer, chanting and traditional music (e.g. Celtic drumming), together with the administration of herbal, and occasionally orthodox, remedies.

Evidence

Scientific evidence is available only for the many uses of acupuncture, some herbal medicines and some of the manual therapies. Further research is urgently needed to ascertain the efficacy and safety of several other practices and medicinal plants.

The limited scientific evidence about the safety of traditional medicine and its efficacy, as well as other considerations, make it important for governments to:[2]

- formulate national policy and regulation for the proper use of traditional medicine/CAM and its integration into national healthcare systems in line with the provisions of the WHO strategies on traditional medicines
- establish regulatory mechanisms to control the safety and quality of products and of traditional medicine/CAM practice
- create awareness about safe and effective traditional medicine/CAM therapies among the public and consumers
- cultivate and conserve medicinal plants to ensure their sustainable use.

Safety

The globalisation of traditional medicine has important implications for both the quality control of medicaments and the training and competence of practitioners.[31] Furthermore, when traditional healthcare procedures are incorporated into complementary and alternative medicine in industrialised countries there is an increased need for vigilance. The WHO has issued a number of documents relevant to the safety of traditional healthcare (available at http://tinyurl.com/pgog8f).

Factors affecting safety

The following safety matters are a source of concern in ethnic medicine: training, uncontrolled products and concurrent therapy.

Training

Practitioners' training varies widely, raising concerns for the quality of the treatment being offered. Little is being done currently to regulate the delivery of traditional healthcare.

Uncontrolled medicinal products

Large amounts of traditional medicines are imported into the UK, legally and illegally, and use of such medicines is frequently not admitted when serious illness forces patients to consult western medical practitioners. These medicines carry with them a risk of adverse reactions; the risk needs to be quantified and as far as possible minimised. Examples of intrinsic toxicity and quality issues associated with traditional Chinese and ayurvedic medicines are described in detail in Chapters 6 and 7. Kava-kava (see Chapter 10) is a recreational herb used widely by Pacific Islanders. It has been banned in Europe, the UK and Canada due to concerns over liver toxicity, although the link has not been proved irrefutably. There are an estimated 250 million people around the world using the herb each year. However, it is claimed that, in almost all cases, the adverse effects have not been definitely attributed to kava-kava and in most cases they were associated with liver damage from alcohol or pharmaceutical drugs. Kava-kava has been reported by researchers at the University of Queensland as being safe and effective at reducing anxiety and improving mood.[32] These results may prompt a future reassessment of the drug by regulatory authorities.

An issue under discussion by European regulatory authorities is whether the proposed herbal medicines directive (see Chapter 6) should extend to traditional medicines containing non-herbal ingredients, such as those used in Chinese and ayurvedic medicine.

The UK Medicines and Healthcare products Regulatory Agency (MHRA) established an ethnic medicines forum to encourage and assist the UK ethnic medicines sector to achieve improvements to safety and quality standards in relation to unlicensed ethnic medicines, in advance of any improvements to the statutory regime that might emerge from current policy initiatives. Representatives of ayurvedic and traditional Chinese medicine suppliers, manufacturers and practitioners in the UK form part of this forum, as well as the MHRA and other bodies in the herbal medicines sector with experience of operating self-regulatory arrangements.

One issue identified by the forum is the lack of understanding of existing law by some of those operating in the ethnic medicines sector. The document

Traditional Ethnic Medicines: Public health and compliance with medicines law, published on the MHRA website, highlights problem areas.[33] It aims to help consumers make an informed choice and seeks to assist businesses and practitioners to understand certain aspects of medicines law.

Concurrent therapy

Patients with chronic or recurrent conditions are particularly vulnerable because they tend to lose confidence in conventional medicine and resort to self-medication without informing their general practitioner.

What needs to be done to ensure the safety of traditional medicine?

There can be no doubt that safety issues are of extreme concern as the use of traditional therapies increases in a largely uncontrolled manner. Travel by tourists and business people to long-haul destinations has brought increasing numbers of people into contact with other cultures.

Immigration brings different cultures to enrich our own. Whether you consider traditional medicine to have a part to play in modern medicine is for you alone to decide.

The risks of participating in traditional Chinese medicine or ayurveda are certainly outweighed by the many benefits that are reported. Adverse reactions are relatively rare, although when they do happen they can be very severe. Perhaps the best solution is to control the practice, improve training and license the medicines. However, there are problems in establishing these ideals.

Practitioners of traditional medicine certainly need to be more aware of the problems of toxicity. In particular, they must learn that infrequent adverse drug reactions will not be recognised without a formal system of reporting. They must participate in such a scheme, and consideration should be given by the MHRA in the UK to making such reporting compulsory, as it is in Germany and China. This is a significant deficiency and, until a formal mandatory system of reporting adverse reactions for traditional medicine becomes available, healthcare providers should be aware of the potential difficulties, advise the public of the dangers whenever necessary, and record and report any problems promptly in the mainstream literature.

Practitioners of orthodox and traditional medicine need to be aware of the occurrence and dangers of dual treatment. Patients need to appreciate that they must disclose exactly what they are taking; such information should be recorded carefully because, as stated above, there is a risk that patients will receive simultaneous western and traditional treatments, particularly when self-treating. This may require a sympathetic non-judgemental approach to questioning. Purchasers of traditional medicines should be advised accordingly.

All practitioners who offer traditional medicines need thorough training and continuing education.[2] Great attention has been paid to the quality of training and further education in orthodox western medicine, and it is time to police more carefully the practice of traditional medicine in the UK. For European herbal medicine this should be easy. The training establishments are situated in the UK, which makes guaranteeing standards and limiting the right to practise to those who are thoroughly trained relatively straightforward. It is much more difficult in the case of traditional Chinese and Indian medicine, because full training cannot currently be obtained in the UK. Verifying the quality of the training given in China and India by identifying appropriate qualifications and recognising them seems prudent. Practitioners who are not qualified should be barred from practice in the UK, and policing this would clearly require a powerful registration body. Ultimately, the creation of academic establishments in the UK, where such training could be given under appropriate regulation, should be considered.

Traditional medicine and the orthodox healthcare provider

Many healthcare providers may not relish the thought of taking a proactive interest in traditional medicine. However, given their role within the multicultural society in which most of us live, the possibilities of coming into contact with traditional Chinese medicine and ayurvedic medicine is possible for a number of reasons:

- concern over interactions between traditional remedies and orthodox medicines
- concern over using traditional remedies during pregnancy
- concern over intrinsic toxicity of traditional remedies and cosmetics, and the safety of some procedures
- the necessity of considering and understanding a patient's total healthcare status when designing pharmaceutical care plans.

The practice of traditional medicine involves concepts with which people in the west are generally unfamiliar. It may be that, with more understanding of the therapies involved, some can be incorporated into our own procedures, e.g. our focus on treating illness could be shifted more towards maintaining health – a process that has already started. We may be able to understand better the needs of our immigrant communities and perhaps use approaches with which they feel more comfortable. A three-step process to assist orthodox healthcare providers in their approach to traditional medicine is presented in Chapter 3.

Biodiversity and sustainability[34]

Environmental awareness

It is estimated that up to 40% of all pharmaceuticals in industrialised countries are derived from natural sources. In the USA about 2% of prescriptions written by healthcare providers are for drugs that have natural ingredients, are synthetic copies or have artificially modified forms of natural chemicals. The search continues for more therapeutically active plant-sourced materials, not always to the satisfaction of host communities.

Two centuries ago, orthodox medicine was offering digitalis and laudanum, but now there are thousands of powerful, efficacious drugs that save lives somewhere almost every second of the day.[35] However, modern drugs struggle to make much impact on the rise in cancer, heart disease and other afflictions of the industrialised world.

This lack of efficacy, together with patients' growing unease over side effects of synthetic drugs, has coincided with an international growth in environmental awareness, particularly concern about the depletion of natural resources. In turn, this has led to a greater sensitivity to the delicate symbiotic balance that exists in nature.

Disappearing rainforests

Unfortunately the rain-forest is being destroyed at such a rate that thousands of species may become extinct before their medicinal potential can be examined. Five thousand years ago the rainforest covered 2 billion hectares, or 14% of the earth's land surface. Now only half remains, but it is inhabited by 50% of all the plants and animals found on the globe.[36] Humans are continuing to destroy an area equivalent to 20 football fields every day, a rate that if maintained will cause the rainforest to vanish by 2030. Slash-and-burn agriculture accounts for 50% of the annual loss. This is a primitive system that involves cutting down a patch of forest and setting the timber alight to release phosphorus, nitrogen, potassium and other nutrients. The resulting ash fertilises the sod, which will then support crops for 2 or 3 years. After this time the land becomes barren, necessitating the clearing of another patch of forest. Logging is a second major cause of forest destruction. In 1990, 3.5 billion cubic metres of tropical wood were felled throughout the world, more than half for fuel sources.

Trees are also consumed for their important products, e.g. India earns US$125m annually from its production of perfumes, essential oils, flavourings, resins and pharmaceuticals. The petroleum nut tree (*Pittosporum resiniferum*) yields oil that can power engines as well as provide a homoeopathic remedy. Other examples are the bark of the Cinchona tree which gives the antimalarial quinine (also known as *china*), products of immense historical significance to homoeopathy. In Madagascar, common *Cantharanthus* (Vinca) species are exploited for the anti-cancer drugs vinblastine and vincristine, two naturally occurring alkaloids isolated in the early 1960s by the pharmaceutical company Eli Lilly. Although there is no fear of these particular plants becoming extinct, serious damage has been done to the ecosystem of which they are a part.

Growing demand

Curare, the South American poisonous vine extract, is a muscle relaxant. In fact, the Amazon Indians use at least 1000 plants medicinally. In Malaysia and Indonesia more than twice this number of plant materials are used to make *jamu*, the traditional medicine. But it is not only in the developing world where there are problems. Germany, the largest European medicinal plant importer, is also a major exporter of finished herbal products, accounting for at least 70% of the European market.

A patent taken out by a US company in 1999 angered Indian scientists and ecology experts greatly. They were furious at what they considered to be the raiding of their country's storehouse of traditional knowledge.[37] The Americans were granted a patent on a composition of bitter gourd, eggplant and jamun, the fruit of the rose-apple tree, which is abundant all over India during the summer months. The use of these substances to treat diabetes dates back many centuries and is mentioned in many ancient texts on healing. Other indigenous Indian herbal products on which patents have been taken out include mustard seeds (used for bronchial and rheumatic complaints), Indian gooseberry (coughs, asthma, jaundice and wounds) and neem (pesticidal, dermatological and antibacterial properties). The last has attracted dozens of patent applications. It is probably the most celebrated medicinal tree in India.

A World Wide Fund for Nature (WWF) report warns that the enormous market demand could have an irreversible impact on many species unless action is taken to regulate trade,[38] e.g. the terpenoid taxol can be made semi-synthetically from one or more of the constituents of *Taxus baccata*, a yew tree that grows among pine forests at around 3000 m in the Himalayas. Taxol is of use in the treatment of ovarian and breast cancer. Pharmaceutical companies have stripped forest areas of this species and available trees in a bid to meet the demand for this drug. One cause of the problem was an earlier unconsidered arbitrary decimation of the yew tree population. In 1977 the plant was not considered important enough even to be included in a book on trees, but within 15 years it had become an endangered species.

According to a newspaper report, more South Africans are using traditional muti made from plants or animals, driving some species to extinction and pushing up prices.[39] The traditional medicine trade in South Africa is a large and growing industry, the authors of the report said. There are 27 million consumers of traditional medicines and the trade contributes an estimated ZAR2.9bn (£0.23bn, €0.27bn, US$0.39bn) to the national economy. At least 771 plant species are known to be used for traditional medicine, including scarce species that fetch up to ZAR4800 (£387, €441, US$637) a kilogram. It is estimated that 86% of the plant parts harvested will result in death of the plant with significant implications for the sustainability of supply.

The WWF report reviews the data available on medicinal plant trade and cites the urgent need for further investigation. One problem is that it is often difficult to decide whether the medicinal plant imports are derived from cultivated or wild specimens. Brazil, China and Nepal have conservation programmes, but India and Pakistan still harvest from the wild, and little is known of the ecological impact of such trade.

Climate changes

As well as the direct threat to plants from humans through their actions on the habitat or by exhausting the plant stock, there are other more natural factors such as climate, although it has to be said that this may well have been changed as a result of human action also. Scientific tests at Canberra's Australian National University have proved a link between stunted plant growth and higher ultraviolet radiation caused by depletion of the earth's protective ozone layer. This depletion is being caused by synthetic chemicals, especially chlorofluorocarbons (CFCs) found in products such as air-conditioners and foam packaging.[40] Since the late 1970s the use of CFCs has been heavily regulated. In 1990, diplomats met in London and voted to call for a complete elimination of CFCs by the year 2000. By the year 2010 CFCs should have been completely eliminated from developing countries as well.

Changes in climate from global warming as a result of the greenhouse effect are also important. However, it is unclear how long-term changes in the composition of the mix of atmospheric gases, soil structure, or pest and disease patterns will affect the capacity of plants to manufacture the important active principles for which we currently rely on them. There are some successes; after the increased use of natural gas and low-sulphur fuels, the amount of sulphur dioxide in the atmosphere has fallen. Some plants may adopt a different habitat, e.g. *Arnica montana* usually grows in alpine regions, but has been known to flourish in milder climates too.

At the same time, ammonia concentrations have risen, with the effect of changing the pH of rootwater and directly affecting the chances of plants to survive in some habitats.[41]

Tackling the problem

Awareness

In Britain, John Evelyn (1620–1706) was the first to warn about the fact that its native trees were disappearing faster than they could grow. Evelyn's *Sylva* published in 1664, became the tree growers' handbook for two centuries.[42] Collecting is a threat to some rare plants; others are affected by the trampling feet of hikers or climbers. At risk from this danger are plant species on the sea coast and hilly areas. The greatest number of endangered species (38) are those of lowland pasture, open grassland and other natural open habitats.[43] Examples of UK endangered or vulnerable species with herbal or homoeopathic applications include species of rock cinquefoil *(Potentilla rupestris)*, Jersey cudweed *(Gnaphalium luteo-album)*, gentians *(Gentians* spp.), rough marshmallow *(Althaea officinalis)* and purple spurge *(Euphorbia peplis)*.

Working with local population

Perhaps the most important way to conserve resources is to work closely with the people who live in and use the forest, the indigenous population, rubber tappers, ranchers, loggers, etc. to strike a balance between the extremes of conservation and exploitation that will protect species and threatened environments while still fostering economic development and reducing poverty. Finding alternative uses for crops is one solution – the town of Aukre in Brazil is making money harvesting Brazil nut oil for the Body Shop set up by the late Anita Roddick.

Redevelopment

Another solution is finding use for the deforested areas. The return of large-scale cattle ranching is even a possibility, provided that grass can be grown for fodder, and programmes of continuing education to encourage better forestry management and appropriate legislation, such as the US Endangered Species Act 1973 and the British Wildlife and Countryside Act 1981. A total of 332 plants were either listed or proposed for listing, under the latter, from 1985 to 1991. It has been suggested that companies should fund forest protection schemes by putting cash up in exchange for exploitation rights. US$1m has been invested by an American drug company in a pilot scheme in Costa Rica. However, the costs are enormous, running into billions of dollars just to preserve resources solely for the pharmaceutical industry. Some of Britain's rarest wild flowers are likely to be encouraged to make a return as a result of an EC Set Aside scheme.[44] The reduction in the cropped area of over 450 thousand hectares between 1992 and 1993 was mainly as a result of the impact of EC Set Aside schemes, which were established to reduce the amount of agricultural land in arable production. The first of these schemes, the Five-Year Scheme, was introduced in 1988. This scheme was superseded in 1992 by the Arable Area Payments Scheme (AAPS), which included a compulsory set-aside requirement except for the smallest farmers. A reduction in the area of land set aside in the UK in 1996–7 was generally attributed to the reduction in payments made to farmers under the Set Aside scheme; however, between 1998 and 1999 the amount of land set aside increased by over 250 000 hectares as a result of the reintroduction of the grants. Other agri-environment schemes make payments for the adoption of agricultural practices to conserve wildlife habitats, and historical, archaeological and landscape features, and to improve opportunities for countryside enjoyment. Support is also provided for a variety of capital works.

Strategic approach

The WHO launched its first-ever comprehensive traditional medicine strategy in 2002 (see earlier).

Plant alternatives

Chemical synthesis would cut down the amount of plant material consumed in extraction processes. Ideally, pharmaceutical companies require novel, single, active molecules that can be made in a laboratory. Although this may be possible for some allopathic drugs, the activity of most crude extracts can seldom be attributed to a single molecule, but is usually the result of several compounds acting in synergy, making production of synthetic copies extremely difficult. Medical herbalists are obliged to use the original source material to protect this unique mix of active principles. Furthermore, the holistic principles of herbal medicine suggest that the relative concentrations of useful plant chemicals achieved by mixing different species together in individualised prescriptions are important in treating patients despite the general lack of standardisation. We know little about the interactive abilities of naturally occurring chemicals, much to the consternation of our orthodox colleagues whose demands are for purified, fully characterised medicines given in regulated doses. Homoeopaths need to use naturally occurring source materials too, complete with any inherent impurities, so that modern drug pictures can be assumed to match exactly with Hahnemann's own work.

There is also the possibility of creating a problem of another kind by following the synthesis strategy. The isolation of the chemical diosgenin, from the Mexican *Dioscorea* species in the 1940s, led to a booming steroid industry in that country. As sophisticated isolation, separation and elucidation techniques developed, the requirement for this particular raw material fell away completely and with it went the accompanying industry, causing widespread local social deprivation. *Dioscorea* continues to be used by homoeopaths.

There is some irony in the fact that the largest pharmaceutical companies in the world are scouring the South American rainforests increasingly, seeking natural sources for drug products.[45] Estimates of the 'hit' rate from random screening programmes vary widely, but are put between 1 in 1000 and 1 in 10 000. The chances of finding active plant extracts is greatly increased by studying the use of plants by various cultures, and the discipline of 'ethnobotany' is growing slowly. Table 1.1 lists a number of orthodox drugs that originally came to scientific attention as a result of ethnobotanical studies

Success story

Ginkgo biloba (Figure 1.3) is a unique survivor from the Jurassic dinosaur era some 190 million years ago; all of its related species have long since died out. The tree has survived in cultivation because of its valuable fruit and wood and possibly because it was planted in temples. It was introduced to Europe from its native China in 1730 and was heading for extinction until fortuitous intervention saved it. Extracts are used in Chinese herbalism under the name *baguo* to treat hypertension.

Table 1.1 Orthodox drugs derived from plants	
Medicine	**Plant**
Atropine	*Atropa belladonna*
Cocaine	*Erythroxylum coca*
Colchicine	*Colchicum autumnale*
Digoxin	*Digitalis purpurea*
Ephedrine	*Ephedra sinica*
Hyoscyamine	*Hyoscymus niger*
Morphine	*Papaver somniferum*
Pilocarpine	*Pilocarpus jaborandi*
Quinine	*Cinchona legeriana*
Strychnine	*Strychnos nux vomica*
Theobromine	*Theobroma cacao*

It is no consolation that complementary practitioners are the cause of the problems, for our uses are but a fraction of the total requirements. It would be unforgivable if future generations were to suffer because remedies disappeared due to the actions of others. We must work out a compromise in plenty of time.

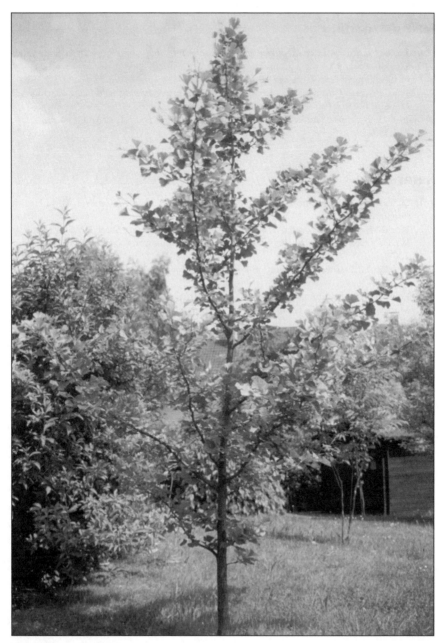

Figure 1.3 *Ginkgo biloba* tree.

More information

Botanic Gardens Conservation International: www.bgci.org
European Herbal and Traditional Medicine Practitioners Association: www.ehpa.eu

Further reading

Hawkins B. *Plants for Life: Medicinal plant conservation and botanic gardens*. Richmond, London: Botanic Gardens Conservation International, 2008. Available at: www.bgci.org/medicinal/medplants (accessed 10 May 2008).

Waylen K. *Botanic Gardens: Using biodiversity to improve human well-being*. Richmond, London: Botanic Gardens Conservation International, 2006.

Williamson E. Systems of traditional medicine from South and South East Asia. *Pharm J* 2006; **276**:539–40.

References

1. Bannerman RH. *Traditional Medicine and Healthcare Coverage*. Geneva: World Health Organization, 1983.
2. World Health Organization. *Traditional Medicine*. WHO Fact Sheet No. 134. Geneva: WHO, revised 2003. Available at: http://tinyurl.com/5mrd5 (accessed 11 December 2008).
3. Bodeker G. Lessons on integration from the developing world's experience. *BMJ* 2001; **322**:164–7.
4. Edinburg TL. Traditional medicines in South Africa. *Pharm J* 1998;**261**:242–4.
5. Marstedt G, Mochus S. *Gesundheitsberichte Bundes – Heft 9 Inanspruchnahme Alternativer Methoden in der Medicin (Health Report by the Federal Government Issue 9 – Use of Alternative Methods in Medicine)*. Berlin: Robert Koch Institut StatischesBudesamt, 2002.
6. Health Canada. *Perspectives on complementary and alternative health care*. A collection of papers prepared for Health Canada. Ottawa: Health Canada, 2001.
7. Thomas KJ, Nicholl JP, Coleman P. Use and expenditure on complementary medicine in England: a population based study. *Complement Ther Med* 2001;**9**:2–11.
8. Kayne SB, ed. *Complementary and Alternative Medicine*, 2nd edn. London: Pharmaceutical Press, 2008.
9. Okpako D. African medicine: Tradition and beliefs. *Pharm J* 2006;**276**:239–40.
10. Geest S van der. Anthropology and the pharmaceutical nexis. *Anthropol Q* 2006; **79**:303–14.
11. Bode M. Taking traditional knowledge to the market IIAS. *Newsletter* Autumn 2007. Available at www.iias.nl/nl/45/IIAS_NL45_23.pdf (accessed 10 May 2009).
12. Declaration of Alma-Ata International Conference on Primary Health Care, Alma-Ata, USSR, 6–12 September 1978. Available at: www.who.int/hpr/NPH/docs/declaration_almaata.pdf. (accessed 16 January 2009).
13. WHO. Traditional Medicine WHO Highlights 2003, Assembly. Available at: www.who.int/features/2003/05b/en (accessed 17 December 2008).
14. Langlois-Klassen D, Kipp W, Jhangri GS, Rubaale T. Use of traditional herbal medicine by AIDS patients in Kabarole District, western Uganda. *Am J Trop Med Hyg* 2007;**77**:757–63.
15. Atherton DJ. Towards the safer use of traditional remedies. *BMJ* 1994;**308**:673–4.

16. Waldheim A. Diaspora and health? Traditional medicine and culture in a Mexican migrant community. *Int Migration* 2008;**46**:95–117.
17. Loizzo JJ, Blackhall LJ, Rabgyay L. Tibetan medicine: a complementary science of optimal health. *Ann N Y Acad Sci* 2007 e-Pub. Available at: http://tinyurl.com/nnc9qt (accessed 17 June 2009)
18. Fourth World. *Eye Traditional Medicine Policy*. Available at: http://tinyurl.com/6h3e38 (accessed 14 January 2009).
19. Bodeker G. Traditional (i.e. indigenous) and complementary medicine in the Commonwealth: new partnerships planned with the formal health sector. *J Altern Complement Med* 1999;**5**:97–101.
20. Conference for the Midterm Review of the Decade on African Traditional Medicine (2001–2010), Yaounde, Cameroon, 31 August 2008. Concept note. Available at: http://tinyurl.com/6coq2p (accessed 17 December 2008).
21. Chaudhury RR. Commentary: challenges in using traditional systems of medicine. *BMJ* 2001;**322**:167.
22. European Parliament. *The Collins Report, Resolution on the Status of Non-Conventional Medicine*. European Parliament: Strasbourg, 1997.
23. Low T. *Bush Medicine*. North Ryde, NSW: Collins/Angus & Robertson, 1990.
24. Riley M. *Maori Healing and Herbal*. Paparraumu: Viking Sevensen NZ, 1994.
25. Cohen K. Native American medicine. In: Jonas WB, Levin J (eds), *Essentials of Complementary and Alternative Medicine*. Baltimore: Lippincott/Williams & Wilkins, 1999: 233–51.
26. Nauman E. Native American medicine. In: Novery D (ed.), *Clinician's Complete Reference to Complementary Alternative Medicine*. St Louis, MO: Mosby, 2000: 293–308.
27. Sofowora A. Plants in African traditional medicine – a review. In: Evans WC (ed.), *Trease and Evans' Pharmacognosy*, 14th edn. London: WB Saunders, 1996: 511–20.
28. van Wyk B-E, van Oudtshoorn B, Gericke N. *Medicinal Plants of South Africa*. Pretoria: Briza Publications, 1997.
29. Weiner MA. *Secrets of Fijian Medicine*. Berkeley, CA: Quantum Books, 1983.
30. Feldman J. Traditional medicine in Latin America. In: Novery D (ed.) *Clinician's Complete Reference to Complementary Alternative Medicine*. St Louis, MO: Mosby, 2000: 284–92.
31. Shia G, Noller B, Burgord G. Safety issues and policy. In: Bodeker G, Burford G (eds), *Traditional Complementary and Alternative Medicine Policy and Public Health Perspectives*. London: Imperial College Press, 2007: 83–4.
32. Sarris J, Kavanagh DJ, Adamsc J, Bone K, Byrnea G. Kava Anxiety Depression Spectrum Study (KADSS): A mixed methods RCT using an aqueous extract of *Piper methysticum*. *Complement Ther Med* 2009;**17**:176–8
33. Medicines and Healthcare products Regulatory Agency. Traditional ethnic medicine: public health and compliance with medicines law. London: MHRA. Available at: http://tinyurl.com/2olbvg (accessed December 31 2008).
34. Kayne SB. Plants, medicines and environmental awareness. *Health Homoeopathy* 1993;**5**:12–14.
35. Huxtable RJ. The pharmacology of extinction. *J Ethnopharmacol* 1992;**27**:1–11.
36. Holloway H. Sustaining the Amazon. *Sci Am* 1993 **269**:77–84.
37. Orr D. India accuses US of stealing ancient cures. *The London Times* 31 July 1999.
38. World Wide Fund for Nature. *International Report – Booming medicinal plant trade lacks controls*. Godalming, Surrey: WWF 1993.
39. Ferreira A. Muti is killing off South Africa's flora and fauna. *South Africa Times* 7 December 2007. Available at: http://tinyurl.com/2sbpkn (accessed 31 December 2008).
40. Anon. Ozone hole cuts plant growth. *Independent* 11 June 1993.
41. Dueck ThA, Elderson J. Influence of ammonia and sulphur dioxide on the growth and competitive ability of *Arnica Montana* and *Viola canina*. *New Phytol* 1992;**122**:507–14.

42. Bellamy D. Something in the air. *BBC Wildlife* 1993;**11**(7):31–4.
43. Sitwell N. *The Shell Guide to Britain's Threatened Wildlife*. London: Collins, 1993.
44. Anon. Threatened wild flowers saved by EC's arable farm policy. *Independent* 19 July 1993.
45. Fellows L. What can higher plants offer the industry? *Pharm J* 1993;**250**:658.

2

Traditional European folk medicine

Owen Davies

Introduction

The study of folk medicine has a long history that reflects on the wider development of healthcare in European society. Over the last 500 years and more, medicine has been defined largely by who has practised it, rather than its theoretical basis or efficacy. It is the medical profession, created by official secular and ecclesiastical sanction, that has determined how folk medicine has been written about and understood in the past. Much of what we know about the history of 'unofficial' medicine derives from prosecutions under laws designed to restrict provision, and from attempts by the European medical establishment to assert a monopoly on healthcare. Bear in mind that we know with hindsight that the treatments provided by professional medicine were, until the last century, often little better than those offered by many unlicensed healers. In the nineteenth century, the rise of the folklore movement tempered the educated condemnation with a more detached curiosity in the perceived 'relics' of the medical 'ignorance' of the past. Although the early folklorists were not usually sympathetic to the remedies that they collected, there was sometimes a recognition that they probably did no more harm than those provided by the general practitioner. As to historians, up until the 1980s they were largely preoccupied with charting the 'progress' of biomedicine and institutional health care, and rarely gave much thought to the nature and continuance of other healing traditions. But now, just as some of the last links with this alternative history of medical experience are disappearing, a range of relatively new disciplines, namely medical anthropology, ethnobotany, phytotherapy and ethnopharmacology, have provided an impetus for looking again at the nature and value of Europe's old medical traditions. By examining the research of these various scholarly endeavours, new and old, we can begin to piece together the significance of European folk medicine in the past and present, and what this tells us about its future.

Folk medical concepts

Influence of supernatural forces

For much of recorded history, folk medicine shared theories and practices with the 'official' medicine of the mediaeval clergy and licensed physicians. In terms of the aetiologies of folk illness, however, there was, perhaps, a greater emphasis on the influence of supernatural forces. This certainly became one of the clearest differences between the two traditions by the eighteenth century, when across much of Europe the intellectual rationale for the existence of witchcraft was undermined. As is evident from trial records from the late fifteenth to the mid-eighteenth centuries, and folklore sources and court cases in the modern era, the diagnosis and cure of witchcraft were an important element of the popular understanding and experience of medicine. Witches were blamed for a wide range of illnesses and accidents, from causing people to break their legs to infesting them with fleas. Conditions, such as cancer, tuberculosis, malaria and epilepsy, which either developed slowly or were recurrent and did not have obvious external symptoms, were particularly likely to attract suspicion of witchcraft. Across Europe illness and disability were also blamed on various types of supernatural being. In Ireland, for instance, fairies remained a significant element of popular aetiology right into the nineteenth century. Here, as well as in Scotland, Wales and elsewhere, sickly wizened babies exhibiting such features as wrinkled skin, stunted growth and oversized heads, which can be identified with various congenital disorders, were thought by some to be fairy children, substitutes for human infants abducted by the fairies.[1] Similar beliefs were held in Norway where the deformities caused by childhood rickets were commonly blamed on the *huldrefolk* (hidden people).[2]

Numerous other folk aetiologies were based on incorrect but nevertheless reasonable observation and deduction about natural associations. These often still required a magical remedy. For example, in Sicily in the 1980s, there still existed a healing tradition based on the notion that a fright or shock could agitate intestinal worms out of their usual 'normal' position in children's intestines, leading to their spread and consequent illness. Herbal healers or *ciarmavermi* treated the condition using a mixture of natural remedies and spells.[3] In Lucania, southern Italy, it is still believed by some that mastitis can be caused by a baby sucking a hair from its mother's head and accidentally pushing it into the breast through the nipple. One reason for the continuance of the belief is that folk medicine not only provides what seems a clear causal explanation for the illness but also a dedicated remedy, which involves placing a hairbrush in the woman's brassiere while a healer recites the following charm:

'Good morning [or good evening], Saint Miserano.'
There was a woman who washed.
'What do you have, my mother, that you are always crying?'
'The hairs above my breasts.'
If you don't say San Sini' San Sena
Three from the mouth and three from the nose.

In Sardinian folk belief mastitis is similarly believed to be caused by a lactating woman swallowing a hair.[4]

Doctrine of signatures

For people who had little or no awareness of the chemical structures of plants and their compounds, the key to curing both naturally and super-naturally inspired diseases lay in various rules that helped make sense of the hidden or occult properties of the plants and animals around them. The doctrine of signatures, the notion that the physical appearance of a plant is indicative of its healing properties, was one of the enduring lega-cies of ancient Greek medicine. Through the writings of the Roman physi-cians Dioscorides (c.AD 40 to c.90) and Galen (c.AD 129 to c.216), it became an integral part of 'official' medicine in the mediaeval west, was widely adhered to in the early modern period despite increasing criticism, and continues today in some alternative and folk medical traditions.[5] Colour and shape are important diagnostics in the doctrine of signatures. So, in parts of Catalonia, thyme-leaved speedwell (*Veronica serpyllifolia*) is known as *herba dels ulls* (eye herb) and used as an antiseptic eyewash because black lines on the inner petal were popularly thought to resemble eyelashes.[6] In the Russian province of Vologda the long-leaved hounds' tongue (*Cynoglossum officinale*) was considered an antidote against the bite of rabid dogs and was applied by baking the roots in bread. More obscure was the use of common storksbill (*Erodium cicutarium*) for convulsions in Kaluga province because the petioles were 'drawn together like elbows, as if in convulsions'.[7]

The doctrine of signatures is one aspect of a more general ancient notion regarding the laws of sympathy in the natural world, and between the natural and supernatural realms. Hidden symbolic and physical associations exist between people and other living things, spirits and inanimate substances, and this means that actions affecting one also influence the other. The classic example is the hair of the dog, whereby rabies was thought to be cured by putting hair from the offending dog on the bite wound. There are many other examples in European folk medicine, such as the cure of congenital hernia by splitting the trunk of a tree, usually oak or ash, passing the affected infant through it and binding the tree up again. As the tree healed so would the ruptured muscle in the child's groin. Although the process was roughly the same across Europe, nineteenth- and twentieth-century folklorists have recorded a diverse range of associated rituals. In Portugal the rite had to be performed at midnight on St John's Eve by three men named John, while three women named Mary spun thread and recited a charm. In Somerset, England, a virgin had to pass the child through the tree.[8,9] Sympathetic magic was commonly employed to cure witchcraft – so taking the heart of a dead bewitched cow, sticking it with pins and thorns, and then baking it, would cause the witch responsible to have excruciating heart pains and force her or him to desist from further malicious acts. Taking the urine of a bewitched patient, placing it in a vessel along with some sharp objects, and boiling it, would similarly affect the witch.

Until the development and acceptance of theory about germs in the nineteenth century, folk medicine and orthodox medicine again shared similar or the same conceptions of contagion and how to deal with it. One significant difference between the two, however, concerned the folk medical notion that some diseases could not be destroyed and so cures could be achieved only by ritually transferring the illness to someone or something else.[10] Several examples can be found in the archives concerning healers prosecuted under Scottish law against witchcraft. In the early seventeenth century Issobell Haldane explained how she cured a child by washing its shirt in some water in the name of the Trinity. She then took the shirt and water to a stream and threw them in. On the way, however, she was cross with herself for having spilt some of the water because, if anyone passed over it, the disease would be transferred to them rather than being washed away in the stream.[11] The same concept, until very recently, still underpinned healing traditions among, for example, the ethnic Albanian communities of northern Basilicata in southern Italy. Here hepatitis is known as the *mal d'arco* or 'rainbow illness' and is thought to be contracted by looking at a rainbow while urinating outdoors, or by walking along a crossroad contaminated with the disease. It is cured by the patient urinating for several nights in a pot containing the plant common rue (*Ruta graveolens*). This is then poured at a crossroads at night while reciting a magical formula. The next person who passes the crossroad will then contract the illness.[12]

In historical terms certain medical concepts, such as the doctrine of signatures, became definable as 'folk' or 'popular' once they had been discarded by orthodox medicine. The most obvious example of this concerns humoral theory. Ancient Greek physicians believed that health was governed by the balance of four substances or humours, namely yellow bile, black bile, blood and phlegm. Illnesses were caused by the imbalance of these substances, which led to excessive heat/cold, moistness/dryness in the body. Cures required the ingestion of foods, liquids or herbs that had hot/cold, wet/dry properties, which counteracted the identified imbalance, or methods such as bleeding, which reduced humoral excesses. In European popular culture people did not necessarily conceptualise health in humoral terms, but their practices and aetiologies were based on the theory as much as legitimatised medicine. Once the European medical community had rejected it by the end of the eighteenth century, however, its continued influence became a marker of scientific backwardness. But we need to be careful. We should not label folk medicine as merely the rump of outmoded medical ideas. In its myriad manifestations it had its own distinct identity in local, regional and national contexts.

Influence of religion

Many aspects of folk medicine were and are inseparable from popular or practical religion. The sacrament of ordination was thought to imbue the Catholic priesthood with the healing power of God's grace, while in Protestant communities ministers and pastors continued to play an important role as healers, using prayer and their literary knowledge of medicine. Jewish Folk Medicine is covered in Chapter 11. The Bible was a source of personal spiritual and physical succour, a prophylactic against illness, and the source of numerous written and oral healing charms. In Catholic communities sacramentals, holy water, blessed herbs, crosses, rosaries and relics had powerful healing properties, and continue to be employed by millions in Europe today. Take, for example, the *Loretokind* tradition in Switzerland, which concerns a small ivory figure of the infant Jesus displayed in the Capucin convent in Salzburg. Large numbers of replicas and pictures are consecrated by touching them against the original, and then sold at the convent or via mail order along with a blessing prayer. The image or replica is placed on the head or the spot on the body that hurts while reciting the accompanying blessing.[13]

In Catholic and Orthodox Europe pilgrimage is an essential aspect of the role of faith in healing strategies. A major survey conducted in the 1980s found that over 6000 shrines in western Europe were still active pilgrimage sites.[14] Many pilgrimages were orchestrated and managed by the clergy, but many others were generated by the lay community and largely autonomous from the churches. To give just one example of the many that could be cited, in Croatia there has been a long history of worshipping St Lucia to cure eye complaints. Fifty years ago, people flocked to a house in the Istrian peninsula in Croatia where a gold ring with an image of St Lucia was kept. Its guardian closed the eyelids of patients and made the sign of the cross over them three times with the ring, which had been dipped in consecrated water. In the region today people with eye problems still make vows to St Lucia on her feast day.[15]

Healing wells, which were often associated with the saints, were key targets of religious reformers in Protestant countries, but the authorities failed to suppress the continued resort to them just as they failed to extirpate the worship of saints and other aspects of Catholicism engrained in the ritual framework of popular belief and practice. While some renowned pilgrimages sites were suppressed, many, such as Holywell, the 'Lourdes of Wales', survived the Reformation. It remained a centre of Catholic activity despite its illegality, and generated numerous accounts of the miraculous healing properties of its waters.[16,17] Thousands of more humble healing springs also continued to function as an integral aspect of the geography of folk medicine, many losing their saintly associations but retaining their healing reputations. It has even been suggested that in Denmark the popular resort to holy springs and wells, mostly for eye complaints and rickets, became even more widespread after the Reformation, despite the condemnation of the country's Lutheran church.[18] The authorities eventually tolerated them as long as no 'superstitious' rites accompanied their use, while the country's medical establishment, as elsewhere, attempted to rationalise the properties of these healing waters by analysing their mineral and metal content.

The vogue for spas in the eighteenth century gave a boost to some old healing wells. The reputation of St Elian's Well in north Wales, described in 1700 as being resorted to by 'papists and other old people' who offered 'either a groat or its value in bread', was, 60 years later, exploited by the building of a 'respectable' medicinal bathing house close by. Around the same time, the well curiously began to attract a reputation in folk culture of having the power to curse as well as cure, generating a thriving trade for its custodians.[19] By the early nineteenth century, however, the role of healing wells in folk medicine had attenuated considerably across much of Catholic and Protestant Europe. The fate of Mag's Well in Surrey, England, was probably shared by many. It went from being widely resorted to for a range of human skin complaints in the seventeenth and eighteenth centuries, to its final use for washing dogs to cure the mange, before falling into complete neglect by the twentieth century. In western and central western France some 850 holy springs were resorted to for their healing properties at the beginning of the twentieth century, but by 1980 only around 50 were still in use.[20] Yet the picture is not one of inexorable decline in the face of secularisation and modern medicine. At the end of the nineteenth century numerous holy healing wells in Ireland were reinvigorated as part of a wider discourse on national identity fostered by the Catholic Church, politicians and folklorists.[21] With the emancipation of Catholicism in nineteenth-century England, the healing waters at Holywell also experienced a massive boom in attendance thanks to the concerted efforts of the Church to invigorate its influence.

Herbalism

The use of plants is the most enduring aspect of folk medical practice. Studies of contemporary traditional herbalism in some parts of Greece indicate that much of the current usage is still based on the ancient Greek understanding of herbs, as described in Dioscorides' founding text of herbal science, *De Materia Medica*.[22] It has even been suggested that ancient Greek knowledge that has long been lost in the written record has survived orally.[23] Botanical remedies were a key element of folk medicine across the whole of Europe, with plants used not only for their natural properties but also for their ritual significance. Some widespread species such as elder (*Sambucus*) were widely used in both natural and supernatural healing contexts. Others had more regional and local cultural significance. Broad regional differences are also apparent regarding the use of fungi, which are, of course, not members of the plant kingdom. Evidence for the use of fungi for medicinal purposes is rare in much of western and northern Europe, but more is known about their use in south-eastern Europe. A study of fungi in Hungarian folk medicine, for instance, found that Judas's ear (*Auricularia auricula-judae*) was used to cure eye complaints by placing it against the eye, and various puffballs (*Lycoperdons*) were thought to be efficacious against bleeding and diarrhoea.[24]

The medicinal use of herbs was bound by a rich ritual lore about when and how they should be gathered and applied. Much depended on astrology. The potency of plants was thought to be influenced by their being picked and administered according to the waxing and waning of the moon. On a more sophisticated level, herbs were associated with certain planets and used to counteract diseases generated by opposing planets. Plants were also picked on specific religious days depending on regional traditions. Southern Czechs used to place St John's wort on their beds on St John's Eve in the hope that the saint would lay upon it at night and bless the herb with curative powers.[7] In Spanish folk medicine there is a long tradition of herbal remedies being administered in periods called '*novenes*', mimicking the Catholic practice of saying prayers on nine consecutive days. So remedies are taken in increasing or decreasing doses for 9-day periods followed by 9 days without treatment. A recent study of medicinal plants in the Pallars region of Catalonia found that 109 of 410 herbs were administered in such *novenes*.[25,26] Three was another important number, representing the holy trinity as well as reflecting earlier pagan preoccupation with the significance of triplication. The number 7 was also widely employed. In the mountainous Molise region of central southern Italy, for example, the practice of winding old man's beard (*Clematis vitalba*) seven times around the necks of nervous sheep has been recently recorded.[27]

Practitioners and their powers

Everyone could practise some elements of folk medicine, but certain sections of the population were seen to have more experience, knowledge or ability than others. Within family groups, women were usually the main practitioners and principal repositories of healing knowledge. Recent studies have found that they make up most of the remaining few traditional folk healers. Women were thought to possess natural abilities for dealing with certain problems, particularly those associated with childbirth and children. As literacy levels were much lower among women than men in much of Europe, until the advent of compulsory education, women were also more associated with oral traditions of medical knowledge, such as obtaining healing gifts from the fairy realm. Furthermore, the fact that, until the late nineteenth century, women were largely excluded from licensed medical practice meant that as healers they were systematically classified both at the time and by later historians as belonging to unofficial categories of medicine, labelled variously as 'unqualified', 'alternative', 'casual', 'popular' or 'folk'.[28,29] Certain male occupations, particularly shepherds, cowherds and blacksmiths, also accrued healing reputations from the knowledge that they were thought to gain through their experience and intimacy with animals and natural forces.

Healing skills could be a birthright. Seventh sons and daughters, for example, were commonly thought to have an innate healing ability, as were those born in a caul. In Catalonia those born on certain saints days were given specific powers. So those born on St Judas's Day could heal wounds by sucking on them.[30] Secret knowledge and skills could also be inherited. The tradition of charming, an integral aspect of European folk medicine based primarily on verbal or written charms containing biblical passages, apocrypha and stories of mythical encounters, was passed down through families from generation to generation, sometimes contrasexually, in other words from male to female and vice versa.[31,32] Folk medical knowledge could also be acquired from outside the oral tradition of families and close-knit communities.

Although the folk medicine of some societies on other continents has been, and still is, a purely oral tradition, the history of its development and nature in Europe cannot be understood without recognition of the influence of print culture. The importance of ancient medical writings has already been noted. With the advent of print in the late fifteenth century, and the significant growth of literacy across much of northern and western Europe in the following centuries, access to medical literature spread far beyond the libraries of the clergy and licensed physicians. Some of the earliest secular books to be printed were herbals. The *Herbarius*, published in Mainz in 1485, was particularly influential, being the source of numerous subsequent texts, such as the first printed Polish herbal, Stefan Falimirz's *On Herbs and their Power*, published in 1534.[33] Astrology was an integral aspect of the print herbal manuals just as it was in oral tradition, and trying to unpick the influence of one on the other is an almost impossible task.

The medical recipes and notions of the ancient physicians also found their way into hugely popular manuals containing the 'secrets' of the natural world. One of the most influential of these books was falsely attributed to the mediaeval German Dominican friar and scientist Albertus Magnus (about 1193–1280), though most of its contents were culled from Pliny and works alleged to have been written by Aristotle. *Le Grand Albert*, as it came to be known in France, began to be sold in a cheap format in the eighteenth century, and its spread to French colonies in the Caribbean and Indian Ocean region had a considerable influence on folk medical traditions there.[34] The almanac, which was the most popular literary format from the late seventeenth to the twentieth century, was another important source of medical knowledge that both informed and borrowed from folk medicine. Almanacs published in Estonia between 1731 and 1900 included information about the use of around 55 medicinal plants.[35]

In the eighteenth century there was also a boom in 'rational' self-help medical manuals for the home.[36] This domestic medicine was, in part, an attempt to eradicate the influence of 'superstitious' oral folk medicine, but it was also a response to the widely recognised inadequacies of formal medical provision in servicing the poor. As Christian Mangor noted in his Norwegian *Lande-apothek* (*Country Apothecary*), first published in 1767 and reprinted numerous times over the next century, such works were important as 'few can afford medicines from the apothecary, let alone the cost of a doctor's travel, time, and trouble'.[2] Mangor recommended various garden herbs and was particularly keen on the healing powers of elderberry. Some authors were also inspired by concerns over the quality of officially prescribed medicines. In the 1760 edition of his *Primitive Physic*, John Wesley said of the apothecary: 'perhaps he has not the drug prescribed by the physician, and so puts in its place "what will do as well." Perhaps he has it; but it is stale and perished'. Better to trust one's own ingredients and experience in cases of minor ailments. Wesley was, of course, the founder of Methodism, and we see elsewhere the evangelical Protestant impulse for self-help in bodily as well as spiritual care. In Estonia, for example, several German pastors produced influential health guides for the common people, such as Otto Jannau's *Country People's Home Doctor or a Short Guide how Every Reasonable Person in His House and Family Can Help if Somebody is Sick, but Doctor is Unavailable* (1857).[33]

Medical print culture was by no means devoid of the magic woven into the oral tradition of medicine. In nineteenth- and twentieth-century France numerous editions of the cheap self-help guide *Le Médecin des pauvres* contained traditional healing charms. Its popularity may have created a certain degree of uniformity in the charming tradition as the print versions of the charms seeped into the oral and manuscript record of healing knowledge.[37,38] Literacy and literature were also important to the success and influence of two important categories of European folk healer. The 'quack doctor' or *charlatan* was defined, in part, by the entrepreneurial exploitation of newspaper advertising, handbills and bogus certificates of official sanction. Quacks vaunted their scientific credentials, but in practice often relied on what were seen by the eighteenth-century medical establishment as either fraudulent facsimiles of orthodox medicine or miraculous, herbal or sympathetic modes of folk medical cure.[39,40] The reputations of many 'cunning-folk', who offered a wide range of magical solutions for everyday misfortunes in matters of health, love and money, made considerable play on their possession of books of magic, astrology and herbalism. In folk culture books were thought to contain secret knowledge otherwise unobtainable in the oral medical tradition.

Cultural exchange

We need to be aware of the non-European influences on the history of European medicine. The importance of Arabic science and medicine during the mediaeval period is well recorded. In Europe much knowledge of classical medicine was lost for centuries after the collapse of the Roman Empire, and so the Arabic world became the main repository of ancient Greek and Roman medical theory. Most of Galen's writings had been translated into Arabic by the tenth century, and it was largely thanks to mediaeval Arab and Jewish scholars in Spain and Constantinople that Galenic theory came to dominate European medicine until the eighteenth century. As well as this crucial role in the development of orthodox western medicine, the Moorish populations of Spain, and Jewish communities across Europe, maintained distinctive folk medical traditions, the practitioners of which were also consulted by Christians. During the sixteenth century the secular authorities and the Inquisition in Spain made a concerted effort to suppress Muslim physicians and Arabic texts, denigrating Arabic–Galenic medicine. As a consequence, over the next few centuries Moorish medical practitioners largely operated within the magical–medical context of *curandismo*, practising herbalism, using charms, and curing and diagnosing based on the Islamic tradition that diseases were embodied by demons or djinns.[41] The influence of this Moorish cultural heritage is still clearly evident in Spanish magical healing traditions today. As a study of folk medicine in Murcia in south-eastern Spain observed, the Latin, Moorish and Jewish medical traditions in the region's folk belief and practice are so entwined that it is a difficult task to disentangle them.[42]

Numerous small-scale population movements have also taken place within Europe over the centuries. Studying folk medical knowledge provides one of the few ways of mapping the cultural experience of these different migrant populations and their adaptation to new environments. Take, for example, the Tabarkins of south-west Sardinia. They are the ancestors of Genoese migrants who, in the sixteenth century, colonised the small island of Tabarka off the Tunisian coast. After two centuries they were forced to flee to Sardinia where they founded their own communities. Researchers recently studied their folk phytotherapy and found that nothing significant remained of their north African experience. But, while they had evidently adopted Sardinian herbal medical traditions, their Genoese heritage was still apparent in their names for local plants.[43] A study of the remnant elderly Istro-Romanian community, the origins of which date back to the four-teenth-century migration of people from the Carpathian basin to the Istrian peninsula in Croatia, found evidence of the survival of some distinctive ethnic folk medical practices, including the prominent use of vinegar from wild apples in a variety of remedies, and houseleek (*Sempervivum tectorum*) for ear pain.[44] Comparisons with the ethnobotany of the diverse mix of Slovenian, Croatian, German and Italian peoples in and around the penin-sula suggest that the acculturation process, and consequent loss of ethno-botanical diversity, might be more 'intense than in other "less multi-cultural" migration contexts', such as the aforementioned Albanian communities in Basilicata in southern Italy.[45]

The history of medicine and colonialism has until recently usually consisted of a narrative of, first, the influence of Galenic medical theory on indigenous folk medicine, and then the spread of western medical bioscience. Yet the path of transmission of medical knowledge was by no means all one way. In eighteenth-century Portugal, healers of African descent, who were brought to the country as slaves either directly from Africa or more commonly from Brazil, attracted considerable renown for their curative powers. The Portuguese Inquisition tried between 15 and 20 healers in the period, among them Maria Grácia, a 40-year-old Angolan slave owned by a wool contractor in Evora. She was tried in 1724 for curing witchcraft-inspired illnesses and the 'malady of the moon'. Her Christian charms did not owe anything to her Angolan homeland, however, but the exoticism of her skin colour and African heritage lent her and other Luso-African healers, women in particular, popular esteem among the Portuguese for their possession of occult knowledge.[46]

As is being increasingly realised, the study of European folk medicine also needs to consider the experiences and practices of those overseas migrant communities that have settled in significant numbers over the last 50 years. Research has recently been conducted, for example, on folk medicine among Thai women in Sweden, Surinamese immigrants in Amsterdam and Sikh communities in London.[47,48] In France over the last three decades immigrant west and north African cunning-folk or *marabouts*, primarily from Senegal, and most of whom adopted the trade after arriving in France, have been successful in carving a niche in the commercial world of folk medicine, magic and alternative healing by playing on their 'unique' ethnic knowledge.[49,50] Surprising historical connections emerge between the medical heritage of migrants and their host communities. A study of traditional medicines used by a Pakistani migrant community in Bradford, England, reveals that, although most of the herbal remedies used are not known in the western tradition, the interviewees subscribe to the *Unani* medical tradition, which developed in mediaeval Persia but was based on ancient Greek humoral theory (*Unani* means Greek).[51]

As well as the influence of population movements, European medicine has also incorporated ingredients and substances imported through trade. Even before European colonial expansion from the sixteenth century onwards, ingredients had long arrived from the east. Cloves, mace and nutmeg were being traded across Europe by the thirteenth century.[52] They were expensive, of course, and largely the preserve of monastic medicine rather than lay medical practice, but they would eventually find their way into the domestic pharmacopoeia and onto the shelves of urban druggists servicing industrialising populations. In nineteenth-century England the popularity of nutmeg as a carminative for flatulence and dyspepsia created a trade in portable nutmeg holders and graters. These were made of silver for the wealthy, while rural craftsmen sold little wooden boxes in the form of an acorn and the like for the humble.[53] Today, of course, ginseng and *Ginkgo biloba* have became an important part of self-medication in Europe.

Now little used in Europe, dragon's blood, the blood-red resin of various non-European trees, was used in the ancient world for medicinal purposes and its use has spread to folk medical traditions around the world.[54] According to one Renaissance Florentine doctor its expense was such that most dragon's blood in apothecaries' workshops was actually a mix of sulphur and mercury boiled together.[55] It was used in ritual healing contexts as well. One of the remedies for relieving the possessed suggested by Florian Canale, an early modern Italian exorcist, involved a distillation including dragon's blood, ground glass, wax and turpentine.[56] The doctrine of signatures dictated that the resin would be efficacious for bleeding, as several popular eighteenth-century medical texts suggested. Editions of *Aristotle's Compleat Master-piece*, for instance, provided several remedies for 'spitting of blood', usually associated with tuberculosis, including one that mixed dragon's blood with 'frogspawn water', 'plantain water' and syrup of roses. It became a staple ingredient of chemists and druggists in the nineteenth century, although often purchased by the poor for use in love divination rituals rather than medicine.[57]

Adaptation and transformation

There has been, and continues to be, a tendency to consider European folk medicine, as well as other aspects of 'folklore', as bound to rural cultures. But, as numerous studies of folk medicine in contemporary urban societies in the Americas, Asia and Africa have shown, this is certainly not the case. In a historical context the same applies to Europe. Britain was the first industrial urban nation and, although little work has been done on the issue, there is sufficient evidence that folk medicine served an important function in this new way of life. The industrial urban population may not have had the natural environment around them to furnish the herbal ingredients of many traditional remedies, but it did generate the huge expansion of herbalists, chemists and druggists shops, which supplied herbs and substances for folk medical use along with dispensing for licensed doctors.[58,59] Thanks to the frequent injuries that were the lot of factory and mill workers, traditional medical arts, such as bone-setting, essentially folk osteopathy, also thrived in the northern towns of England.[29]

As to the continuation of traditional folk medicine today the pattern is difficult to ascertain, and varies significantly within as well as between countries. In terms of the survival of an oral tradition, folk medicine remains strongest in Mediterranean and south-eastern European countries. But the trend everywhere is undoubtedly one of considerable decline, with older people now the last repositories of long-held knowledge. In Italy, recent scholarly interest in the biomedical value of traditional herbal remedies provides some sense of the continuation and decline of this aspect of folk medical tradition in the early third millennium. In one mountainous region of central southern Italy, researchers found that practical knowledge of traditional natural remedies for human ailments was quickly being lost, and the last in a long line of local folk healers had died in 2001. Elderly female family members were still using a few remedies, such as administering stinking tutsan (*Hypericum hircinum*) for colds. They gathered the plant from the surrounding area and dried and stored it for winter.[60] Otherwise, modern pharmaceuticals have almost entirely replaced traditional medicines in much of Italy. Yet older people still know of and reminisce about the great efficacy of well-known remedies even if they are no longer used, remedies such as the latex of sea spurge (*Euphorbia paralias*) used by fishermen in central Italy for assuaging the bite of weever fish.[61] The rate of erosion is by no means uniform and is highly localised. In the hilly Molise region of central southern Italy, for example, folk veterinary medicine had apparently disappeared by 2003, whereas it has recently been described as 'alive and well' in some communities in the Alto Tirreno Cosentino area of southern Italy.[62]

In rural Spain too, the knowledge is restricted largely to older people, with a study in 2007 warning that the loss of popular knowledge was becoming 'an alarming reality, particularly among the younger generations'. The oral repository of folk medicine is not being passed on.[6,63] Still, the impression is that the cultural changes that have eroded oral transmission proceed more slowly in Spain, or at least differently, so that the rump of traditional medicine remains in better health than in Italy.[27] In Murcia, south-east Spain, *'yerberos'* or traditional herbalists continued to sell their herbs and medicines on certain market days in the 1990s.[42] The importance of pastoral farming is probably an important factor in influencing this pattern of continuance. A study of mountain communities in Galicia in the 1990s found that traditional plant remedies were primarily used by stockfarmers distrustful of veterinarians.[64]

The magical aspects of folk medicine should also not be confined to the past – a subject only for historians. In the 1980s French ethnographers found 'charming' alive and well in Brittany and other parts of the country,[65] and it was also being practised in the farming communities of Lower Saxony, Germany.[66] Closer to the present, fieldwork has shown that charming is still employed in parts of Italy, and is a significant aspect of folk medical provision in eastern Europe.[4,32]

This leads us to the question of why some aspects of folk healing continue in Europe today. At this point it is important to stress the distinction between folk *illness* and folk *medicine*.[67] Folk illness (concepts of cause, aetiology and manifestation) usually requires folk medicine (concepts of cure, practices and practitioners), but folk medicine can function independently, and has proved itself eminently adaptable to modern healthcare. Postwar Norway developed one of the best healthcare systems in the world, but, as research in the 1970s and 1980s shows, this by no means usurped some folk medical therapies. In Norway layers-on of hands, religious healers and herbalists continued to be consulted.[68,69] A survey of alternative medicine uptake among inpatients at one German hospital in 2004 revealed that 13% of the sample had used herbal remedies for their condition.[70] What has happened, of course, is that during the twentieth century aspects of traditional European folk medicine have been redefined and gained widespread acceptance as part of the package of complementary and alternative medicines, which are now an integral part of healthcare in the contemporary western world.

Old factors for the preservation of folk medical traditions, such as geographical isolation, cost and the impotence of the 'official' alternative, are no longer as relevant. That said, with regard to the last, numerous people today continue to cope with incurable and terminal illnesses by resorting to alternative therapies. The importance of print for understanding the history of European folk medicine was highlighted earlier, and it needs to be stressed again in relation to the continuance of folk tradition in our modern, highly literate society. Although the oral tradition may be on the verge of extinction, and with it the loss of much unrecorded local knowledge, more generalised published accounts of the oral medical tradition provide an enduring record that is easily accessible to all. Fieldwork in Estonia in 1999 found that healers and wise-folk said that all their knowledge was taken directly from books, and consequently that they could not provide information about the oral tradition of folk medicine.[35] Folk medical texts are easily found in the eclectic mind, body and spirit sections of high street bookshops and authoritative surveys of ethnobotany sell well to the general public.[71,72] In Thessaloniki, herb traders continue to sell in the city centre market much as they have done for over 500 years, and traditional empirics continue to set up their stalls in open-air markets, while modern health food shops run by university-educated people whose knowledge is largely book based also trade in them.[22] The viability of the former is now surely increasingly tied to the influence of the latter.

The cultural distance between patient and official practitioner is no longer as great is it was a century or more ago, and healthcare providers have become more sensitised to patients' conceptions of illness and cure.[73] But the distance has grown between consumers and the biomedical industry.[74] The undercurrent of distrust in the absolutist position of the biosciences is one reason why some people turn to reformulations of folk medicine, whether they be European or borrowed from the traditions of other continents. Concerns are amplified when scientific authority is period-ically and often sensationally exposed as flawed. The growing influence of the green movement has helped shape how Europeans respond to this. The perceived benefits of the purity of self-made or natural remedies over pack-aged, synthetic compounds are weighed up by many medical consumers – an echo of the concerns expressed by John Wesley 250 years ago. Faith-based healing strategies also continue to have a significant influence.

One recent factor affecting interest in and uptake of folk medicine, the collapse of communism and the Eastern Bloc, highlights just how complex the relationship is between conceptions of healing and broader social, economic and political developments. One consequence has been the freeing up of the medical market. In Poland, for instance, the state enterprise monopoly on herbal drugs, 'Herbapol', was dismantled leading to the rapid growth of private and cooperative herbal producers.[33] In post-Soviet Russia there was a huge boom in magical and religious healers, with many adver-tising their 'traditional' status in newspapers and on television. The religious emancipation that also occurred has boosted this appeal to lay healing, despite the condemnation of an increasingly influential Orthodox Church.[75] These trends have also been influenced by the growth of nationalist impulses that promote notions and sentiments regarding the 'traditional' and an idealisation of the rural past. In other words, healing traditions have been used in the process of creating national identity. So folk medicine's rich past is also what continues to ensure its future.

References

1. Eberly SS. Fairies and the folklore of disability: changelings, hybrids and the solitary fairy. *Folklore* 1988; **99**:68–77.
2. Stokker K. *Remedies and Rituals: Folk Medicine in Norway and the New Land*. St Paul, MI: Minnesota Historical Society Press, 2007.
3. Guggino E. Uomini e vermin. Credenze e pratiche medico-magische in Sicilia. *La Ricerca Folklorica* 1983;**8**:71–83.
4. Quave CL, Pieroni A. Ritual healing in Arbëreshë Albanian and Italian communities of Lucania, Southern Italy. *Journal of Folklore Research* 2005;**42**:57–97.
5. Richardson-Boedler C. The Doctrine of Signatures: A historical, philosophical and scientific view (I). *Br Homeopath J* 1999;**68**:172–7.
6. Rigat M, Bonet MÀ, Garcia S, Garnatje T, Vallès J. Studies on pharmaceutical ethnobotany in the high river Ter valley (Pyrenees, Catalonia, Iberian Peninsula). *J Ethnopharmacol* 2007;**113**:267–77, 276.
7. Kolosova VB. Name-Text-Ritual: The role of plant characteristics in Slavic Folk Medicine. *Folklorica: Journal of the Slavic and East European Folklore Association* 2005; **10**(2): 44–62.
8. Hand WD. 'Passing through': Folk medical magic and symbolism. *Proceedings of the American Philosophical Society* 1968;**112**:379–402.
9. Mead FH. On a widely spread superstition in connection with hernia in young children. *Somerset Archaeological and Natural History Society Proceedings* 1892;**38**:362–8.
10. Hand WD. The magical transference of disease. In: *Folklore Studies in Honor of Arthur Palmer Hudson*. Chapel Hill, NC: North Carolina Folklore Society, 1965: 83–109.
11. Davies O. A comparative perspective on early-modern Scottish Cunning-folk and charmers. In: Goodare J, Martin L, Miller J (eds), *Witchcraft and Belief in Early Modern Scotland*. Basingstoke: Palgrave, 2007: 185–206.
12. Pieroni A, Quave C, Nebel S, Heinrich M. Ethnopharmacy of the ethnic Albanians (Arbëreshë) of northern Basilicata, Italy. *Fitoterapia* 2002;**73**:217–41.
13. Lussi K. Magic-religious healing rituals in Central Switzerland. In: Gottschalk-Batschkus CE, Green JC (eds), *Handbuch der Ethnotherapien*. Munich: Institut für Ethnomedizin, 2002: 87–96.
14. Nolan ML, Nolan S. *Christian Pilgrimage in Modern Western Europe*. Chapel Hill, NC: University of Carolina Press, 1989.
15. Skrobonja A, Muzur A, Culina T. The cult of St Lucia, patroness of the eyes: Some examples from Croatian ethnomedical tradition. *Int Ophthalmol* 2004;**25**:37–41.
16. Walsham A. Holywell: Contesting sacred space in post-Reformation Wales. In: Coster W, Spicer A (eds), *Sacred Space in Early Modern Europe*. Cambridge: Cambridge University Press, 2005: 211–37.
17. Seguin, CM. Cures and controversy in early modern Wales: The struggle to control St. Winifred's Well. *North American Journal of Welsh Studies* 2003;**3**(2):1–17.
18. Johansen, JCV. Holy springs and Protestantism in early modern Denmark: A medical rationale for a religious practice. *Medical History* 1997;**41**:59–69.
19. Suggett R. *A History of Magic and Witchcraft in Wales*. Stroud: The History Press, 2008.
20. Audin P. Un example de survivance païenne: le culte des fontaines dans la France de l'ouest et du centre-ouest: du Moyen Age à nos jours. (An example of pagan survival: the cult of springs in western and central-western France: from the Middle Ages to the present day.) *Annales de Bretagne et des Pays de l'Ouest Rennes* 1980;**87**:679–96.
21. ó Giolláin D. Revisiting the Holy Well. *Éire-Ireland* 2005;**40**:11–41.
22. Hanlidou E, Karousou R, Kleftoyanni V, Kokkini S. The herbal market of Thessaloniki (N Greece) and its relation to the ethnobotanical tradition. *J Ethnopharmacol* 2004; **91**:281–99.
23. Brussell DE. Medicinal plants of Mt. Pelion, Greece. *Economic Botany* 2004;**58**: 174–202.
24. Zsigmond G. Les champignons dans la médecine populaire Hongroise. (Fungi in Hungarian popular medicine.) *Bull Soc Mycol Fr* 1999;**115**:79–90.

25. Gavilanes E. El número nueve en la medicina popular. (The number nine in popular medicine.) *Revista de Dialectología y Tradiciones Populares* 1995;**50**(1):243–62.
26. Agelet A, Vallès J. Studies on pharmaceutical ethnobotany in the region of Pallars (Pyrenees, Catalonia, Iberian Peninsula). Part I. General results and new or very rare medicinal plants. *J Ethnopharmacol* 2001;**77**:57–70.
27. Guarrera PM, Lucchese F, Medori S. Ethnophytotherapeutical research in the high Molise region (Central-Southern Italy). *J Ethnobiol Ethnomed* 2008;**4**:7.
28. Blécourt W de, Usborne C. Women's medicine, women's culture: abortion and fortune-telling in early twentieth-century Germany and the Netherlands. *Medical History* 1999; **43**:376–92.
29. Davies O. Female healers in nineteenth-century England. In: Goose N, ed. *Women's Work in Industrial England: Regional and local perspectives.* Hatfield: Local Population Studies Society, 2007: 228–50.
30. Perdiguero E. Magical healing in Spain (1875–1936): medical pluralism and the search for hegemony. In: de Blécourt W, Davies O (eds), *Witchcraft Continued: Popular magic in modern Europe.* Manchester: Manchester University Press, 2004: 133–51.
31. Davies O. Charmers and charming in England and Wales from the eighteenth to the twentieth century. *Folklore* 1998;**109**:41–52.
32. Roper J, ed. *Charms, Charmers and Charming.* Basingstoke: Palgrave, 2008.
33. Kuźnicka B, Wysakowska B. Comparative study on the use of medicinal plants in Poland (16th century and today). *Médicament et nutrition: L'approche ethnopharmacologique.* (*Medicine and Nutrition: The ethnopharmacological approach.*) Proceedings of the 2nd European Colloquium of Ethnopharmacology, Heidelberg, 24–27 March. Paris: ORSTOM-SFE, 1993: 149–52.
34. Davies O. *Grimoires: A history of magic books.* Oxford: Oxford University Press, 2009.
35. Söukand R, Raal A. Data on medicinal plants in Estonian folk medicine: Collection, formation and overview of previous researchers. *Electronic Journal of Folklore* 2006; **30**:171–98.
36. Porter R, ed. *The Popularization of Medicine, 1650–1850.* London: Routledge, 1992.
37. Davies, O. French healing charms and charmers. In: Roper J (ed.), *Charms and Charming in Europe.* Basingstoke: Palgrave, 2004: 91–113.
38. Ebermann O. Le Médecin des Pauvres. (The doctor of the poor.) *Zeitschrift des Vereins für Volkskunde* 1914;**2**:134–62
39. Ramsey M. *Professional and Popular Medicine in France, 1770–1830.* Cambridge: Cambridge University Press, 1988.
40. Gentilcore D. *Medical Charlatanism in Early Modern Italy.* Oxford: Oxford University Press, 2006.
41. Ballesta GL. *Medicina, ciencia, y minorías marginadas: Los Moriscos.* (*Medicine, Science and Marginalized Minorities: The Moriscos.*) Granada: University of Granada, 1977.
42. Rivera Núñez D, Obón de Castro C. Ethnopharmacology of Murcia (SE Spain). In: Schröder E, Balansard G, Cabalion P, Fleurentin J, Mazars G (eds), *Médicaments et aliments: approche ethnopharmacologique.* Paris: ORSTOM, 1996: 215–39.
43. Maxia A, Lancioni MC, Valia AN, Alborghetti R, Pieroni A, Loi MC. Medical ethnobotany of the Tabarkins, a Northern Italian (Ligurian) minority in south-western Sardinia. *Genetic Resources and Crop Evolution* 2008;911–24.
44. Pieroni A, Giusti ME, Münz H, Lenzarini C, Turković A. Ethnobotanical knowledge of the Istro-Romanians of Žejane in Croatia. *Fitoterapia* 2003;**74**:710–19.
45. Pieroni A, Giusti ME. The remedies of the folk medicine of the Croatians Living in Ćićarija, Northern Istria. *Collegium Antropologicum* 2008;**32**:623–7.
46. Walker TD. The role and practices of the curandeiro and saludador in early modern Portuguese society. *História, ciências, saúde – manguinhos* 2004;**11**:223–37.
47. Pieroni A, Vandebroek I, eds. *Travelling Culture and Plants: The ethnobiology and ethnopharmacy of migrations.* New York: Berghahn Books, 2007.
48. Sandhu DS, Heinrich M. The use of health foods, spices and other botanicals in the Sikh community in London. *Phytotherapy Research* 2005;**19**: 633–42.

49. Davies O. Witchcraft accusations in France, 1850–1990. In: de Blécourt W, Davies O, eds. *Witchcraft Continued: Popular magic in modern Europe*. Manchester: Manchester University Press, 2004: 107–33.

50. Bacou M, Biebuyk B, Campion-Vincent V. Les marabouts s'affichent in Paroles urbaines. The Marabouts display themselves in urban terms.) *Cahiers de literature orale* 1988;24:193–200.

51. Pieroni A, Sheikh Q-Z, Ali W, Torry B. Traditional medicines used by Pakistani migrants from Mirpur living in Bradford, Northern England. *Complementary Therapies in Medicine* 2008;16:81–6.

52. Donkin RA. *Between East and West: The Moluccas and the traffic in spices up to the arrival of Europeans*. Philadelphia, PA: American Philosophical Society, 2003.

53. Newman LF. Some notes on the nutmeg graters used in folk medicine. *Folklore* 1943;54:334–7.

54. Gupta D, Bleakley B, Gupta RK. Dragon's blood: Botany, chemistry and therapeutic uses. *J Ethnopharmacol* 2008;115:361–80.

55. Henderson J. *The Renaissance Hospital: Healing the body and healing the soul*. New Haven, CT: Yale University Press, 2006.

56. Sluhovsky M. *Believe not Every Spirit: Possession, mysticism and discernment in early modern catholicism*. Chicago: University of Chicago Press, 2007.

57. Thompson CJ. *The Mystery and Romance of Alchemy and Pharmacy*. London: Scientific Press, 1897.

58. Marland H. *Medicine and Society in Wakefield and Huddersfield 1780–1870*. Cambridge: Cambridge University Press, 1987.

59. Brown PS. Herbalists and medical botanists in mid-nineteenth-century Britain. *Med Hist* 1982;26:405–20.

60. Pieroni, A, Quave, CL, Santoro RF. Folk pharmaceutical knowledge in the territory of the Dolomiti Lucane, inland southern Italy. *J Ethnopharmacol* 2004;95:373–84.

61. Guarrera PM. Traditional phytotherapy in Central Italy (Marche, Abruzzo, and Latium). *Fitoterapia* 2005;76:1–25.

62. Leporatti ML, Impieri M. Ethnobotanical notes about some uses of medicinal plants in Alto Tirreno Cosentino area (Calabria, Southern Italy). *J Ethnobiol Ethnomed* 2007;3:34.

63. Dopico E, San Fabian JL, Garcia-Vazquez E. Traditional medicine in twenty-first century Spain. *Human Ecology* 2008;36:125–9.

64. Blanco E, Macía MJ, Morales R. Medicinal and veterinary plants of El Caurel (Galicia, northwest Spain). *J Ethnopharmacol* 1999;65:113–24.

65. Camus D. *Paroles magiques: Secrets de guérison*. Paris: Imago, 1990.

66. Pérez JM. Encountering the irrational: some reflections on folk healing. *Folklore* 1988;99:178–85.

67. Press I. Urban folk medicine: a functional overview. *American Anthropologist* 1978; 80(1):71–84.

68. Alver BG, Selberg T. Alternative medicine in today's society. In: Kvideland R, Sehmsdorf HK (eds), *Nordic Folklore: Recent studies*. Bloomington, IN: Indiana University Press, 1989: 207–21. (The article was first published in *Temenos* (1984).)

69. Bruusgaard D, Efsking L. Befolkningens syn på og bruk av folkmedisin. (The population's views on and use of folk medicine.) *Tidsskrift for den Norske Lægeforening* 1977; 98:1385–8.

70. Huber R, Koch D, Beisner I, Zschocke I, Ludtke R. Experience and attitudes towards CAM – a survey of internal and psychosomatic patients in a German University Hospital. *Alternative Therapies in Health and Medicine* 2004;10(1): 32–6.

71. Allen DE, Hatfield G. *Medicinal Plants in Folk Traditions: An ethnobotany of Britain and Ireland*. Portland, OR: Timber Press, 2004.

72. Milliken W, Bridgewater S. *Flora Celtica: Plants and people in Scotland*. Edinburgh: Birlinn Ltd, 2004.

73. Hufford DJ. Folk medicine and health culture in contemporary society. *Primary Care* 1997;**24**:723–41.
74. Bakx K. The 'eclipse' of folk medicine in western society. *Sociology of Health & Illness* 1991;13(1): 20–38.
75. Lindquist G. Wizards, gurus, and energy-information fields: wielding legitimacy in contemporary Russian healing. *Anthropology of East Europe Review* 2001;**19**(1):16–28.

3

Aboriginal/traditional medicine in North America: a practical approach for practitioners

John K Crellin

We still use plants from the land to heal some of our cut fingers or aching bones. But in taking plants from the land to use for medicine, we have to do it in such a way that we leave a gift behind. We leave tobacco, or offerings, a gift of respect for some of the things that the Creator has given us. When we do that, that's a healing of our own minds, our own bodies, our own souls.

Saqamaw Misel Joe[1]

If a patient really has confidence in me, then he gets cured. If he has no confidence, then that is his problem. If a person gets bitten by a snake, for example, certain prayers can be used, but if the patient doesn't have enough confidence, then the cure won't work.

Medicine man (quoted in Sandner[2])

One difficulty in preparing a short chapter is the complexity of the North American scene with vastly different geographical/economic/political/cultural regions. The geographical contrast between aboriginal peoples of the south-western USA and the isolated Inuit of the Canadian Arctic hints only at a diversity of traditional practices. Clearly, this can contribute to regional differences in the questions that healthcare practitioners commonly face; some may field questions over magico-religious/ceremonial practices more than do others, although nowadays, with the promotion of herbs as 'dietary supplements', all practitioners can expect questions on 'aboriginal' herbs. In anchoring this chapter on current issues, information from a Saqamaw (chief) of a Canadian aboriginal reserve is noted in a number of places (the reserve is the Conne River Reserve [the Miawpukek First Nation] in Newfoundland, Canada); however, it reflects the efforts among many aboriginal peoples to revitalise traditions and values, while situating them in the development of modern communities.[3] Any approach to aboriginal healthcare needs to understand the revival of interest in recent decades in traditional customs and practices.

In considering topics that healthcare providers in the USA and Canada face with aboriginal patients, this chapter is directed primarily at practitioners who are generally unfamiliar with native concerns and practices.[4] The focus is also on questions from aboriginal patients living off reserves, commonly in urban locations, rather than on the medical services on reserves.[5] One reason for this is that, since the 1960s to 1970s, aboriginal people living off as well as on reserves have been taking increasing interest in their traditional ways of healing that embraced magico-religious/spiritual ceremonies, herbs and lifestyles. Today's rediscovery of many traditions and values only minimally rebalances a long history of aboriginal acculturation driven by North American governments, church policies and broad social changes.[6]

The reinvigoration of aboriginal traditions, alongside continuing social hardships for many aboriginal people in North America, has coincided with a new focus – albeit not consistent – on educating health professionals about multicultural issues and cultural sensitivity.[7] Unfortunately, however, cultural sensitivity does not necessarily lead to easy, non-judgemental decision-making. Dilemmas can arise for healthcare practitioners when non-conventional practices fail to meet the standards of efficacy and safety acceptable to 'evidence-based medicine' (EBM), which, since the 1990s, has been commonly accepted as a new era in healthcare. Although the thrust of the chapter is directed at practitioners of conventional healthcare – in a doctor's surgery, hospital ward, pharmacy, etc. – it also applies to the growing numbers of practitioners of complementary and alternative medicine (CAM) who increasingly face the challenges of EBM and meet the same cultural issues as other practitioners.

There is no doubt that EBM, with critical and systematic approaches to evaluating clinical practice and research, has sharpened opinions that much of traditional medicine (and of CAM) is merely anecdotal and at best placebo. As a result of this, conventional practitioners are known to sidestep discussion with patients on any 'unproven', 'alternative' or 'unscientific' practice by peremptorily dismissing it as being outside the scope of their practice. Other practitioners, however, in being 'pragmatic', tell a patient (unless safety concerns are obvious): 'If it helps, it's OK with me.' Unfortunately, this response, often as a result of 'sitting on the fence', can appear glib and dismissive to a patient.

The healthcare provider and a three-step approach to patients using aboriginal medicine

Amid such a background including tensions between practitioners and between practitioners and patients, this chapter suggests *practical guidelines* for approaching usage by or questions from patients about aboriginal ways. A three-step strategy is offered. By using general approaches to patients' questions and practices (covering herbal medicines and magico-religious or spiritual approaches), this also focuses on the importance of reflecting on conventional medical thinking and attitudes. Although accounts of aboriginal (and other traditional) practices directed at conventional healthcare providers invariably concentrate on belief systems, the premise of this chapter is that effective communication in our increasingly complex multicultural communities also demands an awareness of how conventional thinking shapes professional attitudes to 'unproven' therapies.

Gathering and processing information and responding non-judgementally to patients' questions about aboriginal use is not easy for a number of reasons. One could even be a practitioner's recognition that he or she is being compared with a traditional healer whom the patient is visiting for the same problem. Hence, the three-step strategy is offered to facilitate a working approach and effective communication, an approach that applies to traditional medicine in general and to CAM.

A three-step approach

Step 1

Step 1 is preparation (background education). To be able to respond to aboriginal practices, conventional healthcare providers need not only to understand belief systems, social circumstances and attitudes (perhaps including uncertain trust in conventional practitioners), but also, as indicated, to appreciate the factors that can shape professional attitudes toward non-conventional treatments. As the latter is more for formal education (undergraduate, continuing professional, etc.), some readers may feel that it is out of place to notice even briefly some of the factors in this chapter. However, mention is made of the importance of reflecting on, for example, topics from EBM to the historical background of herbs and placebo actions as a reminder that they are often overlooked as aids to effective communication. Moreover, having the relevant knowledge is important when negotiating different viewpoints between practitioner and patient.

An appreciation of the history and concepts of self-care is also of use, e.g. after European colonisation in the seventeenth century, aboriginal people faced new information from the home and professional medicine of immigrants. No health tradition is entirely static, and it is clear that information was often consciously shared so that it is difficult to say whether or not an aboriginal practice is 'indigenous'. Modern compilations of traditional practices commonly straddle aboriginal and Euro-North American self-care traditions.[8] This applies to, for example, 'high blood pressure' – a condition that emerged in the aboriginal and European-derived traditional medicine literature – after it became a widely used diagnosis in conventional medicine in the early twentieth century. It is easy to speculate that, as an increasingly common medical term, high blood pressure was seen to fit with the long history of popular medicine (aboriginal and other) of blood purification, and so was added to lists of uses for 'blood purifiers' (alder, considered below, is an example). Blood purification continues to be a popular notion; it extends into the complementary/alternative medicine literature, and merits the attention of conventional practitioners.[9]

The greater the level of background knowledge when approaching a patient, the more a practitioner will feel comfortable in making generalizations if there is uncertainty over a treatment, as with alder for headache; at the very least it falls within a *very* weak tradition of usage.

As William Osler reminded physicians: 'The greater the ignorance, the greater the dogma.'

Step 2

Step 2 of the strategy comprises:

- ensuring that a culturally sensitive case history is taken[10]
- when necessary, quickly accessing pertinent information in computerised databases or reference books to help develop, along with background knowledge, a dialogue with a patient about efficacy and safety. Quick assessments are difficult and demand some evaluation of the record of published and other information from practitioners and of the popularity of usage over time.

If, for example, a weak tradition is indicated by a database (and confirmed by a comprehensive literature search), there is no 'scientific' justification for encouraging, say, the use of a compress of alder leaves as a generally effective treatment for a headache (see below). On the other hand, given the safety and absence of known allergic reactions of alder leaves as a traditional external application to relieve or 'cool' insect bites and inflammation, a practitioner may well support a patient wanting to try the treatment. Understanding the reason may be helpful. Maybe the query comes from an aboriginal person who is comfortable following a traditional aboriginal regimen that includes a spiritual component, e.g. acknowledging a connection between the plant and the spirit world during the harvesting of glossy (or new) leaves (compare Joe's remarks in the opening quote to the chapter). Other aspects of a regimen may be important such as changing the leaves frequently to maintain a 'cooling' action, which may well provide comfort and a feeling of relief; an active role by patients in any therapy is often recognised as helpful.

Step 3

Step 3 is not always necessary and runs on from step 2. Occasions arise when differences of opinion between patient and practitioner need to be brokered so as to develop or maintain an effective relationship. This is facilitated, partly through background knowledge (step 1), both by uncovering and understanding a patient's own circumstances and beliefs towards non-conventional approaches, and by critically evaluating published information.

A three-step strategy implies one step after the other; however, this may change in practice depending on a particular situation (e.g. a patient's level of education and knowledge), and shortcuts may be taken. Moreover, the understanding of a specific concept (step 1's preparation) may need to be revisited or learned for the first time after a case history has been taken (step 2). In this situation, admitting lack of knowledge to a patient is often appropriate. Although this is problematic for many practitioners, they can be reassured that patients accept practitioners' frank statement that they need to research a topic outside their customary practice before giving advice. The three-step strategy is therefore intended primarily to ensure that all relevant information is considered when responding to issues of efficacy and safety in the context of cultural sensitivity.

The strategy for evaluating remedies used empirically

Practitioners (and nowadays many patients) want 'scientific' evidence to support effectiveness and safety. Indeed, it is noteworthy that some aboriginal peoples are backing scientific research in the hope of marketing their traditional medicines.[11] As already indicated, the currently accepted standards for robust evidence should meet the principles of EBM. However, just what this means needs reflection because there are tendencies to stereotype EBM as the application of clinical trial data to patients as if one medication, one regimen, fits all. In fact, EBM should be viewed as it was by its early pioneers, namely: 'EBM is the integration of best research evidence and clinical expertise and patient values.'[12] For this reason, many practitioners prefer the term 'evidence-informed practice' to make clear that it focuses on the needs and situation of *each* patient; this may mean that a practitioner – depending on the values and wishes of a patient – supports the trial of a therapy (perhaps an aboriginal practice) even though the evidence for efficacy is relatively low in the hierarchical levels that have become part of the EBM movement.

Such levels are generally along the lines, from top to bottom, of meta-analyses of randomised controlled trials (RCTs), systematic reviews, limited evidence from RCTs, cohort studies, case-controlled studies, case series, case reports, expert opinion and anecdote drawn from one or a few isolated observations.[13] What is missing from hierarchical lists is a place for 'anecdotal knowledge' at a level higher than 'anecdote' and 'expert opinion'. Anecdotal knowledge (or evidence) is that which has been built up over an extended period of time among generations of practitioners and others who develop a specialised knowledge (e.g. herbalists, 'wise women'), through their own experiences, and from comparing these with others of colleagues, in either consultations or published reports. Anecdotal knowledge not only is a feature of much aboriginal/traditional medical practice, but also has long been a key element of conventional medical practice.[14] Although constantly diminishing as a result of the development of modern pharmacology and clinical trials, anecdotal knowledge for treating individual patients remains an everyday part of conventional medicine; even so it is commonly overlooked by those – perhaps more by younger practitioners still close to their medical education – who fail to see an existing paradox, namely conventional medicine's claim to be a positivist science despite the uncertainties of clinical practice in interpretation, flexibility and practicality.[15]

Judgement of the robustness of evidence embedded in anecdotal knowledge is problematic, even though evaluation is more at the level of evidence accepted in civil prosecutions, namely 'more likely than not', rather than the criminal standard of 'beyond a reasonable doubt'.

Examples of applying the three-step approach to herbal remedies in aboriginal usage

Selection of examples of herbs out of the vast armamentarium of aboriginal/traditional remedies (with much regional variation) is not easy. The two chosen (alder and black cohosh) have been selected to illustrate different challenges in response to questions about aboriginal usage. Alder, unlike black cohosh, has not become a major dietary supplement and few scientific data are available to assist in evaluation. In contrast, the top-selling black cohosh has been subjected to many laboratory and clinical studies, albeit with inconsistent findings. At least both herbs reflect a widespread belief that a core of empirical knowledge, long held by herbalists (some called *yerberos*), lies behind the use of herbs – a view that underpins much research on constituents of aboriginal and other traditional medicinal plants. On the other hand, whether or not some form of ceremony or ritual accompanied the administration and contributed to therapeutic benefits is not always clear (see below).

Alder

Alder has been chosen because it was the subject of a question to a general practitioner in 2003, a type of query that might come from anyone interested in 'natural' remedies. On hearing about its use by Mi'kmaq people in Newfoundland, a patient asked whether it was good for headache – better than aspirin which upset the questioner's stomach. It is also an example of one of many herbs about which the busy practitioner has difficulty finding useful information to confirm whether or not it has some general value.

Uses

Well-established databases are not helpful with information on alder, e.g. one of them gives only the following information:

- **People use this for**: pharyngitis and intestinal bleeding
- **Safety**: there is insufficient reliable information available about the safety of smooth alder
- **Pregnancy and lactation**: insufficient reliable information available; avoid using
- **Effectiveness**: there is insufficient reliable information about the effectiveness of smooth alder.[16]

No reference is given to headache. In fact the above information is for *Alnus serrulata*, a related species of *A. viridus* spp. *crispus* which is harvested in Conne River for headache – a reminder that correct botanical identification is essential in evaluating data.[17] *A. serrulata* is commonly noted in the US medical literature; one example gives a lengthy list of reputed uses recorded for the aboriginal Cherokees of North Carolina: for 'pains related to birth; swellings and sprains; skin eruptions; ingredient in tea to clear milky urine; ingredient in tea for menstrual period; an emetic and purgative; rub and blow infusion of bark in eyes for drooping';[18] other recommendations include 'cold bark tea to purify blood or bring down high blood pressure'.[18] It is appropriate to note that such lists, in being unwieldy and unfathomable, are valueless as a clinical aid for most conventional practitioners without some preparation as in step 1 to consider how such lists have evolved.[19]

A check on an indispensable source of information on aboriginal herbs, namely Dan Moerman's database *Native American Ethnobotany* (available on the internet) offers relatively little help in the use of alder for headache.[20] A search for '*Alnus* and headache' in the compilation of information drawn from publications on aboriginal ethnobotany finds two different entries (out of 355 hits for '*Alnus*'). One is to *Alnus rubra* (a different species) as an 'emetic and purgative for headache and other maladies', and the other is to an infusion of the twigs as a 'liniment for pain of sprains, bruises, backache and headache'. However, citing Moerman's work to support any specific usage needs a critical appraisal of the sources of information culled by Moerman; these, variable in quality, commonly raise questions over, for example, the correctness of plant identification, type of preparation used or other details, some of which Moerman felt necessary to omit given the scope of the database.

Such limited information strongly suggests that the use of alder for a headache is a local reputation – all the more so as published accounts of Mi'kmaq usage do not record 'headache'.[21] On the other hand, the oral tradition includes:

> Well an old man had a bad head one time, a headache and I used to go out and pick glossy alder leaves for him and he put it on a rag and tied it around his head and in a half hour or so them alder leaves would turn brown and I would change them. I kept doing that for about all one day, four or five hours I suppose.[22]

Limited or local usage of any medicine is especially difficult to evaluate and is invariably labelled as anecdotal. However, to avoid a minimal response to questions (e.g. 'there is no evidence to support it'), which patients may well perceive as judgemental, practitioners will find it useful to do some preparation/education (step 1) on the different levels of evidence noticed.

Black cohosh

This second herb for consideration, black cohosh, offers a different set of circumstances for discussion with patients. As a top-selling dietary supplement – largely because of a reputation for relieving menopausal symptoms (and, to a lesser extent, menstrual symptoms, e.g. cramps) – it has been subjected to many laboratory and clinical studies. However, although traditional aboriginal knowledge has seemingly been superseded by modern scientific/clinical studies, practitioners may well face queries on at least two matters: (1) the aboriginal reputation and (2) efficacy and safety.

Uses

Published accounts of both the herb and its commercial promotion commonly refer to a history of aboriginal usage, e.g. 'American Indian groups of eastern North America were using the root of black cohosh to treat female conditions and for rheumatism, long before Europeans landed on American shores'.[23] Such statements, commonly offered without documentation or context, generally serve to bolster confidence in recent scientific/clinical data that suggest benefits. Aboriginal women have specifically asked practitioners about how it was used by their people before modern natural healthcare products marketed it in capsules.

Safety and efficacy

Questions/concerns arise because recent research studies offer conflicting conclusions. Aboriginal women today are among the women who are concerned about hormone replacement therapy; many look to such 'natural remedies' as black cohosh.

As mentioned, assessing the evidence of whether a herb reaches the level of anecdotal knowledge is not easy. Two topics are noted here as illustrations, both pertinent to an evaluation of black cohosh.

Evaluating recorded information

In addition to issues already noted in Moerman's *Native American Ethnobotany*, step 1's preparation also needs to examine the often glib claims that a herb has been used for 'hundreds of years' by 'Indians' and others. Careful historical study is often required to determine whether this is justified.

Information on aboriginal treatments published up to the early nineteenth century generally came from travellers who, often with some knowledge of medicine, were curious about aboriginal ways. However, understanding aboriginal therapeutic practices was far from easy given the limited time and opportunities; thus early observations, although in many ways invaluable, have to be treated cautiously. Moreover, because of copying by one author from another, the frequency of references to a particular usage cannot be accepted, without careful review, as providing the level of evidence that reaches, say, anecdotal knowledge.

Specifically, with regard to black cohosh, early observers undoubtedly found it more difficult to assess emmenagogue action and effects on menstruation among aboriginal women than, for example, the obviously vigorous purgative action of mayapple (*Podophyllum peltatum*). Yet emmenagogue activity quickly became noted as an aboriginal usage; it persists in current promotions that do not necessarily take information from the most reliable of sources. One is a quote found in Virgil Vogel's still widely used, if somewhat dated, *American Indian Medicine* (1970); it states that Indians introduced black cohosh to early American medicine and that no early non-aboriginal writers on materia medica 'added anything not given by the Indians as far as the field of action of the drug is concerned except for some nineteenth-century instances of the use of the plant for treating smallpox'.[24] However, even a cursory look at nineteenth-century writings on black cohosh suggests that not only was copying of information from one source to another commonplace, but also physicians and, especially, the practitioners of the eclectic school of botanic medicine contributed to black cohosh becoming a virtual panacea for countless conditions within both conventional and domestic medicine. Recently compiled lists of uses by, for example, North Carolina Cherokees continue to reflect this with all the appearance of information taken from non-aboriginal sources: 'roots in alcoholic spirits for rheumatism; tonic; diuretic; anodyne; emmenagogue; slightly astringent; tea for colds; coughs; consumptions; constipation; tea for rheumatism; fatigue; hives; to make baby sleep; backache' (Hamel and Chiltosky,[18] page 30).

As already indicated, practitioners generally find such lists problematic and difficult to interpret. Moreover, they offer no sense of the differences of opinion that have existed among practitioners over time. In the nineteenth century, some physicians who questioned or expressed caution over efficacy for 'female conditions' were widely recognised medical 'authorities' at a time of widespread usage of herbs, e.g. Robley Dunglison in the USA made no mention of black cohosh's emmenagogue action in his *New Remedies* of 1843, while noting that it was employed 'chiefly in domestic practice, as a remedy in rheumatism, dropsy, hysteria and in various affections of the lungs'.[25] On the other hand, in his popular *General Therapeutics and Materia Medica* of 1850, Dunglison did raise cautions in stating that the testimony of 'pharmacological writers in regard to its action is sufficiently imprecise'.[26] He noted another authority when indicating that, although some practitioners consider it to have a 'practical affinity for the uterus', that was not the case because 'it probably exerts some influence over the nervous system of the nature not exactly understood'. Questioning comments about its effects on the uterus were in line with doubts about the general value of the herb for female complaints, although it was felt that a tonic action – as with many other medications – might be helpful. Further instances of questioning comments cannot be given here, although they do support an ongoing uncertainty about effectiveness for women's complaints.

Lay (sometimes called social) validation of a treatment: concepts of disease

An important aspect of step 1's preparation is an understanding of why the persistent reputation of many non-conventional therapies over time rests on lay validation. This aspect is multifactorial and complex, and certainly demands effective communication skills for a practitioner to uncover relevant issues for individual patients. They may include:

- popular interpretation of medical advances
- testimonials from relatives and others about successful outcomes
- treatments rationalised on the basis of beliefs about a disease (often popular beliefs current at the time such as blood purifiers)
- treatment by a practitioner (perhaps an aboriginal healer) who supports beliefs that are compatible with those that the person holds, e.g. the connections between plants and the spirit world.

A key issue is the popular concepts of disease. These – often relating to the causative agents acting from both outside and within the body – involve both natural and supernatural explanations. Depending on the demographics of their practice, a practitioner will want to be familiar with aboriginal diagnoses and treatments that confound conventional medicine, e.g. susto, a condition – especially among aboriginal people in south-western USA – viewed as the loss of 'soul' during a fright; it is best treated by an aboriginal healer rather than conventional medicine. Although such diagnoses were once regional, recent migrations of populations throughout the USA and Canada mean that all practitioners should be aware of supernatural explanations. Another noteworthy example is rootwork among African–Americans that generally perplexes those who have not been alerted to its existence.[27]

Whatever the belief or beliefs held by a patient, a conventional practitioner will wonder about, for example, the role of the argument that assumes that an intervention accounts for an effect or outcome and placebo effects. Moreover, less tangible matters must not be overlooked in considering persistence of beliefs, e.g. the mystique that has long surrounded 'Indian' herbs and is partly reflected in such common names as Indian chickweed, Indian hemp, Indian pennyroyal, Indian pink, Indian plantain, Indian sage, as well as squawroot and squawvine. Although such a mystique contributes to a 'pedigree' of empirical knowledge, it must be pointed out that relatively few plants used by North American aboriginal peoples had a lasting impact on North American and European *professional* medical practice – as distinct from domestic usage – which raises doubts about the *general* effectiveness of many of them, even black cohosh.[28]

Depending on the patient and the questions (perhaps about the different views that currently exist over the efficacy and safety of black cohosh), practitioner–patient discussion might notice the uncertain historical record, at least for use for menopausal symptoms. As noted, not only is there a history of uncertainty, even when black cohosh was in fashion, but also there are issues over current promotion that selects information to support a case, or even over 'reading' uses into older texts to support current views on a substance's reputation in menopausal symptoms.[29] It is noteworthy that the uncertainties found in the historical records continue into modern clinical and scientific studies, which led to the title of a 2006 commentary: 'Black cohosh: will there ever be an answer or answers?' In reporting on (1) uncertainty over efficacy for menopausal symptoms (data are mixed) and (2) adverse effects, the article also raised a significant issue, namely whether black cohosh is oestrogenic with potentially analogous concerns to those raised by HRT:

> . . . the bulk of current thought and data do not support the idea that black cohosh is estrogenic. However, [recent] studies . . . which report

a trend toward maturation of vaginal epithelium, persist in raising the question of whether black cohosh acts somehow like estrogen.[30]

Science has not been able to deal convincingly with the possibility, certainly not proven, of oestrogenic effects and theoretical adverse effects, especially for those with a history of hormone-sensitive cancers or a family history. In the current climate of practice, a practitioner has a responsibility to provide the pros and cons for the use of a treatment giving a critical evaluation of non-scientific as well as scientific data.

Magico-religious/spiritual practices

Introductory comments

As problematic as the critical appraisal of information on herbs can be, some practitioners may find greater difficulty in responding to queries about what have long been called magico-religious, magical and spiritual practices. Nowadays, the distinction between these categories is commonly blurred, because they depend on how supernatural forces are viewed by individuals.

Although this chapter is not concerned with Mexican traditional practices, they have become part of other North American countries to which Mexicans migrated.

Magico-religious practices commonly embrace beliefs in supernatural influences; these include shamanism, in which a shaman, in the context of healing, can act as a medium for an entering spirit (maybe the spirit of a renowned ancestral healer) to 'orchestrate' the care through the healer. On the other hand, some will describe, say, the charming away of warts as merely 'magical', meaning a magical circumstance – a view perhaps influenced by a popular idea of a healer as someone who is able to help a person develop their own inherent healing powers, or, as some might say, enhancing 'the power of the mind over the body'. The 'power' (or skill) of some such healers may be viewed as a result of a deep knowledge of traditions, perhaps including the ability to make spiritual connections – in other words, divorced from being able to control supernatural forces. Thus ceremonies and their healing powers for individuals and communities, e.g. the sweat lodge, sweetgrass and smudging, and talking circles, are cast in different ways (magico-religious, spiritual or relatively secular, perhaps invoking psychosocial explanations), according to the observer.

It is incumbent on a practitioner responding to the question from a patient about a ceremony (perhaps an aboriginal person looking to reconnect with traditional ways) to appreciate the spectrum of ceremonies and how they may help with specific physical, mental or psychological problems. To do so demands reflection on one's own attitudes as well as an appreciation of the nature of the main ceremonies (step 1).

It is certainly as well to remember that conventional medicine has long looked upon magical practices as lacking credibility, certainly since the seventeenth to eighteenth centuries when supernatural practices were increasingly expunged from regular treatments. In fact, this trend joined the growing scepticism, on the part of many practitioners, of the value of numerous herbal treatments including those used by aboriginal peoples. For instance, in 1897 James Mooney indicated that only 25% of an admittedly small group of Cherokee plants were used correctly (see Hamel and Chiltosky,[18] page 6).

Step 1 (preparation): the placebo effect

Before noting some features of healing ceremonies (the sweat lodge as an example) that can be useful for a practitioner in discussions with patients, it is helpful to reflect on a reason commonly heard today for paying little attention to aboriginal treatments, namely that any benefit is 'merely a placebo effect'. Such a dismissal – it also applies to a wide range of other 'unproven' traditional and CAM treatments – invariably overlooks the negative feelings towards a placebo action that became widespread only after the 1950s when placebo controls became a key part of RCTs. With this new role, physicians began to feel that it was unethical to prescribe a placebo consciously – as had previously been fairly common (the proverbial 'bottle of coloured water', although attacked at times) – either as 'fake' treatment or as one unsupported by clinical trial data.[31] This view was bolstered by a new emphasis on the autonomy of patients, such that any deception in information (meaning failure to give full disclosure) became unacceptable. It is noteworthy that the change in attitudes from before the 1950s seemingly occurred without general discussion on the potential to diminish placebo effects that benefited patients.

Having said this, it is as well to appreciate that, since writing this, some change in attitudes might be under way. At least a *British Medical Journal* editorial (3 May 2008) strongly hinted that the placebo effect may be one of the most 'added value' tools in the medical bag.[32] Certainly some practitioners, in remembering that placebo effects are virtually universal in any therapeutic intervention, challenge any quick dismissal of an unconventional therapy – at least a dismissal without careful assessment merely because it has no modern supporting epidemiological or clinical trial data. This applies to healing ceremonies although they are often acknowledged to have potential psychological effects for some participants, perhaps associated with the power of the ritual (see below). Moreover, many facets of healing ceremonies resonate with those viewed as essential for effective therapeutic relationships:

mutually held beliefs between practitioner and patient, a patient's trust, elements of hope and other factors with a potential to foster a placebo effect. Given this, a conventional practitioner may want to consider seriously whether to positively support a healing ceremony, or indeed for it to become a part of integrated care for an aboriginal person living in an urban situation and looking to try a traditional practice.

The sweat lodge: some key points for step 2 discussion

The sweat lodge is chosen to illustrate certain points that can be useful when responding to a patient who asks whether a healing ceremony might be helpful, as well as for exploring their expectations.

> The sweat lodge is where you can talk openly about how you feel about alcoholism, family abuse or whatever. It becomes an important support. Whenever you have difficulty, you know there will always be people in the circle who do care about you, and do care if you survive or not, and do care for your family. And, too, I've heard a lot of talk from older people on how it helps not only the spiritual part, but also aches and pains. It's one of the best medicines for stress.

These words from the chief of a Mi'kmaq reserve, where the sweat lodge ceremony was recently introduced (after being in limbo for generations) as part of the revitalisation of traditional ways and values, reflects both the widespread use of the lodge to help with sociomedical problems (e.g. spousal abuse, drug addiction) as well as specific physical ailments such as rheumatic disorders.

Although details of the sweat lodge and ceremony are generally well known in outline, it is helpful to stress the beliefs and symbolism behind every stage in constructing a lodge and each step in the ceremony. A brief flavour is given in the following summary of the Mi'kmaq chief's description. This is similar to other accounts of sweat lodge ceremonies although there are many variations in detail such as differences in construction (from permanent to small low-level lodges), in details of the ceremony (e.g. whether fasting before and after a ceremony takes place), and whether the conductor of a ceremony is viewed as a shaman or merely one able to help participants find personal and community connections.

Whatever the differences in detail, spiritual connections are borne in mind throughout the construction of a lodge and the ceremony. This begins with choosing the actual site. On one occasion, the chief's brother saw an eagle fly down into a wooded area, but surprisingly it did not reappear. Given the symbolic nature of the eagle in aboriginal spirituality this was considered a sign of a spiritual place suitable for a lodge. Then, each step in construction made connections to the spirit world or to the traditions and values of the past, e.g. starting from the east, searching for 'special' rocks for heating in the sacred fire (possibly rocks from a place associated with grandfathers), smudging the outside of the lodge and the heated rocks before they were taken inside (see next section for discussion of smudging). Subsequent steps after closing the 'door' (flap) include:

- creating steam by pouring water (sometimes a sacred water) on the hot rocks (viewed as helping to effect purification of the body and spirit)
- prayers to the spirits said by the conductor of the ceremony
- the participants – who are seated on the earth in a circle around the rocks – raising in turn personal or community issues.

It is a place where people can express themselves knowing that people listen.

Although the conductor may not be a shaman, special 'powers' may be brought into a ceremony. Sometimes this is done in ways used only occasionally, perhaps throwing a particular herb or medicine on the heated rocks. One instance has been the use of 'seven sorts' medicine in sweat lodge ceremonies at the Conne River reserve. It is a symbolic way of connecting to the past. One oral account reported:

> One of the old-time favourite medicines is seven sorts – it's like molasses. Put it on a cloth, like a plaster, for cuts, and aches and pains, but I've also used in the sweat lodge ceremony in a spiritual way by putting it on the hot rocks to become part of the steam; it helps to link with the traditional healing of the past. It seems to be magical; if the pain moves then the seven sorts follows the pain.[3]

The ingredients were learned from elders (the oral tradition): often cherry bark, pussy-willow bark and aspen or wild wittie bark, the roots of yellow root and beaver root, the entire boughs of ground juniper and the buds of the balsam. They were boiled together, the solid pieces removed, and the liquid boiled down to the thickness of molasses.

The story of seven sorts is of special interest for its associations with magic, a reminder of the persistence of traditional practices generally viewed as folklore. The earliest recorded account of seven sorts is possibly in an 1896 article titled 'Micmac Magic and Medicine'. The author states that it illustrates the 'mystic' of [Indian] medicinal herbs, the 'magical' associations were linked to the way the seven constituents were collected during a particular season (in the autumn), the order of collection, and for the barks to be taken from particular sections of trunk when each was in sunlight; important, too, was the power attributed to the number seven.[33] Although movement of the seven sorts to follow the pain is not mentioned in the article, there is evidence to indicate that it persists in a fairly strong oral tradition in the Conne River community today.[34]

Clinical studies on the benefits of the sweat lodge are limited – to date they point only to positive changes in spiritual and emotional well-being – but the numbers of 'anecdotal' reports of benefits must be considered as reaching the level of anecdotal knowledge with respect to helping with sociomedical problems, if less so for 'rheumatic' aches and pains and skin diseases.[35] Any discussion with patients about the health aspects of the sweat lodge may be helped – at least in a limited way – by the larger body of literature on saunas; this makes clear that advice must take into account a patient's health, especially as sweat lodge ceremonies can be more physiologically stressful to the body than conventional saunas; various contraindications are reported for saunas such as unstable angina pectoris and recent myocardial infarction.[36] It is appropriate to add that those uncomfortable with a sweat lodge ceremony – not always on medical grounds – may benefit from a talking circle in which participants, in turn, raise issues/problems.

Ceremonies and healthcare institutions

In addition to the sweat lodge, practitioners may be called on to comment on other ceremonies that have a strong healing component. Although it is beyond the scope of this chapter to detail these, practitioners should be prepared to follow up on a patient's interest in any ceremony associated with healing. In so doing a practitioner may call on other sources of guidance – maybe programmes focusing on learning traditional ways such as building wigwams, trapping, etc. – from native friendship centres to social workers acquainted with healing programmes. Team care can be important in many ways as when a patient wants a healing ceremony in a conventional healthcare setting (hospital or surgery/clinic). It is not uncommon for an aboriginal person to first express interest in traditional ways when serious medical problems arise. Such a person may be too timid to ask directly for a ceremony, but an empathic practitioner may sense the need. A not uncommon wish is for smudging, a ceremony recognised for 'purification' that can foster, at the very least, feelings of spiritual well-being. Smoke from a burning braid of sweetgrass (other vegetable products, e.g. sage, cedar, tobacco, may be used) is wafted over the body. Although obvious difficulties arise in performing the ceremony with modern smoke detector–sprinkler systems, modifications of the ceremony might be explored that meet a patient's need.

Other requests can be logistically easier to fulfil, given sensitivity and cooperation on the part of healthcare practitioners and administrators, e.g. taking sacred objects into an operating room. Yet difficulties have arisen. Stories, such as the following, of cultural insensitivity among doctors are not uncommon and should be a salutary reminder that cultural issues surrounding death extend to all peoples.

> I seriously believe that if I went to hospital and if I wasn't treated according to some of my beliefs, I would suffer. If I showed up at the hospital with my feather, my sweet grass, the things that I believe in, if I wasn't allowed to keep these things with me as part of my own healing, I believe that a doctor could do serious harm to me. Modern day medicines are fine medicines, but there's something else that goes along with that. Treatment is far more than handing out pills. It's the way the doctor hands you those pills, it's how he receives you in his clinic, how he is able to relate to some of the things you are talking about. When my uncle died, I wanted to talk to the doctor about making sure that he went to his spirit world, that all the things that had been done during an autopsy were all put back and in place. He didn't take any time to talk about my concern. He sort of ushered me out and we ended up having this discussion in a lobby. He had no concern of what I was talking about, or wanted to talk about, except to say that 'when we cut it out we put it back'.[3]

Closing comments

This chapter has touched on various issues that can help a practitioner approach aboriginal/traditional medicine practices with which he or she has little acquaintance. Although sometimes viewed as 'thinking outside the box', understanding the social and historical aspects of medicine can help a practitioner appreciate that quality care involves negotiating the beliefs, values and social situations of individual patients. In so doing, a practitioner needs to appreciate the role of ritual in healthcare, a key factor in understanding not only aboriginal practices, but also the history of therapy in general, a history replete with metaphors and symbolism. Consistency in encounters between practitioner and patient – whether in conventional medical settings in surgeries and hospitals or in aboriginal healing ceremonies – is just one consideration that medical anthropologists point to as significant in effective therapeutic encounters. Examples, which range from a doctor's white coat to the 'purification' from a sweetgrass ceremony – and countless others symbolic of tradition and authority – can contribute to a patient's confidence and hope and thereby enhance a placebo effect in both conventional and non-conventional practices.[37]

As important as sensitivity is to non-pharmacological (non-specific) effects when approaching aboriginal/traditional medical practices in non-judgemental ways, there is an equal challenge in advising patients about the uncertainties surrounding efficacy and safety issues due to pharmacologically active constituents in herbal preparations. It is a challenge that calls on a systematic approach, effective preparation and communication skills which appreciate that, for example, applying EBM to patients is more than the strict application of clinical trial data.

Notes and references

1. Joe M. Healing: a First Nations' perspective. In: *Traditional/Alternative/Complementary Health Care Issues*, vol. 1. Proceedings of the VIIIth International Conference Traditional Medicine and Folklore held in St John's, Newfoundland, Canada, 1994. St John's: Faculty of Medicine, Memorial University of Newfoundland, 1998: 129–36.
2. Quoted in Sandner D. *Navaho Symbols of Healing*. New York: Harcourt, Brace Jovanovich, 1979: 17–18.
3. The reserve is the Conne River Reserve (the Miawpukek First Nation) in Newfoundland, Canada. The information comes from a forthcoming book: Andersen RR, Crellin JK (eds), *Mi'sel Joe. An aboriginal chief's journey*. St John's: Flanker Press, 2009.
4. This note covers terms used in the chapter. (1) *North America*: Mexico, commonly included in the definition of North America, is excluded; much traditional medicine there is closer to that found in South American countries. (2) *Aboriginal*: this has been selected (with 'native' as an occasional alternative) as, it is hoped, being the most acceptable to First Nations' people in the USA and Canada. Some political sensitivity, not necessarily uniform, surrounds the term 'Indian', although it remains acceptable to many. And although 'indigenous' is preferred by others to indicate knowledge in place independent of influences of European or other immigrants, the impact of post-contact European influence is often difficult to determine. (3) *Patient*: the term is still widely used by the medical profession, whereas many other health professionals are tending more to 'client', although for pharmacists – a point of contact for much self-care (including dietary supplements) – the term 'customer' still applies. Patient is preferred because it continues to reflect a special relationship with a practitioner.
5. For the importance of considering aboriginal people in urban locations (and in rural areas off reserve), see Wilson K, Young TK. An overview of Aboriginal health research in the social sciences: current trends and future directions. *Int J Circumpolar Health* 2008;67(2–3):179–89. Statistical returns on aboriginal people living in urban areas show rising numbers in part through a greater readiness to acknowledge aboriginal ancestry. For activities on reserves, some mindful of integrating traditional and conventional health services, one can consult, for example, US Department of Health and Human Services. Indian Health Services. Available at: www.ihs.gov/index.asp (accessed October 2008).
6. The emergence of interest in the USA and Canada has been mostly noted by non-aboriginal observers, e.g. Waldram JB, Herring SA, Young TK. *Aboriginal Health in Canada: Historical, cultural and epidemiological perspectives*. Toronto: University of Toronto Press, 1995: 204. Although this covers aboriginal people in Canada, analogous situations occur in the USA.
7. Much of the interest comes from the discipline of medical anthropology as reflected in books such as Cecil Helman's: Helman C. *Culture, Health and Illness*, 5th edn. London: Hodder Arnold, 2007. This is singled out here as being a book particularly oriented to practitioners.
8. Modern compilations of aboriginal herbal remedies often show significant overlap with lists representative of Anglo-European traditions. Compare Mackey MA, Bernard L. Traditional medicine used by the Micmacs of Conne River, Newfoundland. In: *I eats them like that*. Changing food patterns of the Micmac of Conne River, unpublished manuscript, 1985: 78–87, and Crellin JK. *Home Medicine: The Newfoundland experience*.

Montreal: McGill Queens Press, 1994. Nevertheless many ceremonies are primarily indigenous, e.g. 'The way the peyote ceremony is practiced, I would say about 99 percent of whatever is taking place in there is basically Navajo. Prayers are all in Navajo; many Navajo traditional prayers have been integrated and incorporated into the ceremonies.' (Davies W. *Healing Ways. Navajo health care in the twentieth century*. Albuquerque: University of New Mexico Press, 2001: 181.)

9. It is appropriate to notice that the current promotion of 'old' medicines and practices often fails to consider new safety information, a consideration as in the example given next, namely the issue of pyrrolizidine alkaloids in coltsfoot. Under the internet heading 'Cold and flu formulas. Make your own herbal medicine for your families cold and flu symptoms': 'Garlic Honey Cough and Cold Syrup (Peel garlic cloves, put into a jar. cover with honey. Set in warm place for 2 weeks or more until the garlic turns opaque. Take 1 teaspoonful as needed. Dilute with a little water or lemon juice for children. Or, Cough Combo ('Equal parts of Coltsfoot, Mullein and Licorice. Combine all herbs and use 1–2 tsp. per cup of boiling water. Steep for 10 minutes.)' Available from: www.taoherbfarm. com/herbs/resources/coldflurecipes.htm (accessed October 2008).

10. Inadequacies in history taking, at least with respect to CAM, have been documented, often in the context that patients, fearing ridicule, do not volunteer information to physicians. Compare Cockayne NL, Duguid M, Shenfield GM. Health professionals rarely record history of complementary and alternative medicine. *Br J Clin Pharmacol* 2005; 59:254–8. Published advice and guidelines exist although these – intended either to elicit specific usage during routine history-taking, or to give advice on how to talk to patients (sometimes referred to as holistic interviewing) – tend to be overly detailed for the busy physician. Eisenberg DM. Advising patients who seek alternative medical therapies. *Ann Intern Med* 1997;**127**:61–9. At least one 'decision tree', useful but complex, has also been published to assist doctors who need to search for information on behalf of a patient and/or to decide whether integrated care is appropriate. For the decision tree: www.amsa.org/ICAM/decisiontree.cfm (accessed October 2008). Taken from Frenkel MA, Borkan JM. An approach for integrating complementary–alternative medicine into primary care. *Fam Pract* 2003;**20**:324–32.

11. For example, Health Canada's note on work with the Cree of Eeyou Istchee, Quebec, Canada. The project investigates use of medicinal plants for diabetes in Cree. Available at: www.hc-sc.gc.ca/sr-sr/activ/consprod/cree-cries-eng.php (accessed October 2008).

12. For example, Sacket DL, Straus SE, Richardson WS et al. *Evidence-based Medicine: How to practice and teach EBM*. Edinburgh: Churchill Livingstone, 2000: 1.

13. Various lists of hierarchies, differing in detail and terminology, have been published. Just to mention some, from the Bandolier group, in descending order of validity: 1. Strong evidence from at least one published systematic review of multiple well-designed RCTs. 2. Strong evidence from at least one published properly designed RCT of appropriate size and in an appropriate clinical setting. 3. Evidence from published well-designed trials without randomisation, single group pre–post, cohort, time series or matched case-controlled studies. 4. Evidence from well-designed non-experimental studies from more than one centre or research group. 5. Opinions of respected authorities, based on clinical evidence, descriptive studies or reports of expert consensus committees. Available at: www.jr2.ox.ac.uk/bandolier/band6/b6–5.html (accessed October 2008). Level 5, the lowest level, is not to be confused with simple expert opinion and personal experience that is sometimes called *eminence*-based medicine.

14. For an indication of this pattern of thinking in conventional medicine, most obvious before the rise of protoclinical trials and animal experiments in the eighteenth century, see Crellin JK. Theory and clinical experience in eighteenth-century extemporaneous prescriptions – a reciprocal relationship? *Pharm Hist* 2006;**48**:3–13. The importance of anecdotal knowledge in other fields of endeavour (e.g. in the fishery) is often recognised.

15. See Montgomery K. *How Doctors Think. Clinical judgement and the practice of medicine*. Oxford: Oxford University Press, 2006: 8 for comments about science and clinical practice, although the theme runs throughout the book.

16. Natural Medicines Comprehensive Database. Available from: www.naturaldatabase. com/(S(rwdt5xm035hbik55dg4fkzf0))/home.aspx?cs=mun&s=ND . It is not the purpose to list herbal databases here, but another widely used in North America is Natural Standard. Available from: www.naturalstandard.com (both accessed October 2008).

17. Unfortunately, the majority of sources of information on herbs do not provide evidence that a specific botanical specimen was gathered by or known to an informant.

18. Hamel PB, Chiltoskey MU. Cherokee plants and their uses – a 400 year history. Cherokee: privately printed, 1975: 22. Reference to purgative action seems out of keeping with other uses that can be rationalised on the basis of astringency (see below) and confusion with another 'alder' (in fact, alder buckthorn) has to be considered.

19. To offer just one point: a number of illnesses are listed because of a reputation to relieve a common symptom, although the latter is not specifically mentioned, e.g. the property of astringency seemingly accounts for the use of alder, as noted in the database, for 'pharyngitis' and the associated styptic action for 'intestinal bleeding'.

20. Native American ethnobotany. Available from: http://herb.umd.umich.edu (accessed July 2008).

21. Comments based on a review of occasional publications on Micmac usage. A recent account merits notice to underscore the diversity of reputations. Lacey L. *Micmac Medicines. Remedies and recollections*. Halifax: Nimbus Publishing, 1994: 22, on the use of alder in Conne River relates a case of 'lameness' – the patient recovered despite a doctor saying that there was 'no cure': 'The individual collected a large bag of alder leaves and spent the following night treating the problem. The leaves were placed over the affected areas of the body, and were replaced with a fresh covering whenever they became "too hot." This cured the lameness.' Elsewhere, in Nova Scotia, Lacey records Mi'kmaq people making a tea by steeping the bark and using it for 'stomach cramps, kidney ailments, fever and neuralgic pain . . . diphtheria [and] the bark and leaves were used together in poultice form as a treatment for festering wounds'.

22. This account by Chief Joe has been told to many visitors to the Conne River reserve, especially on a walk through the community's Medicine Trail.

23. For example, from the writings of well-known herb author, Steven Foster: Black cohosh *Cimicifuga racemosa (Actaea racemosa)*. Available from: www.stevenfoster.com/education/ monograph/bkcohosh.html (accessed October 2008) and countless commercial websites. See also Foster S. Black cohosh: a literature review. *HerbalGram* 1999;**45**:35–50.

24. Vogel V. *American Indian Medicine*. Normal: University of Oklahoma Press, 1970: 370.

25. Dunglison R. *New Remedies: Pharmaceutical and therapeutically considered*. Philadelphia, PA: Lea & Blanchard, 1843: 164–6.

26. Dunglison R. *General Therapeutics and Materia Medica*, vol 2. Philadelphia, PA: Lea & Blanchard, 1850: 196–7. Dunglison's reference to Wood was to: Wood GB, Bache F. *The Dispensatory of the United States of America*. Philadelphia, PA: Grigg, Elliot & Co., 1847: 211–12.

27. For an account for practitioners: Lichstein PR. Rootwork from the clinicians' perspective. In: Kirkland J, Mathews HF, Sullivan III CW, Baldwin K (eds), *Herbal and Magical Medicine. Traditional healing today*. Durham, NC: Duke University Press, 1992: 99–117.

28. For discussion of limited impact on professional medicine: Cowen DL. The impact of the materia medica of the North American Indians on professional practice. In: Hein W-H, ed. *Botanical Drugs of the Americas in the Old and New Worlds*. Stuttgart: Wissenschaftliche Verlagsgesellschaft, 1984: 51–63.

29. For some reference to this with regard to black cohosh: Crellin JK. 'Traditional use' claims for herbs: the need for competent historical research. *Pharm Hist (Lond)* 2008;**38**: 34–40.

30. Richardson MK. Black cohosh: will there ever be an answer or answers. *Menopause* 2006;**13**:164–5. The comment is based on a clinical paper in the same issue of the journal: Wuttke W, Gorkow C, Seidlova-Wuttke D. Effects of black cohosh (*Cimicifuga racemosa*) on bone turnover, vaginal mucosa, and on various blood parameters in postmenopausal women: a double-blind placebo-controlled and conjugated estrogens-controlled

study. *Menopause* 2006;**13**:185–96. Relevant, too, a study indicating a small stimulating effect on the growth of the *MCF*-7 breast cancer cell line compared with untreated cells: Nuntanakorn P, Jiang B, Einbond LS et al. Polyphenolic constituents of *Actaea racemosa*. *J Nat Prod* 2006;**69**:314–18.

31. For background to use of placebo in the past: de Craen AJM, Kaptchuk TJ, Tijssen JG, Kleijnen J. Placebos and placebo effects in medicine: historical overview. *J R Soc Med* 1999;**92**:511–15. Kaptchuk TJ. Intentional ignorance: a history of blind assessment and placebo controls in medicine. *Bull Hist Med* 1998;**72**:389–433.

32. Godlee F. Reclaiming the placebo effect. *BMJ* 2008;**336**:966.

33. Hagar S. Micmac magic and medicine. *J Am Folklore* 1896;**9**:170–7. Hagar seemingly did not consider whether or not the 'directions' for preparing the seven sorts incorporated, knowingly or unknowingly, empirical advice long recognised among Euro-North Americans for collecting herbs, e.g. barks are still said to be best collected in the spring time (in part because this is the time when peeling is easiest), and roots to be gathered in the autumn (when before winter, nutrients are at maximum concentration).

34. Specifically for Conne River, a well-known healer Kitty Burke was said to be successful in making the plaster. For details: John J, Benoit S (*c*.1985). Traditional Medicine, unpublished manuscript (copy kindly provided by Dr Margaret Mackey). See also Lucey[21] (pp 111–12). Testimony to an oral tradition can be found in Wallis WD, Wallis RS. *The Micmac Indians of Eastern Canada*. Minneapolis, MI: University of Minnesota Press, 1955: 124.

35. Schiff JW, Moore K. The impact of the sweat lodge ceremony on dimensions of well-being. *Am Indian Alsk Native Ment Health Res* 2006;**13**:48–69.

36. A list of conditions is given by a physician supporting the value of the sweat lodge ceremony: Aung SKH. Brief report – ethnomedicine: the sweat lodge healing experience: an integrative medical perspective. *Rose + Croix J* 2006;**3**:14–27. Available from www. rosecroixjournal.org/issues/2006/New%20Folder/vol3_14_27_aung.pdf (accessed October 2008). Aung generally follows the language commonly used, namely in terms of benefits from physical, mental and spiritual purification that discharges emotional and other forms of pollution.

37. To reinforce that 'ritual events' span all areas of healthcare, the following references are useful: Montagne M. The metaphorical nature of drugs and drug taking. *Soc Sci Med* 1988;**26**:417–24; Kaptchuk TJ. The placebo effect in alternative medicine. Can the performance of a healing ritual have clinical significance? *Ann Intern Med* 2002;**136**:817–25; Green SA. Surgeons and shamanism: the placebo value of ritual. *Clin Orthop Relat Res* 2006;**450**:249–54. This includes quality time with patients, which embraces active listening, empathy, and communication of confidence and positive expectation, for which, see: Kaptchuk TJ, Kelley JM, Conboy LA. Components of placebo effect: randomised controlled trial in patients with irritable bowel syndrome. *BMJ* 2008;**336**:999–1003. For analyses of placebo results in clinical trials of drugs, and theoretical approaches to explaining placebo effects, see: Moerman DE. *Meaning, Medicine and the Placebo Effect*. Cambridge: Cambridge University Press, 2002.

4

Traditional medicine used by ethnic groups in the Colombian Amazon forest, South America

Blanca Margarita Vargas de Corredor and

Ann Mitchell (Simpson)

In this evolving world with its accelerated transformations, the indigenous traditional medical systems in Colombia are currently facing situations of extreme change as a result of outside influences such as beliefs and attitudes brought in by migrants, colonists and others who have integrated into these *pueblos*. They have brought with them their own conceptions of the environment and world, and amalgamated their diverse religious beliefs with those of the native groups. Traditionally, the elders are responsible for transmitting ancestral knowledge to their younger generations, but the Colombian State education system, contrary to that of the indigenous groups, separates the children from their elders. This has resulted in the present generation of indigenous children following a school curriculum with no allowance for a smooth transition between one system and the other.[1] The modern reality is that the ethnic groups remain trapped in two different worlds, without being able to decide to which of these realities they belong. Similarly, there is an enormous gap between the traditional medicine practised widely in Colombia, and that of western medicine. This gap was highlighted in a recent study undertaken by Ceuterick et al.[2] who investigated traditional medical care used by a diverse migrant Colombian population in London. These researchers looked at the process of adaptation to urban medicine while retaining native traditional medicine.

Indigenous peoples of the Colombian Amazon

Approximately a third of the southern part of Colombia is covered by Amazon rainforest which meets the borders of Peru, Ecuador and Brazil. The Colombian Amazon forest is inhabited by numerous native ethnic groups, migrants and colonists. They speak diverse languages and dialects, many of them from totally unrelated linguistic families and they all have their own particular traditions including medical practice. The *sabedores* live mainly in *resguardos* of the departments of Amazonas and Caquetá medio. *Resguardos* are areas protected by the Colombian government for the benefit of the indigenous people and environment. In the department of Amazonas alone there are 26 different ethnic groups recorded who live in 19 indigenous *resguardos*.[3] Examples of these ethnic groups are the Uitoto, Muinane, Nonuya, Yukuna, Makuna, Andoke, Tikuna and Cocama tribes. As these groups live in the tropical forest, they have unsurpassed knowledge of survival and living in this environment. However, also due to living in this highly diverse habitat, the indigenous groups have been exposed to the effects of colonists and outsiders who have come to search for plants, animal skins and minerals. In particular, the Uitoto groups were victims of the rubber trade of the nineteenth and twentieth centuries where their numbers were reduced to a minimum as a result of slave labour and torture. Notwithstanding these influences, many of the ethnic groups have maintained their language and traditions.[4] Some are undergoing a process of recuperation.

We refer to selected examples of traditional medicine used by a few of these Amazon ethnic groups, including indigenous elders who live on the border of Peru/Brazil/Colombia or in the Ecuadorian Amazon forest. Figure 4.1 shows the approximate location of the *sabedores* and ethnic groups represented in this text.

Traditional Amazonian medical practice

The *Historia*

In spite of the problems involved, the elders of the Amazon ethnic groups continue to practise the traditions of their oral *Historia*, a mythical work that contains all the historical actions of the gods of creation of the universe, the world, humanity, origin of the *pueblos* and punishments (illnesses and healing, evilness and how to combat it). It also includes their traditional medical system and botanical knowledge. In this way, the ethnic groups follow their ancestral knowledge to achieve a valid manner for survival and maintenance of their daily lives. The *Historia* is related by means of 'words of power' in a sacred space in the *maloca* – the plurifamilial house for the extended family by the *sabedores* (see below).[5] According to the *sabedores*,

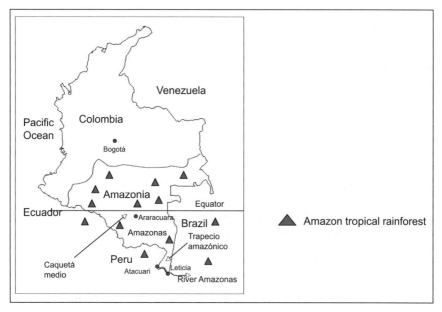

Figure 4.1 Map of Colombia, South America, showing approximate location of Amazonia and the locations referred to in text.

the ritual 'sacred word of power' contains all the knowledge required to cure as well as to cause illness. This includes how to make a diagnosis, look for possible cures, combat and allay spiritual illness, and extract 'bad energies' implanted by 'spells' and revenge, as well those of physical illnesses.[1]

The traditional healers

The true traditional healers (which include the *sabedor*, shaman and *payé*) must be rigorous in their objectives and follow the regimens required – such as evaluations, diets and sexual abstinence – in order to acquire the ability to heal and allay 'bad' or negative energies produced by different illnesses.[6] For this he or she must have great fortitude and energy. To be recognised as a healer capable of managing and applying numerous techniques in the treatment of illnesses, the *sabedor* must demonstrate his powers of healing to his community and beyond.[1]

The sabedores

Abuelo-sabedores(as) or *sabedores(as)* are indigenous wise men or wise women who have gained expert knowledge of plants, traditions such as medicines, and managing the environment by following particular occupations (e.g. dance, medicine, basket making). These occupations are profound and can last as long as 45 years.

From a very young age, the future *sabedor* learns to recognise the diverse types of plants found in the tropical forest environment. He or she must become familiar with the ritual plants, their effects and their results in order to 'extract' illnesses. This can include undertaking highly sacred journeys in which he or she is expected to be able to recover the spirit of the patient completely by investigating how the illness 'arrived'. If thought necessary, the illness or 'bad energy' may be returned to the enemy who sent it in the first place.

The *sabedores* realise that there are illnesses that are outside their social context. By recurring to the entheogens (see below) they are able to find the cause of the illness. When the *sabedores* suspect that the cause of the illness is of viral or bacterial origin they say that these illnesses come from *blancos* or white people. and as such should be treated by their doctors. In the same way serious injuries such as fractures are referred to western medical doctors.

The payé

The *payé* is a person who has achieved the ability to 'see' further than his or her own environment, e.g. a mystic.

The shaman

The word shaman is derived from the Manchu–Tungus word *šaman*, *Sha* or *Sa* (knowledgeable person) and *man* (a being who is dedicated to knowledge).[7] Strictly speaking the term 'shamanism' is considered to describe a Siberian and central Asian religious phenomenon.[8] However, the term 'shaman' has been adopted worldwide. With respect to the indigenous tribes of the Amazon forest, the term is the one that westerners or incomers use – the tribes themselves use their own terminology depending on their respective language and culture. They are the people who maintain the traditional knowledge and who have taken responsibility for the spiritual and material health of their *pueblos*. The knowledge held by these healers is based on ancestral wisdom as well as constant experimentation with plants and other healing materials, and is transmitted by the *sabedores*.

The true shaman is created from birth or, as is the case for the Uitoto ethnic group, the parents and grandparents communicate with the future shaman before birth, caressing and relating the *Historia* to the unborn child.[9] The shaman is considered to be capable of curing both spiritual and material illness by the movement of energies using plants, water, earth, animals or wind depending on the illness presented. They manage sacred plants and the energies of these plants, e.g. *jinaka buinaima*, which is one of the many varieties of *albahaca* (see example below). In addition to these 'true' shamans there are other types of shaman who are not formed from birth. These include, for example, individuals who have managed to survive a serious illness, an animal attack or a lightning bolt, and from that point have dedicated their lives to shamanic rituals. These rituals include learning with the aid of drums, maracas, chanting and body paint. Another variety of shaman is one known as the 'chaman de agua' (water shaman) whose illness has been converted into a piranha tooth, an animal bone or other object such as a plant seed. For all types of shaman, certain costumes and private or secret 'energy protectors' are used that are relevant to their formation. These may be made of a variety of natural materials such as feathers, seeds, bones or minerals.

Approach to healing

The relationship between the traditional healer and his or her patient is not limited to the treatment of an illness, x or y, but is immersed in a socio-cultural context within the environment. The traditional healer considers health in general in an integral form. This includes the spiritual and physical state of the patient's health and how it relates to a specific environment. The latter is almost always associated with sacred spaces or locations such as the *Maloca*, where the transmission of knowledge of the environment and the surrounding forest is narrated. The traditional practitioner is expected to treat both physical and spiritual ailments. The diagnosis and treatment take the form of seeking possible causes of the pain or discomfort that the patient is experiencing – this may be a result of physical causes, illness or disease, or can be suspected because someone has 'sent' it.[1] In general traditional healers exchange knowledge between cultures and recognise different forms of diagnosis and healing in order to cure many illnesses.[1] The same applies to their ability to prescribe and apply remedies and healing techniques.

Diagnosis

As already indicated, there is a vast difference between the medicine practised by traditional medicine practitioners in the Amazon tropical forest and western medicine. In modern or western medicine the initial diagnosis is made by the practitioner listening to the patient's description of symptoms, as well as a physical examination. The causes of the illness or discomfort felt by the patient are related directly to the function of the human body. In contrast, indigenous traditional medicine has other forms of diagnosis because the causes of the illness are variable: sometimes these coincide with modern medicine but in other cases they do not, e.g. 'bad eye' (*el mal de ojo*), 'bad wind' (*el mal viento*) and 'bad air' ('*el malaire*') are believed to be caused by someone, perhaps an enemy or witch, sending the illness to the person concerned. Other conditions may be caused by hunting or fishing to excess. The cure is based on conjuration, or methods such as 'sucking' the bad energy or illness out of the body. The positive energy is restored to the body using water, massage, plants and other natural materials, or a mixture of these techniques. Overall, the mind and the desire to cure exercise their healing power.[1]

The prescription – choosing a remedy

It is important to note that the *sabedores*, shamans, *payés* and traditional medical practitioners approach the plants by 'feeling' or sensing the energies or spirits contained in them, in order to heal. These can be the ordinary curative plants or those of 'extreme' knowledge, such as a diverse selection of entheogenic plants. Entheogen, derived from part of the Greek root *entheos* or god, literally translated means 'which generates the experience of god within us'.[10] The term was invented by a group of ethnobotanists and scholars of mythology including RE Schultes in 1979.[11]

In this way traditional healers extract the necessary information and knowledge to cure spiritual and physical ailments. Within this traditional healing process numerous spirits and energies exercise their power. Equally, the sacred plants *ambil* (tobacco), *ayahuasca*, *mambe* (coca) and *yajé* (also known as *yagé*), to which other substances are added such as the various species of *borrachero* (e.g. *Brugmansia suaveolens)*, act on the mind enabling the individual to 'see further'.[10]

Ritualistic practice

The shaman, other traditional healer or owner of the *Maloca* carries out the daily ritual of the *mambeo*, or the ritual of management of *yajé* or *ayahuasca* in which part of the great *Historia* is narrated. This includes teaching apprentices the necessary knowledge to become a successful healer. During these rituals *mambe* (coca) is prepared and ingested together with *ambil* (tobacco), enabling the *sabedor* to communicate with spirits and the energies of the surrounding environment.

The rituals materialise the myths and *Historia* of the ethnic groups. Within these rituals components of the ethnic groups are not simply being represented (as in a theatre) but the time of the creation of the universe is being reactivated. A rebirth of the world and the entire ecosystem is enacted. At this time, all the energies, spirits and owners of the universe are present. By means of this ritual all types of harassment, aggression and illnesses are eliminated in a form of renovation. This rebirth is managed by the *sabedores* and shamans who are capable of controlling situations of good and evil. Other ethnic groups from near and far are invited to participate in these events and they are celebrated as ritual dances. Figure 4.2 shows a Uitoto ritual dance, in which the creation of the universe, the world and humans is re-enacted – all illnesses

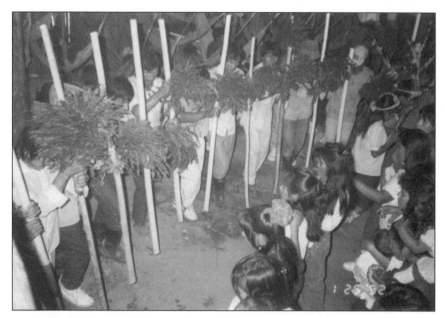

Figure 4.2 Uitoto ritual dance, Caquéta medio, Amazonas, Colombia, 25 January 1992.

and aggressiveness are eliminated during this ritual, which is of great importance to the ethnic group.

Examples of traditional medicines used in ritualistic practice

By agreement of the *sabedores* we are able to present photographs of plant and animal medicines, examples of their identification, preparation and use, and explanations as given by the *sabedores*. Each *sabedor* gave his or her permission to take the necessary photographs and include them together with their healing knowledge.

Ambil (tobacco)

Preparation

Figure 4.3 shows a tobacco plant (*Nicotiana tabacum* L.). The leaves are collected from traditional indigenous gardens or farms known as *chagras* where edible, ritual and medicinal plants are cultivated and cooked in water for at least 24 hours until the volume has reduced to a minimum.

Figure 4.4 shows *Sabedor* Oscar Román Enokaai cooking tobacco leaves in the preparation of *ambil*. Juice from *maraca viche*, a forest fruit, is mixed

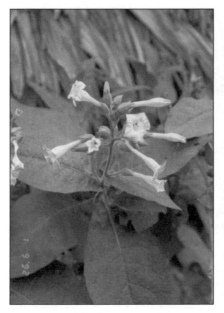

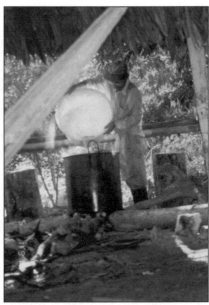

Figure 4.3 Tobacco plant (*Nicotiana tabacum* L.) in flower. *Resguardo* Monochoa, Caquéta medio, Amazonas, Colombia, 1 September 1992.

Figure 4.4 *Sabedor* Oscar Román Enokayaɨ cooking tobacco leaves in preparation of *ambil*, 5 January 1997.

together with vegetable salt (prepared previously from certain forest plants). The proportions depend on the use to which the *ambil* will be put.

Use

Ambil is used to afford protection from, and to allay, negative energies.

Mambe (coca)

Sabedor Rene Moreno Vaneo from the Ethnic group Cocama explained the ritual and medicinal use of coca (*Erythroxylum coca*), Leticia, Amazonas, Colombia. He told the authors in an interview in November 2008 (interview 1 in the addendum).

> Coca is for our ethnic group a plant which our ancestors have used over a period of around six thousand years. It is a native plant, sacred for us in the indigenous *pueblos* including Cocamas, Ingas, and other Amazonian ethnic groups. For us, coca, together with *ayahuasca* form the foundation of our entire traditional medicine. We consume or mambea coca together with *yaje* or *ayahuasca* but in small quantities, only using three or five coca leaves – depending on the size of the leaf.

Preparation

In the *chagra* the coca leaf (*Erythroxylum coca*) (Figure 4.5) is collected in a basket (*Kirige* in Uitoto language), which is taken to the *Maloca*.

The coca leaves are toasted in a clean *tibe* (earthenware tray), taking care not to burn them (Figure 4.6). Once they have been toasted they are transferred to a large, tall mortar and pulverised with a pestle.

Completely dry fallen leaves from the yarumo tree (*Cecropia* spp.) are then collected and burned. The resultant ash is mixed with the pulverised coca to form *mambe* (Antonio Kiriyatɨki: Muina (Uitoto), Cacique of Peñas Negras (Resguardo) Localisation: between: *resguardo* los Monos and above *Resguardo* of Puerto Sábalo; right hand side of the Ríver Caquetá). The yarumo is found in various locations in the Amazon forest and is an invasive, colonising plant. The leaves have the appearance and shape of a human hand (Figure 4.7).

Yajé cielo (*Banesteriopsis caapi*)

Sabedor Rene Moreno Vaneo told the authors in an interview (interview 1 in the addendum):[12]

> *Yajé* is a plant which is fundamental to the ancestral knowledge for us in the Trapecio (Amazonas, Colombia). In my culture (Cocama) we know the plant as *ayahuasca*. In other parts of Colombia such as the Páez and Inga *pueblos*, and other ethnic groups in the Putumayo area, the plant is known as *yajé*. It has almost the same application in all Amazonian cultures. For the Cocama

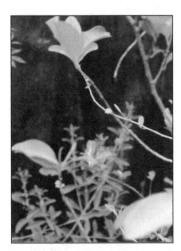

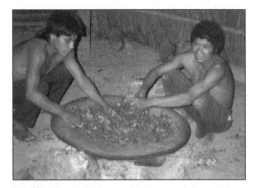

Figure 4.5 Ceremonial coca (*Erythroxylum coca*), Araracuara, Caquéta medio, Amazonas, Colombia, 10 January 1992.

Figure 4.6 Cacique Antonio Kiriyatɨki's grandsons toasting coca leaves in the maloca. Resguardo Peñas Negras, Caquéta medio, Amazonas, Colombia, 22 February 1991.

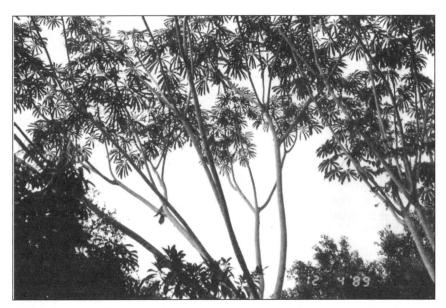

Figure 4.7 Yarumo (*Cecropia* spp.) tree, Araracuara, Caquéta medio, Amazonas, Colombia, 12 April 1989.

group in the area known as Trapecio, *yajé* or *ayahuasca* is a sacred plant and forms the base of the Cocama knowledge in the Trapecio. The variety of *yajé* shown in the photograph is *cielo* (sky) *ayahuasca* or *cielo yajé*. It is called this because when the ritual is carried out with this variety of *yajé* it is possible to travel to infinity.

Uses

Yajé and other entheogenic plants are used in the realisation of powerful and dangerous shamanic journeys of recognition. In the state of trance when people move from normal conscience to altered conscience by means of taking, inhaling or bathing in entheogenic substances, or using other methods under the effect of entheogens, especially *yajé* or *ayahuasca*, conscience and sensations are activated, including: intuition, visionary capacity and amplified sensorial perception, among others; spiritual forms are 'seen' and 'felt' and strange odours and surroundings are experienced. During these journeys the shaman is exposed to a struggle between good and evil which he must overcome using his skills and wisdom. The individual's fears are brought to the surface in such a way that, on returning from the entheogenic trance to the normal state of conscience, the memory of the trance remains.[10] On returning from this 'journey' the shaman should have achieved clarity of an appropriate treatment for each illness. For Uitoto and Muinane ethnic groups the use of *yaje* is used only as a last resource for the solution of problems or illnesses that cannot be resolved using other more commonly used ritual plants such as coca or tobacco or minerals.[12]

Curative medicines of plant origin

The *sabedores* have a profound knowledge of the plants in the tropical forest. They have their own methods of identification, which they describe as identifying the energy of the plant – its power to heal. Identification includes observation, touching, smelling and tasting the plant. The location, identification and collection of the plants require great concentration.

An infinite number of curative plants can be collected from the forest, but the most commonly used are planted very near to the houses to be available for frequent use; others are planted together with the ritual and edible plants in the *chagras*.[13] The close proximity of medicinal and ritual plants to homes is also believed to protect the inhabitants from negative energies and 'enemies'.

The time of collection of medicinal plants is considered to be important and depends on when the plants are sensed to be more powerful or have positive energy to heal. In general the ethnic groups in Amazonia use their medicinal plants fresh because they consider them to have more healing power than when dried. In many cases the plants are used directly in the forest (Figure 4.8). When available the indigenous groups will use western medicine to treat fractures. However, due to the remote location of many of the communities, the *sabedores* use the bark of certain trees as a splint which they say heals the bone as well as acting as an analgesic.

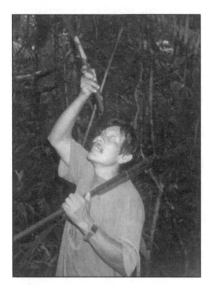

Figure 4.8 *Sabedor* Marceliano Jékonai Guerrero (Uitoto Muina) applying drops from a fine liana directly into his eye, Yarì, Caquéta medio, Amazon tropical forest, Colombia, 1996.

Examples of traditional curative plant medicines

Among the enormous number of plants, below are included a few of those used by *sabedores* from different tribes in the Amazon forest.

Amori (Uitoto language)

Preparation

The *Amori* tree, which has not been botanically identified, is found in primary forest. The part used medicinally is the sap which is collected by making a cut in the bark and allowing it to flow (Figure 4.9) (interview 2 in the addendum).

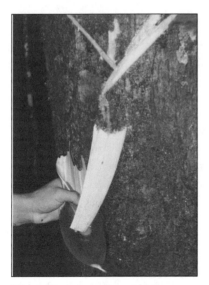

Figure 4.9 *Sabedor* Oscar Román
Enokayɨ collecting sap of medicinal tree
Amori or Am*bil de monte* allowing the tree
sap to flow from the cut in the tree bark;
Araracuara, Caquéta medio, Amazonas,
Colombia, 26 June 1991.

Use

The sap is used to treat internal infections. The *sabedores* record it as having hallucinogenic effects and it is also known as *ambil de monte*.

Albahaca (Ocimum micranthum Willd. + other species negra and blanca)

Also known as wild basil, wild mosquito plant, *Chaiwatu* (Tikuna language).

Use

According to *Sabedor* Rene Moreno Vaneo, *Albahaca* is a basic medicine used to cure numerous illnesses in both adults and children. It is curative for nervous conditions, high blood pressure and for children in the treatment of '*mal aire*' and diarrhoea. This is a plant native to Amazonas and for them is an important medicinal plant. It is also used as a condiment. In Cocama language they call this plant '*Sara taita*.'.

In the Caquetá Media geographical area *Albahaca* is known in the Uitoto language as *Jaibikie*.

According to *Sabedor* Oscar Román, the plant is used to bathe children to improve their mood and to lower fevers caused by influenza and cough. It is used to treat madness or rage by taking the cooked preparation once. To treat diarrhoea the plant is prepared in hot water with cinnamon and lemon (see interview 3 in the addendum).

As a comparison, we include an example of use of the same plant, *Albahaca* (*Ocimum micranthum*), used by the Quichua ethnic group, Amazon forest, Ecuador. In this case, *Sabedor* Gabriel Tapuy explains that the plant can be used to treat '*mal aire*'. The plant is collected and passed over the person repeatedly in the form of a cross in order to extract negative energies or 'clean' them. According to *Sabedor* Gabriel, the person who carries out the treatment will feel the arm become heavy if he or she is successful at extracting the '*mal aire*' (see interview 4 in the addendum).

Badea (*Passiflora quadrangularis*)

Sabedor Hilario Rivero Yukuna, originally from Mirití said in an interview in, Leticia, Amazonas, Colombia (see interview 5 in the addendum):

> Seven leaves of Badea are collected and cooked in water. They are taken in a large cup of warm water before breakfast. Then the patient waits three minutes before vomiting. The plant is used to clean the stomach when suffering painful cramps and diarrhoea.

Members of other ethnic groups or *pueblos* such as Muinas (Uitotos), Muinanes, Andokes, Yukunas and others use the young *Badea* leaves to cure hepatitis A and B in the early stages: on the first day of treatment, the juice of one leaf is taken, and each following day the juice of another leaf is added until nine leaves are being used; the plant is then suspended for 3 days. On resuming the treatment, the number of leaves taken is reduced by one leaf each day until returning to one leaf (see interview 6 in the addendum).

Escama de Pirarucu, Escama de Paichi (Quéchua language) (*Kalanchoe* sp. (aff. pinnata) [syn. *Bryophyllum* sp.]

Sabedor João Costa Rios Filho explained in an interview (see interview 7 in the addendum):

> The leaf of Escama de Paichi crushed with honey is used for cough and whooping cough. It is also used topically as an anti-inflammatory and to control haemorrhage from a wound; the cold leaf is applied directly to the affected area.

Maria Luisa–Hierba Luisa; Santo Cuipa (Quéchua language) (*Cymbopogon citratus* (*DC*. ex Nees) Stapf

Sabedor João Costa Rios Filho said in the interview (see interview 7 in the addendum):

> The Santa Cuipa leaf can be used as a disinfectant as well as to treat insect bites and kill ticks. Internally it can be taken as an infusion made with the leaves, or taken as the pure juice to lower blood pressure. In order to increase hair growth the leaf is crushed and applied to the head without bathing.

Fungus: *Oreja de palo* (*Pycnoporus sanguineus* L. ex Fr.)

The fungus *oreja de palo*, shown in Figure 4.10, grows on fallen, dead trees in the *chagras*. The fresh fungus is red in colour, and at this stage is

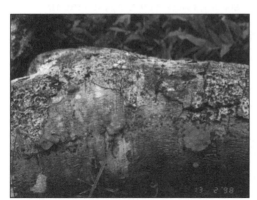

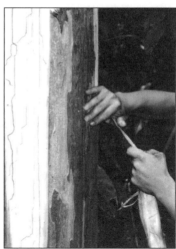

Figure 4.10 Fungus 'Oreja de palo' (Pycnoporus sanguineus) at a young stage, when it is used by Uitotos to treat mouth infections; Caquéta medio, Amazonas, Colombia, 13 February 1998.

Figure 4.11 Collection of Koduiro bark by Tomás Román, Uitoto, Araracuara, Caquéta, Amazon tropical forest, Colombia, 1989.

powdered and used to treat mouth infections – directly applied to the affected area. After 3 or 4 days the fungus begins to turn white in colour and at this stage of ageing is highly toxic (see interview 8 in the addendum).

Koduiro (Eschweilera sp.)

Koduiro or *Eschweilera* sp. is a tree found in primary tropical forest, *Caquetá medio*. The bark is collected (Figure 4.11) and used to prevent and cure infections and to heal wounds. It is also used as a body and hair colorant (see interview 9 in the addendum).[14]

Phytolacca americana L.

Also known as Pokeweed, hierba carmín, tintilla and granilla.

The leaves of *Phytolacca* are heated (Figure 4.12) and applied directly to the affected area to treat inflammation (see interview 10 in the addendum).

Curative medicine of animal origin

Mojojoy larvae (Rhynchophorus palmarum L.)

Mojojoy larvae (Figure 4.13) are found in palms such as Canangucho (*Mauritia flexuosa*). According to *Sabedor* Oscar Roman Enokaɨ (see

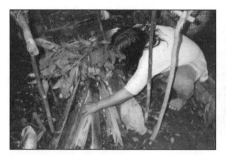

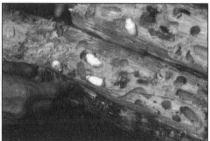

Figure 4.12 *Phytolacca americana* L. plant being heated by Uitoto *sabedora* Alicia Roman Sanchez, for the treatment of swollen ankles; Araracuara, Caquéta medio, Amazonas, Colombia, 4 April 1992.

Figure 4.13 Mojojoy (*Rhynchophorus palmarum* L.), Araracuara, Caquéta medio, Amazonas, Colombia, 27 June 1991.

interview 11 in the addendum) and other sources (see interview 1 in the addendum and Corredor et al.[15]) the fat of mojojoy is used to treat bronchitis, asthma and other pulmonary diseases. The fat is removed from the grub and some of it massaged on to the patient's chest, and the rest is given to the patient to eat. It has also been reported to be used as a cure for haemorrhagic diseases (bleeding).[15]

Final comment

The authors have spent more than 20 years, together with the *sabedores(as)*, researching and documenting their traditional medicine. The limited information presented here is based on research by the authors, and unless otherwise referenced is based on this work. A particular effort has been made to give credit directly to the *sabedores* who have given specific information.

The authors have recorded ancestral knowledge of healing *pueblos* or ethnic groups of the Amazon forest. They do not suggest that the plants and other natural products should by used by anyone in any way. As has been reported the *sabedores* adhere to restrictions and regulations and have a lifetime of experience of survival in tropical forest conditions. Each of these treatments has been used by the *sabedores* following the necessary restrictions, dosage and follow-up by the relevant *sabedor*.

Photography

Unless otherwise stated, photographs were taken by Ann Mitchell and Blanca de Corredor.

Further reading

Eliade M. *El Chamanismo*. (Shamanism.) Mexico: Fondo Cultura Económica (FCE), 1976.

Fericgla JM. ¿Alucinógenos o adaptogenos inespecíficos; Propuesta teórica para una innovación del estudio de los mecanismos cognitivos de adaptación cultural. (Hallucinogens or non-specific adaptogens? Theoretical proposal for an innovative study of the cognitive mechanisms of cultural adaptation.) *Revista de Antropología Social (Journal of Social Anthropology)* 1993: 167–83.

Fericgla JM. *Los jíbaros, cazadores de sueños. Diario de un antropólogo y experimentos con la ayahuasca*. (*The Jíbaros, Dream Hunters. Diary of an anthropologist and experimentation with ayahuasca*.) Barcelona: Integral-Oasis, 1994.

Fericgla JM, ed. *Plantas, Chamanismo y estados de consciencia*. (*Shamanism and States of Conscience*.) Cogniciones collection no. 5. Barcelona: Libros de la Liebre de Marzo, 1994.

Font IQ. *Plantas medicinales. El Dioscorides renovado*. (*Medicinal Plants. The renovated Dioscorides*.) Barcelona: Peninsula Editions, 1983.

Harner MJ, ed. *Alucinógenos y chamanismo*. (*Hallucinogens and Shamanism*.) Punto Omega Collection No. 213. Madrid: Editorial Guadarrama, 1976.

Harner MJ. *The Way of the Shaman*. New York: HarperCollins, 1990.

Reichel-Dolmatoff G. *Rainforest Shamans: Essays on the Tukano Indians of the Northwest Amazon*. Dartington: Themis Books, 1996.

Schultes RE. An overview of hallucinogens in the Western hemisphere. In: Furst de P (ed.), *Flesh of the Gods: The ritual use of hallucinogens*. New York: Praeger, 1972: 3–54.

Schultes RE, Hofmann A. *Plants of the Gods: Origins of hallucinogenic use*. Maidenhead: McGraw Hill, 1979.

Schultes RE, Hofmann A. *Plantas de los Dioses Orígenes del uso de los alucinógenos* (*Plants of the Gods – Origins and use of hallucinogens*). Mexico: FCE, 1982: 120–7.

Schultes RE, Raffauf FR. *The Healing Forest. Medicinal and toxic plants of the Northwest Amazonia*. Portland, OR: Dioscorides Press, 1990.

Schultes RE, Raffauf FR. *El Bejuco del Alma. Los Médicos tradicionales de la Amazonia colombiana, sus plantas y sus rituales*. (*The Spiritual Vine. Traditional medical doctors of the Colombian Amazon, their plants and rituals*.) Banco de la Republica, Colombia: Ediciones Uniandes, Universidad de Antioquia, 1994.

Wasson RG, Paulovna V. *Mushrooms, Russia and History*. New York: Pantheon Books, 1957.

References

1. Rodríguez Rueda A. *Medicina indígena*. (*Indigenous Medicine*.) School series and Amazonia No. 9. Ministry of National Education; Amazon Fund Programme; Coordination of Amazon Education; Fundación Caminos de identidad (Foundation of Paths of Identity), 1996: 12–13, 16–18, 29.

2. Ceuterick M, Vandebroek I, Torry B, Pieroni A. Cross-cultural adaptation in urban ethnobotany: The Colombian folk pharmacopoeia in London. *J Ethnopharmacol* 2008;**120**:342–59.

3. *Diccionario Geográfico de Colombia*. (*Dictionary of Geography of Colombia*, vol. 1.) Codazzi: Agustín Codazzi Geographical Institute, 1996: 84.

4. Schultes RE, Raffauf FR. *The Healing Forest. Medicinal and toxic plants of the Northwest Amazonia*. Dioscorides Press, 1995: 17.

5. Corredor, B de La Maloca. Investigación realizada en un grupo Murui y Muinane, de la Amazonia Colombiana. (The Maloca; An investigation of a Murui and Muinane group in the Colombian Amazon.) Thesis, National University of Colombia), Faculty of Human Sciences, Department of Anthropology, Bogota, Colombia, 1986: vol. 3, 457.

6. Drexler D. *En los montes, si; aquí, no! Cosmología y medicina tradicional de los Zenúes*. (*In the mountains, yes; here no! Cosmology and traditional medicine among the Zenúes*.) Quito, Ecuador: Ediciones Abya-Yala, 2002: 95–6.

7. *Britannica.* Available at: www.britannica.com/EBchecked/topic/538200/shamanism (accessed 20 April 2009).
8. Eliade M. *Shamanism: Archaic techniques of ecstasy.* London: Arkana, 1989: 4.
9. Corredor B de. La Maloca. Investigación realizada en un grupo Murui y Muinane, de la Amazonia Colombiana. (The Maloca; An investigation of a Murui and Muinane group in the Colombian Amazon.) Thesis, National University of Colombia), Faculty of Human Sciences, Department of Anthropology, Bogota, Colombia, 1986: vol. 1, 28.
10. Fericgla JM. *Al trasluz de la ayahuasca.* (*Seen through the Light of ayahuasca.*) Barcelona: Los libros de la liebre de Marzo, SL, 1997: 18–21, 23–4, 27–30, 35, 37, 39.
11. Wikipedia. Entheogen terminology. Available at: http://en.wikipedia.org/wiki/Entheogen#Terminology (Accessed January 18 2009)
12. Corredor B de. Yajé regalo de los dioses. (Yajé a present from the gods.) In: Corredor B de, Torres W (eds), *El chamanismo, un arte del saber.* (*Shamanism, A Knowledge Art.*) Bogotá, Colombia: Anaconda Editores, 1986: 34.
13. Mitchell AM, Corredor B de, Rodríguez NJ, Morales U, Gray AI. Medicinal plant use and domestication by Colombian Amerindian people. In: International symposium on herbal medicine: A holistic approach. International Institute for Human Resources Development. College of Health and Human Services: San Diego State University, 1997: 451–63.
14. Corredor B de, Mitchell AM, Torrenegra RD, Román Enakayi O. Medicina Tradicional-Farmacognosia Plantas medicinales amazonicas. (Traditional medicine – pharmacognosy; Amazon medicinal plants.) In: *Symposio de plantas medicinales.* (*Symposium of Medicinal Plants.*) Publication No. 3. Santafe de Bogotá, Colombia: Fundación Joaquín Pineros Corpas, 1989: 193–7.
15. Corredor B de, Mitchell A, Corredor A. *Chagras de los espíritus. Sabedores, Sabedoras: Metodos de recuperación, preservación y manejo de la selva y de la várzea.* (*Chagras of the Spirits. Wisemen, wisewomen: Methods of recuperation, preservation and management of the forest and varzea.*) Bogotá, Colombia: Escala Ltd, 2006: 93.

Addendum: Interviews

1. Interview with *Sabedor* Rene Moreno Vaneo, Cocama ethnic group, Leticia, Amazonas Colombia 23/11/08.
2. Interview with *Sabedor* Oscar Román Enokayɨ, Araracuara, Caquetá medio 26/6/91
3. Interview with *Sabedor* Oscar Román Enokayɨ, *Sabedora* Alicia Sánchez Román, Tomás Román 9/4/89
4. Interview with *Sabedor* Gabriel Tapuy, ethnic group: Quichua del Napo, Amazon forest, Ecuador 26/11/94.
5. Interview with *Sabedor* Hilario Rivero Yukuna, Yukuna ethnic group from Mirití, Amazonas, Colombia.
6. Interview with *Sabedores*: Placido Mendoza Ethnic group Uitoto Muina, Araracuara, Amazonas; Oscar Román Enokayɨ Ethnic group Uitoto Muina Araracuara, Amazonas; Cacique Eduardo Pakɨ, Muinane, del Resguardo Villa Azul, Caquetá medio, heart of the Colombian tropical forest.
7. Interview with *Sabedor* João Costa Rios Filho, Ethnic group Quichua, Leticia, Amazonas, Colombia 22/11/08.
8. Interview with *Sabedor* Isaias Román Sánchez, Muina, Uitoto ethnic group, who has inherited the career of his father: elder: Oscar Román Enokaɨ 19/2/98.
9. Interview with *Sabedor* Oscar Román Enokayɨ and his son Tomás Román, Uitoto, Araracuara, Caquetá medio, Colombia 1989.
10. Interview with *Sabedora* Alicia Román Sánchez, Uitoto, Araracuara, Caquetá medio, Amazonas, Colombia 7/4/92.
11. Interview with *Sabedor* Oscar Román Enokayɨ and his son Tomás Román, Uitoto, Araracuara, Caquetá medio, Colombia 27/6/91.

5

Traditional medical practice in Africa

Gillian Scott

Introduction

Continental Africa currently comprises some 52 states. This chapter focuses on traditional medical practice (TMP) in states comprising the eastern, western and southern African regions (Figure 5.1), roughly equivalent to the World Health Organization (WHO) African region. These 46 states lie between 20°N and 32°S and support vegetation ranging from lowland rain forest to semi-desert succulent scrubland (Figure 5.2).

The 10 most common causes of morbidity in the WHO African region are HIV/AIDS, malaria, lower respiratory tract infections, childhood diseases, diarrhoeal diseases, perinatal conditions, unintentional injuries, neuropsychiatric disorders, maternal conditions and road traffic accidents. Of these, the first seven are also among the ten most common causes of mortality in the region, together with malignant neoplasms, cerebrovascular disease and ischaemic disease. In most states of the region, patients seeking treatment with traditional medicine (TM) generally present with conditions related to morbidity, including malaria, HIV/AIDS and associated opportunistic infections, diarrhoeal disease, childhood illnesses, reproductive health problems, asthma, disorders of the gastrointestinal tract, diabetes, hypertension, sickle cell anaemia and epilepsy.[12]

With two exceptions (Liberia and Ethiopia), all African states have at some period of their history been governed by European powers. One of the products of colonial occupation was the introduction to Africa of the western allopathic system of medicine. The traditional medical practices of the continent, despite their ancient origins, were largely ignored by colonial authorities. Traditional practitioners (TPs), although highly respected members of their communities, played almost no role in the establishment of formal healthcare systems in Africa. This state of affairs can, in part, be

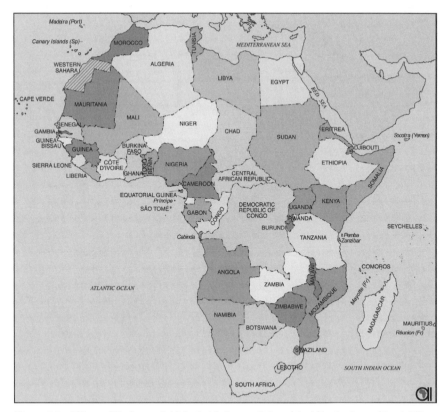

Figure 5.1 Africa: political map. *Published with the permission of the Africa Institute of South Africa.*

attributed to the fact that African indigenous medical systems have always been an oral tradition, whereby knowledge is passed from healer to trainee by word of mouth during a long apprenticeship and no written record is maintained. The effect has been to render African TMP inaccessible to practitioners trained in the western allopathic system and to retard the entry into formal healthcare of potentially useful therapeutic agents derived from African plant species. This is borne out by the fact that only a handful of African indigenous remedies have found their way into western pharmacopoeias (Table 5.1), in contrast with the many European, American, Asian and Oriental TMs that have merited monographs in earlier and current editions of the British, European and US pharmacopoeias.

Definitions

The WHO has defined[26] indigenous healers as 'a group of persons recognised by the community in which they live as being competent to provide health by using vegetable, animal, and mineral substances and other methods based on the social, cultural and religious backgrounds as well as on the

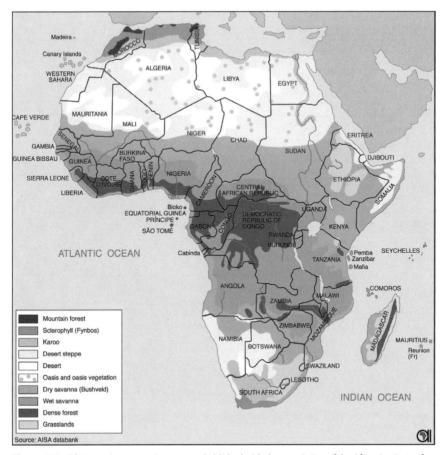

Figure 5.2 Africa: main vegetation zones. *Published with the permission of the Africa Institute of South Africa.*

knowledge, attitudes and beliefs that are prevalent in the community regarding physical, mental and social well-being and the causation of disease and disability'. This definition underscores two key elements of TMP, i.e. its holistic approach and the fact that TPs are accorded their status by the communities that they serve.

According to Kokwaro:[3]

> ... traditional medicine is the sum total of all the knowledge and practices, whether explicable or not, used in diagnosis, prevention and elimination of physical, mental or social imbalance and relying exclusively on practical experience and observation handed down from generation to generation, whether verbally or in writing ... a solid amalgamation of dynamic medical know-how and ancestral experience. Traditional African medicine is also considered to be the sum total of practices, measures, ingredients and procedures of all

Table 5.1 Pharmaceutical monographs for African plant species in current and earlier editions of the *British Pharmacopoeia* (BP), *British Pharmaceutical Codex* (BPC) and the *European Pharmacopoeia* (EP)

Plant species	Plant family	Monograph	Crude drug	Country of origin	Medicinal use
Aloe ferox Mill.	Aloaceae	Aloe capensis (Cape aloes) EP 2008 (6th edn) and BP 2009	Dried leaf juice	South Africa	Purgative
Agathosma betulina (P.J. Bergius) Pillans	Rutaceae	Buchu BPC 1963	Dried leaf	South Africa	Diuretic and urinary antiseptic
Harpagophytum procumbens DC and *H. zeyheri* Decne.	Pedaliaceae	*Harpagophyti radix* EP 2008 (6th edn) and BP 2009	Dried tuber	Namibia, Botswana	Analgesic/anti-inflammatory in the treatment of arthritis
Rauwolfia vomitoria Afzel.	Apocynaceae	African rauwolfia BPC 1963	Dried root	East Africa	Antihypertensive
Physostigma venenosum Balf.	Fabaceae	Physostigmine BPC 1963	Fruit (Calabar bean) as a source of physostigmine	West Africa; mainly Nigeria	Cholinesterase inhibitor used mainly as a miotic
Cola nitida (Vent.) Schott & Endl. and *C. acuminata* (Pal.) Schott & Endl.	Sterculiaceae	Cola BPC 1949	Dried cotyledon	Tropical West Africa	Source of caffeine in the treatment of migraine

kinds, whether material or not, which from time immemorial had enabled the African to guard against disease, to alleviate his sufferings and to cure himself.

Traditional African practice

African traditional health systems

A prominent South African TP has stated[4] that 'although it is not possible to find a single African traditional healing system, the differences between cultures south of the Sahara are sufficiently small for generalisations to be made within certain limits'.

This is especially true of neighbouring states, between which ethnic ties may be very strong and political boundaries quite artificial.[5] There are, however, two groups of people to which this statement does not apply:

- San hunter–gatherers (referred to in earlier literature as Bushmen) who are the true First Nations of the Southern African region, having become established there more than 20 000 years ago.[1]
- Khoe-khoe/Khoi-khoi pastoralists (formerly referred to as Hottentots) who settled in the same region at some point in the last 2000 years.[6]

Later migrations from the north brought to southern Africa the Nguni and other Bantu language-speaking peoples whose TMP is now dominant in the region. There is evidence to suggest that the different groups lived side by side for several centuries, interacting and intermarrying.[7] By virtue of their superior numbers, the Bantu language groups slowly assimilated their San and Khoi-khoi neighbours. After the arrival of European settlers in South Africa in 1652, the inexorable process of cultural disruption continued, to the point where only small isolated groups of San and Khoi-khoi peoples are to be found in southern Africa today. Little remains of their traditional medical practices and there is a real risk that much of their medical knowledge will be lost to modern science. This is regrettable because the San in particular are widely acknowledged as having been exceptional economic botanists.[8,9] To the San hunter–gatherer, familiarity with the medicinal properties of plants has always been a matter not merely of utility but also of survival. It is likely, however, that, through intermarriage and cultural exchange, much San medicinal plant lore has been subsumed into modern traditional medical practice in southern Africa.

Perceptions of ill-health

The single unifying theme in African TMP is an enquiry into the causality of ill-health. The patient consulting a TP will ask 'Why am I ill?', in contrast to his or her counterpart in the western allopathic system whose question is 'What is the nature of my illness?' In African traditional medical practice, disease is considered to be due to several possible agencies, the most important being:

- natural causes, e.g. normal developmental processes, life stages and seasonal changes
- behaviour offensive to the patient's ancestral spirits, e.g. an immoral act or the transgression of a social code
- supernatural forces, e.g. witchcraft or intervention by evil spirits.

In a detailed study of traditional medical practice in Zimbabwe, it was found that the greater part of the TPs' practice was concerned with the treatment of illnesses recognisable in terms of scientific medicine, and that almost 50% of patients presented with complaints that were diagnosed by the TP as being due to natural causes.[10]

The traditional practitioner

In African culture, in order to become a TP, one must first experience a call to priesthood. This is recognised as an illness, the symptoms of which are caused by ancestral spirits seeking to possess the future healer. It is a holy calling that comes from God via ancestral spirits. The sickness may come at any age but is most prevalent during adolescence. Once the call to priesthood is diagnosed, the patient is immediately placed under the care of a traditional healer and enters training as an initiate. Training can last from a minimum of 7 years to 15 years, depending on culture, religion, ethnic group and custom.[4] Figure 5.3 shows TP Philip Kubukeli, head of a large TP association in South Africa, addressing a meeting of TPs and Figure 5.4 shows members of the Western Cape Traditional Healers and Herbalists Association in South Africa.

The role of the African TP, apart from establishing the cause of illness and directing its cure, is also that of intercessor between patient and his or her ancestral spirits, religious, legal and political adviser, marriage counsellor and social worker. The TP thus plays a pivotal role in the stability and social cohesion of the community in which he or she lives.

Specialist categories of TP are recognised, e.g. surgeons, herbalists, bone-setters and diviners. Traditional birth attendants (TBAs) oversee pregnancies, prescribe TMs in order to maintain maternal and fetal health, and ensure a trouble-free delivery, and also advise on the care of the newborn

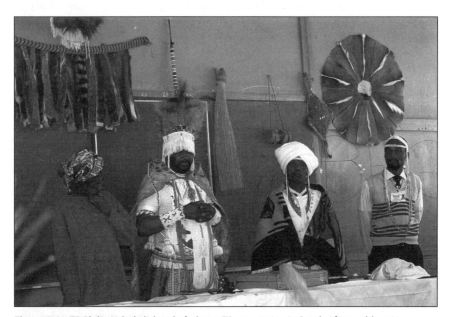

Figure 5.3 TP Philip Kubukeli, head of a large TP association in South Africa, addressing a meeting of TPs.

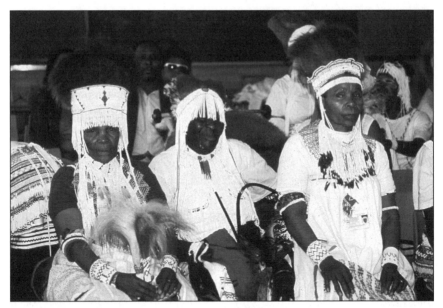

Figure 5.4 Members of the Western Cape Traditional Healers and Herbalists Association, South Africa.

infant. Certain herbs and procedures may be reserved for this purpose, e.g. among the Zulu people of South Africa, particular herbs prescribed during pregnancy are known as *isihlambezo* (cleansing agents) or *umsekelo* (a support or prop).

TP–patient relationship

The special relationship that exists between traditional healer and patient throughout Africa is reflected in the fact that, even in the most sophisticated of today's urban African societies, the healer is often the first port of call in times of trouble. More importantly, in the rural areas of the continent, where state healthcare provision is often minimal, the TP may be the only reliable source of relief in ill-health. Favourable healer:patient ratios (an estimated 1:200 in some African states) ensure that traditional healthcare is accessible to most, usually at affordable rates. Indeed, many healers will accept payment (or a gift) only when the patient has been cured.

Three factors – affordability, accessibility and cultural acceptability – together account very largely for the fact that some 80% of Africa's people today utilise traditional systems of medicine.[12,26] This is not to say that state healthcare systems are altogether avoided, but that traditional medical practice is deemed preferable in some situations and in others represents the only available option.

Treatment

Once the cause of ill-health has been established (by divination if necessary), its treatment may comprise only herbal remedies or may call for additional measures, e.g. behavioural adjustment, cleansing or appropriate ritual procedures.[13] In this way, the physical, mental and spiritual needs of the patient are all met, and health (defined by the WHO as a complete state of physical and mental well-being, rather than the mere absence of disease or infirmity) is achieved.

The use of indigenous plants

History

Despite a lack of formal recognition, the potential of TM as a source of useful therapeutic agents was not entirely overlooked by early colonial governors, physicians, botanists and missionaries working in Africa. In South Africa, one of the first African states to come under colonial rule (1652), frequent comments are to be found in the literature of the seventeenth and eighteenth centuries concerning the medical application of locally available plant species.

An early account (1785) of the traditional uses of 28 African plants, entitled *De Medicina Africanorum*,[14] was made by the Swedish botanist and physician Carl Peter Thunberg (1743–1828), a student of Linnaeus. Thunberg had been granted permission by the Dutch East India Company (VOC) to spend some time (1772–4) at the Cape, which served at the time as a VOC supply station. Botany and medicine being closely allied professions at that time, Thunberg was keenly interested in the medicinal uses of the plants that he encountered at the Cape and clearly saw a role for them in healthcare. The VOC itself, soon after its establishment in 1602, had encouraged its governors in Africa, India and the East to undertake ethnomedical research with a view to providing effective healthcare to the staff employed at its various stations.[15] This was a matter of necessity, because the herbal medicines despatched from the VOC apothecary shop in Amsterdam deteriorated rapidly during long sea voyages and were often ineffective against tropical diseases. As Smith[9] noted 'In the field of medicinal remedies, far from the original centres where the standard remedies grew, the colonists turned to the lore of the natives and adapted the native medicines to their own pharmacopoeias'.

The most comprehensive account to date of the traditional medicines of Africa was published in 1932, followed by a second edition in 1962.[16] The authors of this work were two medical officers employed by the then South African Chamber of Mines in Johannesburg. In the course of treating mineworkers who had come from all parts of Africa to seek employment in the rich gold fields of the Witwatersrand, these scientists were able to record information about the traditional medical uses of plants in their patients' countries of origin. All information published from about 1800 onwards in respect of the species' chemistry, pharmacology, toxicology and ethno-medical use was included, as was an index of vernacular names in each of the major languages of southern and eastern Africa. These indices have proved to be essential tools for the modern pharmacognosist, ethnobotanist and ethnopharmacologist, while the work itself remains the starting point for much current ethnomedical research on African plant species. With remarkable foresight, the authors wrote, in the preface to the second edition: 'These remedies are still in common use, but much of the folk medicine of the indigenous peoples of Southern and Eastern Africa is disappearing before the advancing tide of civilization with its synthetic medicines. There is little doubt that the greater part of it will have disappeared within measurable time and the recording of it has seemed to us to be not only a matter of urgency but one of necessity.'

The *African Pharmacopoeia*

During the period 1900–75 there were several other important contributions to the documentation of African traditional medicines. This endeavour has, in the last 30 years, greatly accelerated, at continental, regional, national and provincial level. Major published works on this topic are listed in Box 5.1. In 1985 the then Organisation of African Unity (OAU), now the African Union (AU), published Volume 1 of the *African Pharmacopoeia*,[17] an initiative financed by the WHO.

Box 5.1 *Major publications since 1940 (chronological order) dealing with African traditional medicines at continental, regional, national or provincial level*

Githens TS. *Drug Plants of Africa*. African Handbooks: 8. Philadelphia, PA: University of Pennsylvania Press, 1948.

Gelfand M. *Medicine and Magic of the Mashona*. Cape Town, South Africa: Juta & Co. Ltd, 1956.

Ayensu ES. *Medicinal Plants of West Africa*. Michigan, OH: Reference Publications Inc., 1978.

Jansen PCM, Mendes O. *Plantas Medicinais: seu uso tradicional em Moçambique*, vols 1 and 2. Maputo, Mozambique: Minerva Central, 1983.

Gelfand M, Mavi S, Drummond RB, Ndemera B. *The Traditional Medical Practitioner in Zimbabwe*. Gweru, Zimbabwe: Mambo Press, 1985.

Oliver-Bever BEP. *Medicinal Plants of Tropical West Africa*. Cambridge: Cambridge University Press, 1986.

Hedberg I, Staugård F. *Traditional Medicine in Botswana: Traditional medicinal plants*. Gaborone, Botswana: Ipeleng Publishers, 1989.

Iwu MM. *Handbook of African Medicinal Plants*. Boca Raton, FL: CRC Press Inc., 1993.

Kokwaro JO. *Medicinal Plants of East Africa*, 2nd edn. Nairobi, Kenya: Kenya Literature Bureau, 1993.

Sofowora A. *Medicinal Plants and Traditional Medicine in Africa*, 2nd edn. Ibadan, Nigeria: Spectrum/John Wiley, 1993.

Hutchings A et al. *Zulu Medicinal Plants*. Pietermaritzburg, South Africa: University of Natal Press, 1996.

Maliehe EB. *Medicinal Plants and Herbs of Lesotho*. Maseru, Lesotho: Mafeteng Development Project, 1997.

Von Koenen E. *Medicinal, Poisonous and Edible Plants in Namibia*. Windhoek, Namibia: Klaus Hess Publishers, 2001.

Although a welcome addition to the literature, this work cannot claim to be particularly African in character, in that more than 60% of the monographs presented (±100) deal with plant species not indigenous to Africa (although some have become naturalised there). Volume 2, envisaged at the time, has not yet materialised. Few African countries have recognised the *African Pharmacopoeia* as official; in South Africa the *British Pharmacopoeia* and *British Pharmaceutical Codex* are used. In view of the increasing number of scientific papers dealing with African traditional medicines published during the past 15 years in journals such as *Phytomedicine, Planta Medica, Phytochemistry, Phytotherapy Research, Fitoterapia, Pharmaceutical Biology* and *Journal of Ethnopharmacology*,[18] a revival of the *African Pharmacopoeia* project now seems likely.

At the present time, few states in the WHO African Region have a national TM pharmacopoeia although several (Angola, Republic of Congo, Guinea, Guinea-Bissau, Ivory Coast, Niger, Nigeria, Rwanda, South Africa) are in the process of developing one. At national level, pharmaceutical monographs are currently available for Ghanaian,[19] Mozambican,[20] South African[21] and Ugandan plant species[2] used as TMs. Iwu[23] has presented monographs for 152 African plant species used as TMs and a separate collection of 50 monographs for African TM plant species is currently in preparation.[24] These monographs have different emphases; some focus on quality issues whereas others are pharmacognostic profiles. Three monographs dealing with African traditional medicines appear in the WHO series on selected medicinal plants:[25] *Cortex Pruni Africanae*, *Radix Harpagophytum* and *Aloe*.

Materia medica used in traditional medical practice

Many African states have extremely rich floras, often characterised by a high degree of endemicity, i.e. plant species occurring only within the boundaries of that particular state (Table 5.2). Most notable in this regard is the Cape Floristic Region (CFR) of South Africa, which ranks as one of the five floristic kingdoms of the world on account of its exceptional species richness and large number of endemic plants. Africa's botanical wealth provides most of the materia medica that underpins its TMP.[26]

All plant parts are utilised in traditional medical practice: leaf, stem, bark, fruit, seed, subterranean organs, whole plant, gums/resins and fresh plant juices. A list of 1046 plant species (from 150 angiosperm families) considered to be most important to traditional medical practice in Africa is given by Iwu.[23] According to this author, major angiosperm families utilised are: Apocynaceae/Asclepiadaceae (61 species), Asteraceae (45 species), Euphorbiaceae (62 species), Fabaceae (106 species) and Rubiaceae (49 species). This finding is not surprising, given that Asteraceae and Fabaceae are the two largest angiosperm families and also boast a great variety of secondary chemicals with known therapeutic application, including alkaloids, sesquiterpene lactones and saponins. Fabaceae is reputed to have provided more medicinal species than any other plant family.[27] Alkaloids are common in both Rubiaceae and Apocynaceae/Asclepiadaceae, while the latter is also rich in cardiac glycosides. Euphorbiaceae has yielded interesting anti-tumour agents, e.g. phorbol esters.

Preparation of remedies

TPs in rural areas of Africa harvest their own materials from natural stands of vegetation in their neighbourhood, while those practising in an urban setting either obtain their supplies from herb dealers or travel to rural areas to replenish stocks of herbal medicines. Many city-based healers travel long distances in order to get what they need. Cultivation of plants used in traditional medical practice is not widely practised; indeed many TPs regard cultivated plants as less potent than their wild-grown counterparts. Given the extent of intraspecies variation in, as well as the effects of external factors such as fertiliser/water regime, altitude and soil type on, plant secondary chemistry, this view is not necessarily unreasonable. An awareness of seasonal, diurnal or age variation in therapeutic activity is also

Table 5.2 Numbers of plant species

Region/state	No. of species	Area (km²)	Species/area[a]	Endemic species (% of total)
Australia	25 000	7 710 000	3.2	–
USA	20 000	9 360 000	2.1	–
Europe	14 000	5 680 000	2.5	–
Tropical Africa	30 000	20 000 000	1.5	–
West Tropical Africa	7 300	4 500 000	1.6	–
Southern Africa[b]	23 200	2 570 000	9.03	–
Benin	200	112 622	1.78	5
Burundi	2 500	27 834	89.8	–
Cameroon	8 000+	475 500	16.8	2
CFR[c]	8 590	90 000	95.4	68
DRC[d]	11 000	2 345 410	4.69	29
Gabon	8 000	267 667	29.85	22
Ghana	3 600	238 305	15.1	1.2
Ivory Coast	4 700	322 463	14.57	1.3
Kenya	6 000	582 644	10.3	5
Malawi	3 600	94 081	38.26	2
Mozambique	5 500	784 754	7.0	4
Namibia	3 159	824 293	3.83	–
Nigeria	4 614	923 850	4.99	4.3
South Africa	23 000	1 184 827	19.41	–
Tanzania	10 000	939 762	10.6	11
Uganda	5 000	236 578	21.13	0.6
Zambia	4 600	752 617	6.1	4.8
Zimbabwe	5 420	390 310	13.9	2.3

Blanks in the far right-hand column of the table indicate that no data were available for endemic species in the country/region concerned.

[a]Species/area ratios expressed as 10^3 plant species per 10^6 km².
[b]South Africa, Lesotho, Swaziland, Namibia, Botswana.
[c]Cape Floristic Region.
[d]The Democratic Republic of The Congo.
Data from *Plants in danger-what do we know?* Davis SD *et al*. International Union of the Conservation of Nature and Natural Resources (IUCN), Gland, Switzerland. 1986.

evident in the common practice among TPs of collecting some plant species only at certain times of the day, specified times of the year or a particular stage of the plant's development.

Traditional dosage forms

The most common dosage forms used by TPs are aqueous infusions (for both internal and external use), poultices, snuffs, powders (internal/external use), ointments, inhalations, enemas and vaginal washes. These may be prepared using fresh or dried plant material (whole, powdered or in small pieces). Powders for internal use may be mixed with gruel or porridge, whereas ointments are usually prepared using plant oils or animal fats as a base. Inhalations may be moist (plant material added to boiling water and the steam inhaled or directed to specific body parts) or dry (dried herbs placed on heated stones and the smoke inhaled). Both single and multi-component preparations are prescribed.

The WHO Traditional Medicines Programme and Africa

Acknowledging for the first time the potential of traditional medical practice for the expansion of health services, the World Health Assembly (WHA) passed a number of resolutions:

1 Drawing attention (1976) to the personnel reserve constituted by TPs[28]
2 Urging member states (1977) to utilise their traditional systems of medicine[29]
3 Calling for a comprehensive approach (1978) to the subject of medicinal plants;[30] this approach was to include:
    – an inventory and therapeutic classification, periodically updated, of medicinal plants used in different countries
    – scientific criteria and methods for assessing the safety of medicinal plant products and their efficacy in the treatment of specific conditions/diseases
    – international standards and specifications for identity, purity, strength and manufacturing practices
    – methods for the safe and effective use of medicinal plant products by various levels of health worker
    – dissemination of such information by member states
    – designation of research and training centres for the study of medicinal plants.

In 1987, the 40th WHA reaffirmed these points and, amongst other things, urged Member States to:

- initiate comprehensive programmes for the identification, evaluation, preparation, cultivation and conservation of medicinal plants used in traditional medical practice
- ensure quality control of drugs derived from traditional plant remedies, by using modern techniques and applying suitable standards and good manufacturing practices.

In pursuance of these goals, the WHO has since 1987 produced a number of publications on aspects of TMs and in 2002 a comprehensive TM strategy.[26] This strategy focused on four areas in which action was deemed necessary if TMs (as well as complementary and alternative therapies) were to play a meaningful role in formal healthcare:

1 National policy and regulation
2 Safety/efficacy/quality
3 Access
4 Rational use.

In 2002, the WHO identified challenges and problems within each area, which amounted to deficiencies in and/or a lack of, the following.[26]

National policy and regulation

- Regulatory/legal mechanisms
- Integration of traditional medical practice within the national healthcare system
- Equitable distribution of benefits with respect to indigenous knowledge
- Adequate resource allocation for TM development.

Safety/efficacy/quality

- An adequate evidence base for traditional medical practice therapies and products
- International/national standards for ensuring safety/efficacy/quality assurance
- Adequate regulation of herbal medicines
- Registration of traditional medical practice providers
- Research methodology.

Access

- Data measuring access levels and affordability
- Official recognition of the role of traditional medical practice providers

- Cooperation between traditional medical practice providers and allopathic practitioners
- Attention to the unsustainable use of medicinal plant resources.

Rational use

- Training of traditional medical practice providers
- Training of allopathic practitioners in traditional medical practice
- Communication among TPs, allopathic practitioners and consumers
- Public information on the rational use of TMs.

Addressing WHO deficiencies in traditional medical practice in Africa

The following text considers what progress has been made by western, eastern and southern African states in addressing these deficits. Particular emphasis is placed on the quality/safety/efficacy assessment and conservation of plants used as TMs, as well as on issues of intellectual property associated with indigenous knowledge systems.

National policy and regulation

Regulatory/legal mechanisms

During the colonial period, traditional medical practice was discouraged or prohibited in most African countries. Colonial administrations had little faith in the efficacy of TMs and saw the practice as a system that prevented patients receiving effective western medicine.[31,32] Post-colonial governments have sought to redress this situation, and traditional medical practice is now widely accepted.

As can be seen from Table 5.3 progress with the formulation of national policies on traditional medical practice and with the establishment of legal and regulatory mechanisms in respect of traditional medical practice varies between states. According to Kasilo et al.,[12] 61% of states in the WHO African Region have national traditional medical practice policies, 86% have traditional medical practice administrative centres (usually affiliated to the health ministry) and 78% have traditional medical practice research units, demonstrating a commitment to the promotion and development of the scientific basis of African traditional medical practice. An estimated 58% of states in the region have laws or regulations dealing with traditional medical practice, 44% have national expert committees and 19% a system of registration for TPs. A legal framework for the practice of traditional medicine is in place in 53% of states and management bodies for the coordination of matters pertaining to traditional practice in 57%.

Table 5.3 National policy and regulation in respect of traditional medical practice in states of the western, eastern and southern African regions						
Country	Legal framework	National policy	National management/ coordinating body	Regulation	Legal recognition of TM providers	National budget allocation
Angola	In prep.	–	+	In prep.		
Benin	+	+	+	–		
Botswana		In prep.			+	
Burkina Faso	–	–	+		+	
Burundi	In prep.	In prep.	+	In prep.		
Cameroon	–	In prep.	+	In prep.	+	
Central African Republic	In prep.	In prep.	+	In prep.		
Chad	In prep.	In prep.	+	In prep.		
Republic of the Congo	+	–	+	–	+	
DRC	+	In prep.	+	+		
Equatorial Guinea	+	+	+	+		
Gabon	In prep.	+	+	–		
Gambia	–	In prep.	+	–	+	
Ghana	+	+	+	+	+	+
Guinea-Bissau	–	–	–	–	+	
Ivory Coast	+	+	+	–		+
Kenya	In prep.	In prep.	–	In prep.	+	
Lesotho	+		+		+	
Malawi						
Mali	+	In prep.	+	+	+	+
Mozambique	In prep.	+	+	In prep.		
Namibia	+		+		+	
Nigeria	+	+	+	+	+	+
Rwanda	In prep.	–	–	In prep.		+
South Africa	In prep.	+	+	In prep.	+	+

Continued

Table 5.3 *Continued*						
Country	Legal framework	National policy	National management coordinating body	Regulation	Legal of TM providers	National budget allocation
Tanzania	In prep.	+	+	In prep.	+	
Uganda	In prep.	In prep.	In prep.	In prep.		
Zambia	In prep.	+	+	In prep.		
Zimbabwe	+		+		+	

Data from report of WHO global survey: National Policy on TMP and regulation of herbal medicines. Geneva, May 2005.

Empty cells in the table indicate that no data were available.

In 2006, South Africa established a Directorate of Traditional Medicine within the Health Ministry and in 2007 enacted the Traditional Practitioners Act (No. 22 of 2007), which provided for the convening of a Traditional Practitioners Council. In 2008 a Draft National Policy on African Traditional Medicine (*Government Gazette* No. 31271, 25 July 2008) was published for comment. This policy document provides a framework for the institutionalisation of TMP within the state healthcare system.

Integration of traditional medical practice within the national healthcare system

With regard to the integration of traditional medical practice within the national healthcare system of states in the WHO African Region, a comprehensive account of the many challenges posed by such a step is given in Last and Chavunduka.[33] A major challenge is the feasibility of forming national professional organisations of TPs, a prerequisite for their successful integration into the formal healthcare system. As pointed out by Twumasi and Warren,[34] local associations of traditional healers have always existed in Africa, formed along ethnic/linguistic (Figure 5.5), geographical or occupational lines, the last recognising various categories of TPs, e.g. TBAs, herbalists, bone-setters, diviners or traditional surgeons. Amalgamation of these local associations into a single national umbrella body, speaking with one voice and with a uniform code of practice and criteria for registration/accreditation, has proved difficult in many African states.

It must be remembered that African traditional health systems have cultural and spiritual as well as physical components. A cautionary note in this regard has been sounded by MacCormack:[35]

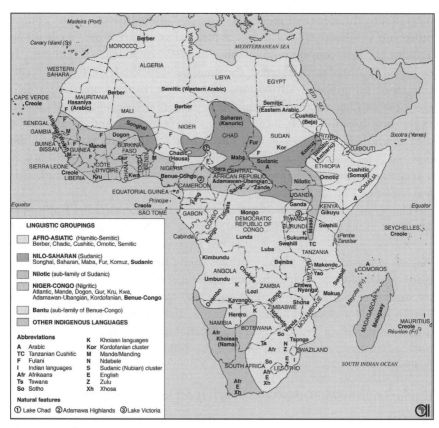

Figure 5.5 Africa: indigenous languages/ethnic groups. *Published with the permission of the Africa Institute of South Africa.*

Healers who practise under a mandate of traditional legitimacy derive their legitimacy from membership in a congregation, sodality or lineage, not necessarily an organisation of the type envisaged by the WHO. Their office in that group and the entire corporate group's role in the local society, must be allowed for in health planning which seeks to achieve health for all through community participation. Plucking the practitioners, or the chemicals from their herbal remedies, out of the context of healing and transferring them to the university, is a gesture of goodwill but it is not truly a collaborative association of plural medical systems.

A similar concern has been expressed by Bodeker et al.[31] as an 'emerging trend for certain elements of traditional healthcare to be removed from their original context and subsequently incorporated into formal health care systems, or developed as part of a parallel complementary and alternative medicine (CAM) sector'. Iwu[23] noted that 'the African medical system does not fall into the sphere of what is known as "alternative medicine", but is rather a complementary but different medical system that uses medicine in a more or less conventional manner for the treatment of diseases. It employs, in a fundamental sense, the same basic methods as Western medicine, with additional contributions from the spiritual dimension, which gives the healing depth and meaning within the African cosmology and experience. It cannot be reduced to simple herbalism . . . and should not be seen as a substitute for qualitative health care for the rural poor, or (in the name of conservation of cultural diversity) be misconstrued by politicians as a social alibi to mask the inadequacies of public health programmes. It is only one possible tool in health care'.

The South African Draft National Policy (2008) on African Traditional Medicine explicitly states that, while aiming at the institutionalisation of traditional medical practice, it does not envisage integration of traditional medical practice within the allopathic system; the intention is that the two systems will function side by side under the state healthcare umbrella. According to Mahunnah et al.[36] Tanzania, with an established National Traditional Practitioners' Association (regulating registered TPs) and a Traditional Health Practitioners' Council (regulating the registration of both practitioners and herbal medicines), offers an example of successful integration.

Equitable distribution of benefits with respect to indigenous knowledge systems

While it is widely acknowledged that indigenous knowledge merits protection and that the holders of such knowledge are entitled to benefits derived from its use, there is no consensus at present as to how this is best achieved. Although a commonly followed route lies via intellectual property (IP) law, it is not generally accepted that patents, trade marks and copyright are appropriate to indigenous knowledge systems (IKSs).[37,38] The IP approach is embodied in Article 27.3 (b) of the WTO (World Trade Organization) Council for Trade-Related Aspects of Intellectual Property Rights (TRIPs) Agreement and is integral to current WIPO (United Nations World Intellectual Property Organisation) discussions.[39] African states seeking to protect IKSs via this route would need to amend their national legislation accordingly. The South African Patents Amendment Act No. 20 of 2005 seeks to address the recognition of indigenous knowledge via IP law, in that it requires patent applications to state whether indigenous knowledge constitutes a component of the application and, if so, whether the applicant has the authority to make use of this knowledge.

Critics of the IP approach argue that western legal and economic definitions pertaining to property in general and intellectual property in particular do not recognise the validity of ancient customary laws, philosophies, values and norms relating to land, resources and knowledge.[40] It is further contended that, while IP instruments rest on the existence of novelty, an identifiable author/inventor, specific delineation and a temporal limitation, these criteria are not applicable to traditional knowledge.

An alternative route to indigenous knowledge protection is via Article 8(j) of the Convention on Biodiversity (CBD), which affirms that indigenous peoples have rights over their knowledge, practices and innovations in respect of indigenous biological resources, whether or not these rights are patentable. Each African state that is a signatory to the CBD is required to put in place the necessary legislation enforcing its terms. The required legislation was enacted in South Africa in 2004 (South African Environmental Management: Biodiversity Act No. 10). The regulations implementing those terms that relate to bioprospecting, access and benefit sharing (section 97(1): d–h) state that permits will be required for all bioprospecting activities (which include those based on traditional knowledge). Benefit-sharing agreements will have to be drawn up between all would-be bioprospectors and stakeholders, according to a specified template. Regulation 10(3) lays down principles for identifying stakeholders, including communities or parts of communities.

The South African Draft National Policy on TM (2008) seeks to draw attention to the inadequate protection afforded indigenous medical knowledge by currently available legal instruments and contemplates legislation that is specific and applicable to African TMs.

An interesting test case in this regard is that of the San peoples in southern Africa, whose claim to intellectual property rights in the use of *Hoodia* (Figure 5.6) species (Apocynaceae) as stimulants and appetite suppressants while on hunting forays has only recently been recognised.

This followed the patenting, by scientists from the South African Council for Scientific and Industrial

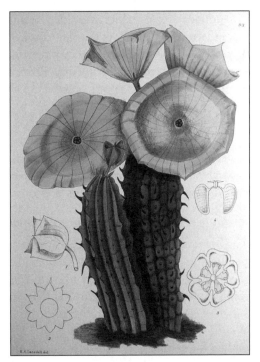

Figure 5.6 *Hoodia* spp. From: Flowering Plants of South Africa Vol. 3, t. 23 (1923). Artist: K.H. Lansdell. Ed. I.B. Pole Evans. L. Reeve and Co. Ltd., London.

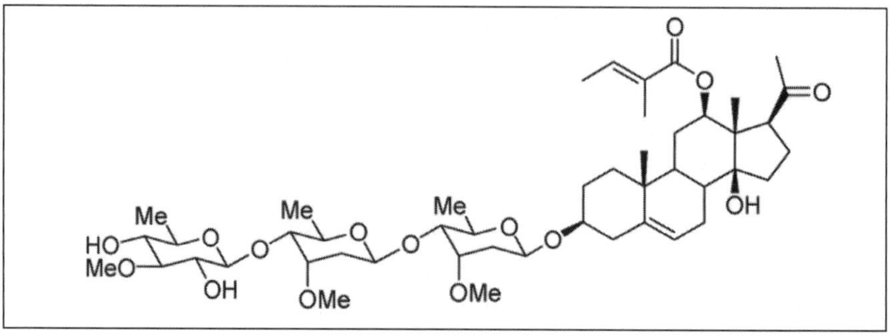

Figure 5.7 Appetite-suppressant pregnane glycoside isolated from *Hoodia gordonii* and *H. pilifera*.

Research (CSIR), of appetite-suppressant extracts prepared from *H. gordonii* (Masson) Sweet ex Decne. and *H. pilifera* (L. f.) Plowes.[41] Two pregnane glycosides, one of which (Figure 5. 7) was shown to have appetite-suppressant activity, have since been isolated from both species.[42] The patenting of extracts of *Hoodia* prompted widespread criticism that San traditional ethnomedical knowledge had been neither recognised nor rewarded.[43] A Memorandum of Understanding, subsequently drawn up and signed by representatives of the South African San Council and the CSIR, now provides for royalties and other financial payments to the San peoples of southern Africa. To date the San Council has received an amount of R560 000 (about £35 000), but further payments will depend on whether multi-national pharmaceutical company Pfizer or UK-based herbal medicines company Phytopharm, both of which have licensing agreements with the CSIR for the development of *Hoodia* products as appetite suppressants, achieve this goal.

With the current drive to bring more San traditional medicines, e.g. cancer bush (*Sutherlandia frutescens* (L.) R. Br.; Fabaceae), into the commercial arena,[44] it has become increasingly important to ensure that the IP of this now-scattered nation is appropriately acknowledged.

Adequate resource allocation for traditional medical practice development

Data for state, non-governmental organisation (NGO) and private sector spending on traditional medical practice development in states of the WHO African Region are scanty. According to Kasilo et al,[12] the percentage of total health expenditure on TPs is 2.19% (Malawi), 4.31% (Rwanda) and 1.46% (Uganda). Research related to traditional medical practice is conducted in 78% of states and local production of TMs in 50%, although the source of funding for neither is specified. In South Africa, the Ministries of Health (via the South African Medical Research Council) and Science/Technology (via the South African National Research Foundation) provide support funding for TM research and development. In most African states, no public financing mechanisms or private insurance programmes exist for traditional healthcare services, the costs of which are paid out of pocket by the patient.

Efficacy/safety/quality

Efficacy – an adequate evidence base for traditional medical practice therapies and products

Considerable research effort on the part of the multinational pharmaceutical industry was devoted during the period 1985–2000 to bioprospecting, guided by ethnobotanical 'leads'.[45] This effort for the most part targeted biodiversity-rich countries in Africa, South America and south-east Asia, where traditional medicines were widely used but had been little investigated as a source of new therapeutic agents. The purpose was new drug discovery for the treatment of essentially first-world health problems, e.g. lifestyle diseases and neurodegenerative disorders. The generally adopted approach was that of bioassay-guided fractionation in order to isolate one or more 'actives' that might lend themselves to laboratory synthesis and/or subsequent structural modification. An example is the isolation of the alkaloid galanthamine from Balkan *Galanthus* (snowdrop) spp. (Amaryllidaceae) and its successful introduction as a treatment for early stage Alzheimer's disease,[46] following reports of its use as a traditional remedy for muscular weakness.

Since the year 2000, the main thrust of ethnomedical screening of African plants appears to have shifted from the domain of the multinational pharmaceutical industry[47] to that of public research institutions or private enterprises within individual African states. The focus of this research has also shifted, with less emphasis on first-world diseases and more on the major causes of mortality/morbidity in Africa, e.g. malaria, tuberculosis (TB) and HIV/AIDS. The research approach has, however, remained essentially the same, i.e. one of bioassay-guided fractionation and a search for individual molecules with therapeutic activity.

An example of a national initiative is the current South African research and development programme for novel drug development from indigenous medicinal plants (see www.sahealthinfo.org/noveldrug/novelpamphlet.htm). The aim of this programme, which brings together a consortium of three government agencies (medical, environmental and agricultural) and four local universities, is the discovery and industrial development of novel therapeutic agents for the treatment of TB, malaria and diabetes mellitus, as well as the identification of new immune modulators and tonics. Initially destined to run over 3 years (2004–6), the programme is on-going and has published some of its preliminary findings.[48,49]

A recent example emanating from African private enterprise is the development of preparations derived from South African *Sceletium* (Figure 5.8)

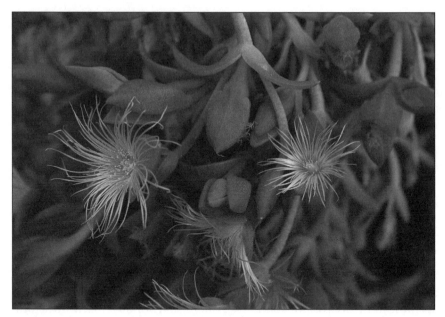

Figure 5.8 One of the *Sceletium* spp. used to prepare *'canna'*.

spp. (Aizoaceae) as antidepressants, by virtue of the reported serotonin reuptake inhibitory activity of a range of alkaloids present in the above-ground parts of the plant.[16,50,51] The traditional preparation concerned is known to the Namaqua people by the vernacular name *canna*. Its use as a mood enhancer was first recorded during a VOC-led expedition in 1685, the journal of which states as follows (see Appendix 1 for original text):

> [In lieu of drink] they mostly chew a certain plant which they call canna, the roots as well as stems being bruised between stones, then stored up and preserved in sewn-up sheepskins. When we came to the Coperbergh in October, it was being gathered from the surrounding hills by everybody (to serve as a supply for the whole year). They use it as the Indians use betel or areck, being in extremely cheerful mood most evenings at their gatherings.

Both usage and mode of preparation of *canna* have continued almost unchanged to the present day. Patented (World Patent 9746234, 1997, Gericke and van Wyk), standardised alkaloid preparations derived from *Sceletium tortuosum* (L.) N.E. Brown and other *Sceletium* species are currently under investigation for the treatment of psychiatric and psychological conditions including depression, anxiety, drug dependence and bulimia. Animal studies have shown promising results.[52]

While the results of new drug discovery programmes may serve to highlight the validity of an ethnobotanical approach, they cannot be said to support the claims for efficacy made by traditional medical systems. The reason is that, in African TMP, almost no organic solvents are used and whole plant products or extracts are administered. Furthermore, it is being increasingly recognised that the efficacy of whole plant extracts may be the product of a complex balance between various secondary chemicals involving synergistic and solubilising effects, as well as a possible mitigation of toxicity.[53] Attempts to isolate one or two 'actives' from traditionally used plants have frequently been disappointing, in that individual compounds have exhibited a loss of activity and/or increased toxicity or presented difficulties in formulation.[54] Many TM plant species have defied identification of individual 'actives' or have been shown to contain mixtures of therapeutically active secondary metabolites that are ubiquitous in the plant kingdom, e.g. tannins, flavonoids and oleanolic acid.[55,56]

A further drawback associated with bioassay-guided fractionation lies in the fact that it has permitted the patenting of isolated molecules for particular therapeutic applications, thus bypassing the need for recognition of IP rights in indigenous knowledge. This legally permissible but ethically questionable practice will persist until such time as all African states have adequate legislation in place for protection of traditional medical systems and practitioners.

With respect to the validation of efficacy of (as opposed to new drug discovery from) African TMs, in vitro assays are widely used, mainly on account of their greater affordability when compared with in vivo models. The most common approach is to prepare plant extracts of varying polarity and test these separately for activity, often using a single in vitro bioassay. There are some flaws in this approach, namely that aqueous infusions are used in African traditional medical practice and, second, that a single bioassay is probably insufficient to demonstrate activity.[57] Consequently, much of the current scientific literature purporting to validate the claims made by TMs does not in fact do so. There have been some studies using traditional dosage forms,[58–60] but few that take into account the effects of genetic or environmental variability on plant secondary chemistry/bioactivity. Box 5.2 lists some recent publications dealing with ethnopharmacological screening programmes for antimalarial/antiplasmodial activity, carried out in various African countries.

A different approach has been taken by the phytomedicines industry, which utilises whole plant products or extracts of plant species used as traditional medicines. Examples of successful introductions of African TMs to this sector of the market are given in Table 5.4 (see also Stewart[61,62]).

Safety

Much benefit is to be gained from the rational use of traditional medicines within the formal healthcare system in Africa.[31] For this reason there is a need

Box 5.2 *Recent screens of African plant species used in traditional medical practice for antimalarial/antiplasmodial activity*

Kenya

Gathwira et al. *In vitro* antiplasmodial and *in vivo* antimalarial activity of some plants used traditionally for the treatment for malaria by the Meru community in Kenya. *J Natural Med* 2007;**61**:261–8.

South Africa

Clarkson et al. *In vitro* antiplasmodial activity of medicinal plants native to or naturalised in South Africa. *J Ethnopharmacol* 2004;**92**:177–91.

Pillay et al. Investigating South African plants as a source of new antimalarial drugs. *J Ethnopharmacol* 2008;**119**:438–54.

Nundkumar, Ojewale. Studies on the antiplasmodial properties of some South African medicinal plants used as antimalarial remedies in Zulu folk medicine. *Methods and Findings in Experimental and Clinical Pharmacology* 2002;**24**:397–401.

Prozesky et al. *In vitro* antiplasmodial activity of ethnobotanically selected South African plants. *J Ethnopharmacol* 2001;**76**: 239–45.

Tanzania

Gessler et al. Screening Tanzanian medicinal plants for antimalarial activity. *Acta Tropica* 1994;**56**:65–77.

Weenen et al. Antimalarial activity of Tanzanian medicinal plants. *Planta Medica* 1990;**56**:369.

Uganda

Kaatura et al. Antiplasmodial activity of extracts of selected medicinal plants used by local communities in Western Uganda for the treatment of malaria. *African J Ecol* 2007;**45**:94–8.

West Africa

Soh, Benoit-Vical. Are West African plants a source of future antimalarial drugs? *J Ethnopharmacol* 2007;**114**:130–40.

Zimbabwe

Kraft et al. *In vitro* antiplasmodial evaluation of medicinal plants from Zimbabwe. *Phytotherapy Research* 2003;**17**:123–8.

Table 5.4 Phytomedicines from African plant species used as traditional medicines

Species	Family	Origin	Plant part	Vernacular name	Application	Preparation
Prunus africana (Hook. f.) Kalkman	Rosaceae	Cameroon	Bark	African prune; Pygeum	Treatment of BPH	Tadenan®
Harpagophytum procumbens (*Burch.*) DC and *H. zeyheri* Decne.	Pedaliaceae	Namibia, Botswana	Tuber	Devil's claw	Anti-rheumatic and anti-inflammatory	Dried tuber Liquid extract Tincture Capsules/tablets
Pelargonium sidoides DC and *P. reniforme* Curtis	Geraniaceae	South Africa	Tuber	Umckaloabo	Treatment of bronchitis	Umckaloabo drops®
Xysmalobium undulatum (L.) W.T. Aiton	Apocynaceae	Namibia, South Africa	Root	Bitterwortel; ishongwe	Treatment of intestinal spasm and diarrhoea	Uzara®

to assess the safety of indigenous traditional herbal remedies and to address the problem of serious adverse events associated with their consumption, particularly by neonates and young children. In many African countries, there is a lack of documented evidence about the safety of TMs, but extensive toxicological study of all traditionally used herbs would be time-consuming, economically unfeasible and probably unnecessary. The WHO guidelines for the assessment of herbal medicines[63] approach the issue of safety by acknowledging that, while a long history of uneventful use does not guarantee absence of risk, 'the guiding principle should be that, if a product has been traditionally used without demonstrated harm, no specific regulatory action should be undertaken unless new evidence demands a revised risk–benefit assessment'.

It is accepted that a proportion of patients treated by western allopathic practitioners will develop iatrogenic complications; by the same token it can be expected that those treated by traditional healers might develop similar complications.[64] Nevertheless it is desirable that adverse events be kept to a minimum. Indeed, concern has been expressed recently in Australia at the unacceptably high number (80 000/year) of allopathic drug-related hospitalisations, which represent a major (but largely avoidable) public health problem.[65]

A review of some of the available data in respect of acute toxicity associated with consumption of South African TMs suggested that these are mostly without harmful side effects, but that some 40 plant species (out of approximately 500 that are in common use nationally and a further ±1000 that are regularly utilised) may be a cause for concern.[66] Inappropriate use of these species appeared to be associated with a high mortality rate, particularly among children. Possible causative factors were identified as:

- inappropriate administration of traditional remedies to neonates and toddlers
- excessive or prolonged self-medication, e.g. during pregnancy
- overdosage by an inexperienced prescriber
- overdosage due to the use of a particularly potent biotype or to seasonal or geographical variation in plant secondary chemistry
- a pre-existing disease that may be exacerbated by the traditional remedy used.

The review noted that there was also a need to give attention to possible interactions between traditional and western allopathic medicines taken concurrently. Pending the outcome of toxicological studies, interim preventive measures (aimed at reducing the number of hospital admissions due to poisoning by traditional remedies) were suggested. These included:

- discouraging long-term use of TMs (>1 month)
- counselling pregnant women about the inadvisability of taking any medication during pregnancy or breast-feeding
- discouraging the use of enemas in neonates and young children
- scheduling those traditional medicines known to be associated with adverse events or fatalities (prescription only, issued by a registered TP) and withdrawing them from the public marketplace
- providing education programmes for healthcare workers, drawing attention to the fact that the clinical picture seen may be modified in patients taking TMs
- conducting public awareness campaigns in clinics in rural areas, advising parents of young children about the known toxicity of certain popular traditional herbs
- implementation of a system for reporting adverse events associated with the use of TMs, as is routinely done for allopathic medicines
- development of methods for the detection of key toxin metabolites in body fluids.[67]

A study of current patterns of TM usage in Africa would assist in establishing to what extent these may have a bearing on the incidence of adverse events associated with TM use. In South Africa some disruption of traditional lifestyle has inevitably accompanied migration from rural to urban milieu. One result is that the traditional healer practising in the city is now obliged either to travel long distances to obtain necessary materia medica or to rely on imported stock, the origin and mode of collection/preparation of which may be unknown to the prescriber. In the latter case, an important component of traditional quality assurance is lost. The establishment of nurseries and farms supplying plant material of consistent quality would help to minimise accidental overdosage due to natural variability in potency.

Another result of urbanisation in South Africa appears to be 'the irresponsible quackery and reckless profiteering racket into which the erstwhile dignified practice of traditional medicine is currently degenerating in the townships and cities' (Zondi, personal communication in Ref. 68). This is a phenomenon of which traditional healers are well aware and which they seek to eradicate (Kubukeli, personal communication). Registration and certification of traditional healers, as is required for their western allopathic counterparts, have been proposed as a solution and may contribute to a reduction in the incidence of poisoning.

A further problem may be that the South African city dweller, driven by constraints of time and money, is now self-medicating with TMs 'counter prescribed' by herb sellers plying their trade in the marketplace. The latter, if motivated by economic necessity alone and lacking the rigorous training of the TP, may provide inadequate or incorrect information. The best of drugs, in the hands of the irresponsible or ignorant, is potentially dangerous. It may be necessary to alert the public, by means of a media campaign, to the hazards of self-medication with traditional herbs known to have deleterious side effects. Although it is not possible to say if the South African experience holds true for other African states, it would be surprising if the effects on traditional medical practice of cultural disruption occasioned by urbanisation, political unrest, war or climate change would not be felt throughout the continent.

A study aimed at investigating the potential hazards associated with the long-term effect of medicinal plants commonly used as TMs in South Africa tested polar and non-polar extracts of some 50 plant species for genotoxic effects using in vitro bacterial and mammalian cell assays, such as the Ames test, VITOTOX test, micronucleus test and comet assay.[69] It was found that most of the 50+ plant species investigated caused either DNA damage (as detected by the comet assay), chromosomal aberrations and/or non-dysjunction or chromosome lagging in human white blood cells (as detected in the micronucleus test). A few plants showed frame-shift mutations in the salmonella/microsome assay. These findings are a cause for concern and further toxicological studies are necessary before the species concerned can be prescribed with confidence.

Quality assurance

Quality assurance of medicines rests on the establishment of standards relating to their identity, purity and potency. This constitutes the first step in the process of bringing traditionally used plant species from the field into the clinic, dispensary and hospital. In African states seeking to promote the rational use of TMs, attention must be given in the first instance to correct species identification, because very few traditional herbs are cultivated and almost all raw material is obtained from the wild. Consequently, misidentification or adulteration can easily occur. Once in the marketplace, TMs are frequently encountered in a form (dried, powdered, comminuted) that renders identification (ID) impossible. Classical microscopy has been used as an aid to the ID of African TMs, as have high-performance liquid chromatography/thin-layer chromatography (HPLC/TLC) fingerprints[21,22] and infrared scans.[24]

Budgets permitting, TLC and HPLC results can be quantified and used as the basis of an assay. Even if the therapeutically active components of a TM are unknown, quantities of major constituents can serve as a preliminary guide to potency, pending identification of 'actives'. Other quantitative procedures, e.g. alcohol- and/or water-soluble extractive values and volatile oil content are useful low-cost indicators of quality.

Access

Official recognition of the role of TM providers

Many treatments prescribed by TPs have proven therapeutic effects and as such are more readily accepted by health agencies and western allopathic practitioners as effective. Indeed, TPs are collaborating with governments in implementing national health programmes in some countries, e.g. Zambia and Zimbabwe.[70] Traditional medical practitioner associations (TMAs) have been formed in most states in the WHO African Region; many have formal links with their health ministries and are recognised as having positive inputs into their healthcare systems. Some TMAs have been formed with the objective of promoting TMs, improving cooperation between TPs and health agencies, and addressing relevant legal issues. The situation with regard to TMAs varies between states; in some cases, e.g. Namibia, Kenya, only one TMA is given official recognition while in others several TMAs exist. Many African TPs do not, however, belong to a TMA, making official recognition of their role difficult.

Cooperation between TM providers and allopathic practitioners

Collaboration between African traditional and western allopathic medical practitioners at the local primary healthcare level may constitute a first step towards integration of traditional medical practice into national healthcare systems. Successful collaboration at this level in the WHO African Region has been driven by the current HIV/AIDS crisis, where the training of TPs in necessary allopathic procedures has been encouraged. In South Africa,[71] information sharing and educational programmes have resulted in TPs providing correct HIV/AIDS advice as well as demonstrations of condom use. An estimated 1510 TPs were trained by these programmes and an estimated 845 600 of their patients reached with AIDS/sexually transmitted infection (STI) prevention messages during the first 10 months of the programme. Similar programmes have been undertaken in Mozambique, Zambia, Zimbabwe, Botswana and Malawi. UNAIDS[72] has observed that, in addition to serving as effective agents in the dissemination of prevention/education messages in respect of HIV/AIDS, TPs are able to offer affordable and effective treatments, particularly for opportunistic infections and STIs. In Uganda, an indigenous NGO known as THETA (Traditional and Modern Health Practitioners Together against AIDS and other diseases) is dedicated to collaboration between traditional and allopathic practitioners in education, counselling and improved clinical care for people with STIs, including HIV/AIDS.[73] According to Marshall,[70] the outstanding feature of Uganda's public healthcare system is the cooperation between western allopathic practitioners and TPs.

Malaria, a second major public health problem in sub-Saharan African, also lends itself to local collaborative programmes between TPs and allopathic practitioners. Primarily a disease of the rural poor in Africa, *Plasmodium falciparum* malaria causes more deaths than any other infectious agent in young African children and is responsible for almost 40% of these deaths. Up to 75% of malaria sufferers use locally available TMs,[74] because these remedies are often the only option in remote rural areas. The efficacy of such remedies has been demonstrated by the successful development of modern antimalarials from traditionally used *Cinchona* and *Artemisia* spp.[75] Traditional preparations of *Artemisia annua* L. have been shown to be effective[76] for the treatment of semi-immune patients (adults and older children) in malaria endemic areas, where complete parasite clearance is probably unnecessary.[77] However, the issue of possible recrudescence after incomplete parasite clearance needs to be taken into account. Evaluation of the efficacy of locally available TMs (as selected by TPs) in the treatment of uncomplicated malaria and involvement of TPs in malaria control programmes at the local level would enable scarce resources to be allocated to dealing with more severe cases. The Research Initiative for Traditional Systems of Health (RITAM) has recently produced a publication dealing with many issues pertinent to the use and evaluation of traditional herbal antimalarials, including a review of clinical trials.[78]

Attention to the unsustainable use of medicinal plant resources

Olayiwola Akerele, former manager of WHO's Traditional Medicines Programme, noted: 'logically, the investigation, utilisation and exploitation of medicinal plants by a country should also include measures for their conservation.'[79] A plea for a global effort directed to the preservation of medicinal plants was issued jointly in 1988 by the WHO, the World Wide Fund for Nature (WWF) and the International Union for the Conservation of Nature (IUCN). Known as the Chiang Mai Declaration, after the city in which the first WHO/IUCN/WWF International Consultation on the Conservation of Medicinal Plants took place, it called upon WHA member states to 'Save the plants that save lives'.

Twenty years later, Africa's fragile oral knowledge systems are threatened by war, famine, political instability and urbanisation (with concomitant loss of the 'ecosystem generation'). Unsustainable harvesting practices, deliberate habitat destruction and climate change threaten the survival of the plant species on which Africa's traditional healers depend. The greatest threat to traditional medical practice, however, is the burgeoning global population, whose growth and consumption of natural resources places plant diversity at risk in most parts of the world. The quantity of wild plant material exported from Africa and destined for the international pharmaceutical trade is enormous, but pales into insignificance compared with that required by the trade in crude drugs used in traditional medical practice, within individual states or across regional borders. Stimulated by high population growth rates, rapid urbanisation, rural unemployment and the value placed on TMs, national and regional commercial trade in TMs is now greater than at any time in the past.

Formerly most TPs gathered their own materia medica, but in an increasingly urbanised and commercialised world this is no longer possible. As a result, a niche has arisen for collectors who often travel long distances to procure plant or animal medicinals for sale to vendors or TPs, for export or for their own use.[70] In African countries with large urban populations, medicinal plant use has changed from being a purely specialist activity of TPs to one involving an informal sector group of medicinal plant gatherers and vendors. Unlike rural TPs who gather plant material in small quantities, commercial gatherers are motivated primarily by profit. This has resulted in a disregard for traditional conservation practices and 'an opportunistic scramble for the last bag of bark, bulbs or roots'. High rates of unemployment and low levels of formal education have also given rise to an increasing number of medicinal plant vendors, plying their trade in the marketplace (Figure 5.9).[80,81]

The link between local poverty and over-collection of many medicinal plants from the wild must be taken into account when formulating conservation strategies. Suggested measures for the conservation of African plant species used as TMs include:

- Empowering local people to protect their natural resources, e.g. establishment of community nurseries for the cultivation of popular TMs, for sale or consumption

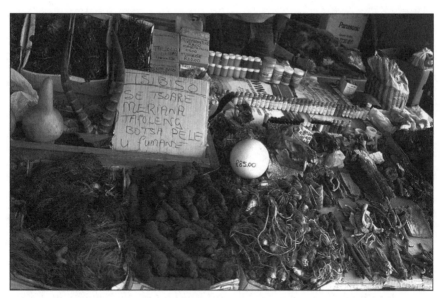

Figure 5.9 Traditional medicines on sale in the marketplace, Maseru, Lesotho.

- Improving control of harvesting from natural stands of vegetation, e.g. permit systems for registered collectors/TMPs
- Improving harvesting methods, e.g. prevention of ring barking of trees.

TPs would be well placed to advise their communities about the need for plant conservation and to coordinate efforts in this regard.

Regional initiatives in respect of traditional medical practice

In addition to the WHA and WHO general recommendations in respect of traditional medical practice outlined above, the WHO African Regional Office has tabled a strategy promoting the use of TMs in reducing morbidity and mortality on the continent and, during a meeting of African Ministers of Health, has taken a decision to celebrate African Traditional Medicine Day on 31 August each year. The African Union (AU) has acknowledged the critical role of traditional medical practice in healthcare provision in Africa and formulated a Plan of Action (AHG/Dec 164 XXXVIII) in this regard. The primary objective of this plan is the institutionalisation, by 2010, of African traditional medical practice in the public health systems of AU member states. The period 2001–10 has been declared the Decade of African Traditional Medicine and an Africa Health Strategy (2007–15) has been formulated, focusing on the strengthening of health systems for equity and development in Africa.

A Southern African Development Community (SADC) inter-ministerial subcommittee on TMs has recommended that member states each provide the legal framework for recognition of African traditional medical practice. The subcommittee has proposed that financial and technical resources be mobilised for the implementation of TM policies in Africa, undertaken to assess the needs and status of traditional medical practice in the SADC region by 2006 and to formulate policy for the recognition, regulation and control of traditional medical practice by 2007.

Conclusion

There is no doubt that Africa's rich botanical biodiversity and well-established traditional medical systems can be harnessed for the provision of better healthcare throughout the continent. Pharmacists in AU states are well equipped to bridge the gap between traditional and western allopathic medical systems through the application of standard pharmaceutical methods to quality assurance, safety assessment and efficacy testing of TMs in use in their countries. Adding value or benefits to TMs as finished products (e.g. tablets, ointments, syrups) may constitute the foundation of a phytomedicines industry and is also the domain of the pharmacist. Much of this work lends itself to postgraduate student research projects. The necessary expertise and infrastructure do not exceed the capabilities of the average African university School of Pharmacy. Consideration might be given by health ministries in neighbouring states to the creation of regional centres of excellence in TM research, if possible with WHO financial and technical support. In this way duplication of facilities and research effort might be minimised, as the use of many TMs straddles country borders.

The domestication of plant species used as TMs as crops and their agricultural improvement are additional steps in the process of bringing TMs from the field to the pharmacy and clinic, with potential benefits to both the health and economies of AU states. Government support in the form of collaboration between ministries of health, agriculture, environment and industry is needed to facilitate the process, ensuring also that the rights of TPs are respected and the plant species concerned properly conserved.[79]

Africa's pharmacists have an additional role: to ensure that whatever TM research is undertaken in their countries is both necessary and relevant, that the results of this research are communicated to TPs, healthcare providers and the public, and that the most cost-effective methods are employed throughout.

Appendix 1

'. . . kouwen meerendeels seeker kruyd by haer canna genoemt, t'welck zy met wortel en stam gesamentlyk tusschen steenen kreusen, en in toegenayde schaaps vellen opleggen en bewaeren. Toen wy in Oktober omtrent den Coperbergh quamen, weird door alle man 'tselvs op d'omliggende bergen (tot voorraad vant geheele jaar) ingesamelt 't welck zy gelijk d'Indianers den betel of areck gebruijcken, synde seer vroolijk van humeur, meest alle avonden in haer 'tsamenkomst . . .'

Photographs

Unless otherwise stated, photographs were taken by G Scott.

References

1. Deacon HJ. An introduction to the fynbos region: time scales and palaeoenvironments. In: Deacon HJ, Hendey QB, Lambrechts JJN (eds), *Fynbos Ecology: A preliminary synthesis*. South African National Scientific Programmes Report No. 75. Pretoria: CSIR, 1983: 1–20.
2. World Health Organization. *The Promotion and Development of Traditional Medicine*. Technical Reports Series 622, Geneva: WHO, 1978.
3. Kokwaro JO. *Medicinal Plants of East Africa*, 2nd edn. Nairobi: Kenya Literature Bureau, 1993.
4. Kubukeli PS. Traditional healing practice using medicinal herbs. *Lancet* 1999;354:24.
5. Sofowora A. Plants in African traditional medicine – an overview. In: Evans WC (ed.), *Trease and Evans' Pharmacognosy*, 15th edn. Edinburgh: WB Saunders Co. Ltd, 2002: 488–96.
6. Soodyal H. *A Walk in the Garden of Eden: Genetic trails into our South African past*. African Human Genome Project Occasional Paper Series No. 2. Cape Town: HSRC Publishers, 2003.
7. Jolly P. Interaction between South-Eastern San and Southern Nguni and Sotho communities c. 1400–1880. *South African Hist J* 1996;35:30–61.
8. Story R. Plant lore of the Bushmen. In: Davies DHS (ed.), *Ecological Studies in Southern Africa*. The Hague: W. Junk, 1964: 87–99.
9. Smith CA. *Common Names of South African Plants*. Botanical Survey Memoir 35. Pretoria: Government Printer, 1966.
10. Gelfand M, Mavi S, Drummond RB, Ndemera B. *The Traditional Medical Practitioner in Zimbabwe: His principles of practice and pharmacopoeia*. Gweru: Mambo Press, 1985.
11. Staugaard F. Traditional health care in Botswana. In: Last M, Chavunduka GL (eds), *The Professionalisation of African Medicine*. International African Seminars New Series No. 1. Manchester: Manchester University Press in association with the International African Institute, 1986: 50–86.
12. Kasilo O, Soumbey-Alley E, Wambebe, C, Chatora R. Regional overview: African region. In: Bodeker G, Ong C-K, Grundy C, Burford G, Maehira Y (eds), *WHO Global Atlas of Traditional, Complementary and Traditional Medicine*. Kobe, Japan: WHO Centre for Health Development, 2005: 3–12.
13. Okpako D. African medicine: traditions and beliefs. *Pharmaceut J* 2006;276:239–40.
14. Thunberg CP. Dissertatio de Medicina Africanorum. Dissertationes academicae sub praesidio C.P. Thunberg. Vol. 1. Göttingen: JC Dieterich, 1785: 269–76.
15. Scott, G, Hewett ML. Pioneers in ethnopharmacology: the Dutch East India Company (VOC) at the Cape from 1650–1800. *J Ethnopharmacol* 2008;115:339–60.
16. Watt JM, Breyer-Brandwijk MG. *The Medicinal and Poisonous Plants of Southern and Eastern Africa*. Edinburgh and London: E&S Livingstone Ltd, 1932, 1962.

17. OAU. *African Pharmacopoeia*, Vol. 1. Lagos, Nigeria: OAU Scientific, Technical and Research Commission, 1985.
18. Light ME, Sparg SG, Stafford GI, van Staden J. Riding the wave: South Africa's contribution to ethnopharmacological research over the last 25 years. *J Ethnopharmacol* 2005; **100**:127–30.
19. WHO. *National Policy on Traditional Medicine and Regulation of Herbal Medicines*. Report of a WHO global survey. Geneva: WHO, 2005.
20. Jansen PCM, Mendes O. *Plantas medicinais e seu uso tradicional em Moçambique*, Vols 1–5. Maputo: Instituto Nacional do Livro e do Disco, 1983–1991.
21. Scott, G, Springfield EP. Pharmaceutical Monographs on CD-ROM for 60 South African plant species used as traditional medicines. Pretoria: South African National Biodiversity Institute, 2004.
22. Springfield EP, Eagles PFK, Scott G. Quality assessment of South African herbal medicines by means of HPLC fingerprinting. *J Ethnopharmacol* 2005;**101**(1–3):75–83.
23. Iwu M. *Handbook of African Medicinal Plants*. Boca Raton, FL: CRC Press Inc., 1993.
24. Association for African Medicinal Plant Standards, 2008. Available at: www.aamps.org.
25. World Health Organization. WHO Monographs on selected medicinal plants, Vols 1 and 2. Geneva: WHO, 1999, 2002
26. World Health Organization. Traditional Medicines Strategy 2002–2005. Geneva: WHO, 2002.
27. Evans WC, ed. *Trease and Evans' Pharmacognosy*, 15th edn. Edinburgh: WB Saunders Co. Ltd, 2002: 25–36.
28. World Health Association. Resolution WHA 29.72. 1976.
29. World Health Association. Resolution WHA 30.49. 1977
30. World Health Association. Resolution WHA 331.33. 1978.
31. Bodeker G, Kronenberg F, Burford G. Policy and public health perspectives on traditional, complementary and alternative medicine: an overview. In: Bodeker, G, Burford G (eds), *Traditional, Complementary and Alternative Medicine: Policy and public health perspectives*. London: Imperial College Press, 2007: 9–39.
32. Chavunduka GL. *Traditional Medicine in Modern Zimbabwe*. Harare: University of Zimbabwe, 1994.
33. Last, M, Chavunduka GL, eds. *The Professionalisation of African Medicine*. International African Seminars New Series No. 1. Manchester: Manchester University Press in association with the International African Institute, 1986.
34. Twumasi PA, Warren DM. The professionalisation of indigenous medicine: a comparative study of Ghana and Zambia. In: Last, M, Chavunduka GL (eds), *The Professionalisation of African Medicine*. International African Seminars New Series No. 1. Manchester: Manchester University Press in association with the International African Institute, 1986: 117–135.
35. MacCormack C. The articulation of Western and traditional systems of health care. In: Last M, Chavunduka GL (eds), *The Professionalisation of African Medicine*. International African Seminars New Series No. 1. Manchester: Manchester University Press in association with the International African Institute, 1986: 151–62.
36. Mahunnah RLA, Uiso FC, Kitua AY et al. United Republic of Tanzania. In: Bodeker G, Ong C-K, Grundy C, Burford G, Maehira Y (eds), *WHO Global Atlas of Traditional, Complementary and Traditional Medicine*. Kobe, Japan: WHO Centre for Health Development, 2005: 3–12.
37. Büchner S. *Protection of traditional and indigenous knowledge*. Trade Law Centre for Southern Africa (TRALAC) discussion document 23/7/2002, 2002.
38. WHO. *Report of the Inter-Regional Workshop on Intellectual Property Rights in the Context of Traditional Medicine*. Geneva: WHO, 2001 (document ref. WHO/EDM/TRM/2001.1).
39. WIPO. *WIPO Intergovernmental Committee on Intellectual Property and Genetic Resources, Traditional Knowledge and Folklore*. Geneva: WIPO, 2007 (document ref. WIPO/GRTKF/IC/11/5(a).

40. Tauli-Corpuz V. *Biodiversity, Traditional Knowledge and the Rights of Indigenous Peoples.* IPRs Series No. 5. Proceedings of an International Workshop on Traditional Knowledge, Panama City, 21–23 September 2005. Geneva: UN Permanent Forum on Indigenous Issues, 2005.

41. Van Heerden FR, Vleggaar R, Horak RM, Learmonth RA, Maharaj VJ, Whittal RD. Pharmaceutical compositions having appetite-suppressing activity. PCT/GB98/01100, 1998.

42. Van Heerden FR, Horak RM, Maharaj VJ, Vleggaar R, Senabe J, Gunning P. An appetite-suppressant from *Hoodia* species. *Phytochemistry* 2007;**68**:2545–53.

43. Swart E. *Hoodia gordonii*: a review. Paper presented at the Indigenous Plant Use Forum (IPUF) meeting, Gaborone, Botswana, July 2006.

44. Van Wyk B-E, Albrecht C. A review of the taxonomy, ethnobotany, chemistry and pharmacology of *Sutherlandia frutescens* (Fabaceae). *J Ethnopharmacol* 2008;**119**: 620–9.

45. Farnsworth N, Akerele O, Bingel AS, Soejarto DD, Zhengang G. Medicinal plants in therapy. *Bull WHO* 1985;**63**:965–81.

46. Wilkinson D, Murray J. Galanthamine: a randomised double-blind, dose comparison in patients with Alzheimer's disease. *Int J Geriatr Psychiatry* 2001;**16**:852–7.

47. Cordell GA, Colvard MD. Some thoughts on the future of ethnopharmacology. *J Ethnopharmacol* 2005;**100**:5–14.

48. Van de Venter M, Roux S, Bungu LC et al. Antidiabetic screening and scoring of 11 plants traditionally used in South Africa. *J Ethnopharmacol* 2008;**119**:81–6.

49. Clarkson C, Maharaj VJ, Crouch NR, et al. *In vitro* antiplasmodial activity of medicinal plants native to or naturalised in South Africa. *J Ethnopharmacol* 2004;**92**:177–91.

50. Smith MT, Field CR, Crouch NR, Hirst M. The distribution of mesembrine alkaloids in selected taxa of the Mesembryanthemaceae and their modification in the *Sceletium* derived 'kougoed'. *Pharmaceut Biol* 1998;**36**:173–9 and references therein.

51. Smith MT, Crouch NR, Gericke N, Hirst M. Psychoactive constituents of the genus *Sceletium* NE Brown and other Mesembryanthemaceae: a review. *J Ethnopharmacol* 1996;**50**:119–30.

52. Gericke N, van Wyk B-E. *Sceletium* – a review update. *J Ethnopharmacol* 2008;**119**: 653–63.

53. Williamson EM. Synergy in relation to the pharmacological action of phytomedicinals. In: Evans WC (ed.), *Trease and Evans' Pharmacognosy,* 15th edn. Edinburgh: WB Saunders Co. Ltd, 2002: 49–54.

54. Houghton PJ. Traditional plant medicines as a source of new drugs. In: Evans WC (ed.), *Trease and Evans' Pharmacognosy,* 15th edn. Edinburgh: WB Saunders Co. Ltd, 2002: 125–34.

55. Bladt S, Wagner H. From the Zulu medicine to the European phytomedicine Umckaloabo®. *Phytomedicine* 2007;**14**:SVI 2–4.

56. Bamuamba K, Meyers P, Gammon DW, Dijoux-Franca M-G, Scott G. Antimycobacterial activity of 5 plant species used as traditional medicines in the Western Cape Province (South Africa). *J Ethnopharmacol* 2008;**117**:385–90.

57. Houghton PJ, Howes M-J, Lee CC, Steventon G. Uses and abuses of *in vitro* testing in ethnopharmacology: visualizing an elephant. *J Ethnopharmacol* 2007;**110**:391–400.

58. Scott G, Springfield EP, Coldrey N. A pharmacognostical study of 26 South African plant species used as traditional medicines. *Pharmaceut Biol* 2004;**42**:186–213.

59. Yimei J, Guodong Z, Jicheng J. Preliminary evaluation: the effects of *Aloe ferox* Mill. and *Aloe arborescens* Mill. on wound healing. *J Ethnopharmacol* 2008;**120**:181–9.

60. Steenkamp V, Fernandes AC, van Rensburg CEJ. Antibacterial activity of Venda medicinal plants. *Fitoterapia* 2007;**78**:561–4.

61. Stewart KM. The African cherry (*Prunus africana*): can lessons be learned from an over-exploited medicinal tree? *J Ethnopharmacol* 2003;**89**:3–13.

62. Stewart K. The commercial harvest of devil's claw (*Harpagophytum* spp.) in Southern Africa: the devil's in the details. *J Ethnopharmacol* 2005;**100**:225–36.

63. WHO. *Guidelines for the Assessment of Herbal Medicines.* WHO Technical Report Series No. 863 (F/S). Geneva: WHO, 1996.

64. Buchanan N, Cane RD. Poisoning associated with witchdoctor attendance. *South African Med J* 1976;**50**:1138–40.

65. Roughead EE. The nature and extent of drug-related hospitalisations in Australia. *J Qual Clin Pract* 2000;**19**:19–22.

66. Scott G. Acute toxicity associated with the use of South African traditional medicinal herbs. *Trans R Soc South Africa* 2003;**58**(1):83–92.

67. Steenkamp V, Stewart MJ, Zuckerman M. Clinical and analytical aspects of pyrrolizidine poisoning caused by South African traditional medicines. *Therapeut Drug Monitor* 2000;**22**:302–6.

68. Bodenstein JW. Toxicity of traditional herbal remedies. *South African Medical Journal* 1977;**52**:790.

69. Elgorashi EE, Taylor JLS, Verschaeve L, Maes A, van Staden, J, de Kimpe N. Screening of medicinal plants used in South African traditional medicine for genotoxic effects. *Toxicol Lett* 2003;**143**:195–207.

70. Marshall NT. *Searching for a Cure: Conservation of medicinal wildlife resources in east and southern Africa.* TRAFFIC International Report. Cambridge: TRAFFIC International, 1998.

71. Bodeker G, Neumann C, Ong C-K, Burford G. Training. In: Bodeker G, Burford G (eds), *Traditional, Complementary and Alternative Medicine: Policy and public health perspectives.* London: Imperial College Press, 2005: 61–81.

72. UNAIDS. *Ancient Remedies, New Disease: Involving traditional healers in increasing access to AIDS care and prevention in East Africa.* UNAIDS/02.16E. Geneva: UNAIDS, 2002.

73. Bodeker G, Kabatesi D, King, R, Homsy J. A regional task force on traditional medicine and AIDS. *Lancet* 2000;**355**:1284.

74. Willcox ML, Bodeker G. Malaria. In: Bodeker G, Burford G (eds), *Traditional, Complementary and Alternative Medicine: Policy and public health perspectives.* London: Imperial College Press, 2005: 239–53.

75. Pillay P, Maharaj VJ, Smith PJ. Investigating South African plants as a source of new anti-malarial drugs. *J Ethnopharmacol* 2008;**119**:438–54.

76. Mueller MS, Karhagomba IB, Hirt HM, Wernakor E, Li SM, Heide L. The potential of *Artemisia annua* L. as a locally produced remedy for malaria in the tropics: agricultural, chemical and clinical aspects. *J Ethnopharmacol* 2000;**73**:487–93.

77. De Ridder S, van der Kooy F, Verpoorte R. *Artemisia annua* as a self-reliant treatment for malaria in developing countries. *J Ethnopharmacol* 2008;**120**:302–14.

78. Willcox M, Bodeker G, Rasoanaivo P, Addae-Kyereme J, eds. *Traditional Medicinal Plants and Malaria.* London: CRC Press, 2004.

79. WHO/IUCN/WWF. *Guidelines on the Conservation of Medicinal Plants.* Gland, Switzerland: IUCN, 1993.

80. Cunningham AB. *An Africa-wide Overview of Medicinal Plant Harvesting, Conservation and Health Care.* WWF/Unesco/Kew People and Plants Initiative, 1999.

81. Lewington A. *A Review of the Importation of Medicinal Plants and Plant Extracts into Europe.* TRAFFIC International Report. Cambridge: TRAFFIC International, 1993.

6

Traditional Chinese medicine

Steven Kayne and Tony Booker

This chapter describes the basic concepts governing the practice of traditional Chinese medicine (TCM) and then focuses on two of the most widely practised disciplines, acupuncture and Chinese herbal medicine (CHM), in greater detail. A brief overview of other similar traditional medicine practices is also included.

All healthcare providers, particularly those who practise in areas with substantial Chinese immigrant populations, will find it useful to have some background knowledge of this topic. However, the reader should appreciate that this chapter is designed only to be a brief introduction to what is a very wide-ranging and complex subject, and it will certainly not equip you to set up as a TCM practitioner!

Traditional Chinese medicine

Definition

TCM is a generic term used to describe a number of medical practices that originated in China but have now spread throughout the world. It includes not only acupuncture and CHM, but also a number of other disciplines such as dietary therapy, mind and body exercise (e.g. tai c'hi), and meditation.

History

The earliest Chinese medical treatise, *Huangdi Neijing,* is attributed to the highly esteemed Yellow Emperor (Huangdi) who, according to legendary history, ascended to the throne of China around 2698 BC.[1] The text, also known as *The Yellow Emperor's Classic of Internal Medicine* or *The Yellow Emperor's Inner Canon*, is considered to be the highest authority on TCM.[2] It comprises two separate works:

1   *Suwen*, a book of simple questions
2   *Lingshu*, a book on acupuncture and moxibustion.

Written in the form of a discourse between Huangdi and his ministers on the nature of health, it contains a wealth of knowledge, including aetiology, physiology, diagnosis, therapy and prevention of disease, as well as an in-depth investigation of such diverse subjects as ethics, psychology and cosmology.[3] It is likely that the book was developed by others over the centuries until a definitive version appeared in the first century BC, but it is, none the less, usually ascribed to Huangdi. The theories of medicine expounded in *Neijing* remain to this day the most authoritative guide to TCM.

Another significant influence on the development of Chinese medicine was produced in the first or second century AD. Entitled *The Classic of Difficult Issues*, it discusses the origins of the nature of illness, describes an innovative approach to diagnosis and outlines a system of therapeutic needling.

The origins of what might be called modern TCM can be traced back to Zhang Ji, who practised in the Qing Chang mountains close to Chengdu, Szechuan province, in the early years of the third century AD, although it was known to have existed in various forms for more than 1000 years before this date.[4] Ji was described as the sage of medicine and probably used traditional methods of healing that were originally linked to Indian practices but were subsequently modified according to Chinese Taoist spiritual philosophy. Another of the famous masters of Chinese medicine active in the third century AD was Hua Tuo, a surgeon and practitioner of a range of therapies.

In the western world TCM, especially acupuncture and CHM, experienced its main expansion during the nineteenth and twentieth centuries as populations moved with developing means of transport. It diffused from immigrant families into host communities and was promoted by subsequent media exposure. The UK's 100-year involvement in Hong Kong led to immigration from the colony and returning merchants, both spawning an interest in all things oriental.

In 1849 the Gold Rush in California brought a large influx of Chinese people to the western USA. They brought their traditional medicine with them and it proved to be popular among the prospectors and their families, particularly as western medicine was largely unavailable in these remote areas. The steady expansion of interest in TCM in the past 30 years in the USA has been attributed to media interest during President Nixon's visit to the People's Republic of China in the early 1970s (see Acupuncture below).

Principles of TCM

TCM is necessarily embedded in a complex theoretical framework that provides conceptual and therapeutic directions.[5] Unlike the earliest Chinese healing, which relied on supernatural guidance or altered states of consciousness, classic Chinese medicine relies on ordinary human sensory awareness. Its fundamental assertion, similar to the kindred philosophical systems of Confucianism and Taoism, is that contemplation and reflection on sensory perceptions and ordinary appearances are sufficient to understand the human condition, including health and illness. This assertion is fundamentally different from the western biomedical viewpoint, which gives privileged status to objective technology and quantitative measurement.

The Chinese approach to understanding the human body is unique. It is based on a highly sophisticated set of practices designed to cure illness and to maintain health and well-being.[6] Ji is reputed to have said:[7]

The superior physician helps before the early budding of disease.

These practices also represent an energetic intervention designed to re-establish harmony and equilibrium for each patient according to the holistic principle.

Whenever the practitioner uses acupuncture or herbal medicine, prescribes a set of exercises or proposes a new diet, his or her activities are all considered to be mutually interdependent and necessary to restore (or maintain) health.

Acupuncture and CHM are considered as separate therapies in this chapter but, in the West, it is common practice to treat patients using a combination approach. This differs somewhat to how Chinese medicine is practised in China where doctors tend to specialise in acupuncture, herbal medicine or tuina massage. This difference is probably due to the fact that there are far more practitioners in China than in the West.

TCM is as much a proactive process as a reactive one – that is to say, the principles of TCM may be applied to daily life to stimulate better health without the presence of an illness to initiate it.

Below is a brief description of the concepts that are fundamental to an understanding of how Chinese medicine is used:

- Yin and yang
- The five phases
- The five substances
- The organs
- The meridians or channels.

Although they are presented in discrete sections, they are all interlinked, like a jigsaw puzzle. In isolation each piece of the puzzle (concept) has little significance.

Yin and yang

According to Emperor Fu His, who lived in the Yellow River area of China, approximately 8000 years ago, the world and all life within it are made up of paired opposites, each giving meaning to the other. They may be viewed as complementary aspects of the whole. Fu His formulated two symbols to represent this idea: a broken line and an unbroken line. These symbols depicted the two major forces in the universe – creation and reception – and how their interaction formed life. This duality was named yin–yang and represents the foundation of Chinese medicine. Thus, the meaning of night is linked to the meaning of day, the ebb of a tide to the flow, and hot with cold. Perhaps the most appropriate link might be that of health and disease, often thought of as being direct opposites. A different view might be that these are both facets of life, each necessary for the other, indeed each giving rise to the other.[8] Thus disease may be thought of as a manifestation of health.

The relationship between the two elements is dynamic: nature constantly moves between the two. An analogy might be provided by considering a cup of coffee that starts as yang; as it cools the yang changes to yin, passing through an equilibrium that is just right for drinking. At any stage the application of heat will cause a flow back into yang. This element of change involving energy flows (see below) is seen as a fundamental quality of life.

Yin and yang are now reflected in the well-known entwined symbol (the tai ji symbol), depicted in Figure 6.1. Thus:

- Yin is a negative state associated with cold, dark, stillness and passivity: its symbol can be represented by the dark side of a mountain.
- Yang is a positive state associated with heat, light and vigour: its symbol can be represented by the sunny side of a mountain.

An example of the yin–yang principle in therapeutics may be provided by considering a patient who has a fever, i.e. an excess of yang. Only when the opposites are in equal balance is life in harmony. Too much or too little of either element results in disharmony. Treatment would therefore be seen as the ability to promote the conversion of excess yang into yin, allowing restoration of the equilibrium between the two and a consequent resolution of the fever.

As the organs of the body were discovered they were deemed to be yin or yang. Yang organs, including the heart, spleen, lungs, kidneys and liver, are hollow and normally referred to as the '*fu*', whereas yin organs, including the stomach, intestines and bladder, are solid and referred to as '*zang*'.[9] Each organ also has a yin and yang element within it, and it is the overall imbalance that leads to disease.

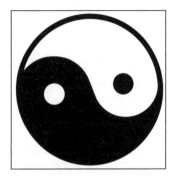

Figure 6.1 Yin and yang symbols.

Rather like the constitutional patient in homoeopathy,[10] many ailments may be described as being yin or yang. Thus, a yin-deficient patient may be hot and feverish, restless and stressed out. A yang-deficient patient will feel cold and be pale and lethargic.

The basic principles of TCM are summarised in Figure 6.2.

The five phases (wu xing)

According to Chinese philosophy, the body organs are related to one of the five phases (or elements): wood, fire, earth, metal and water. These are said to represent the circle of life. The five phases have a flow in which they move, called the 'generating cycle' (Figure 6.3):

- Water generates wood (by nourishing trees)
- Wood generates fire (rubbed together to generate fire)
- Fire generates earth (ashes fall to support the soil)
- Earth generates metal (ore)
- Metal generates water (when molten resembles water).

The five phases are applied to the practice of TCM in a number of different cycles:

- In the *sheng* cycle, organs are considered to be in a familial relationship supporting each other, e.g. the kidney may be considered to be a fire organ (or 'mother' organ) and the liver an earth (or 'son')

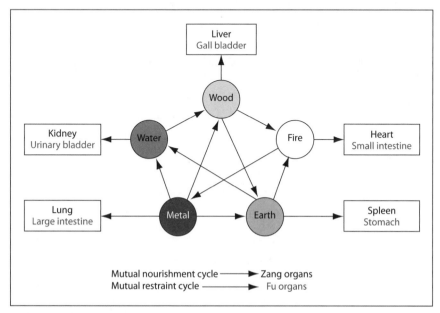

Figure 6.2 Basic principles of traditional Chinese medicine.

organ. Treating the 'mother' organ might provide a route to improving the health of a deficient 'son' organ. This is more of a supportive role: the heart is considered to support the spleen, while the spleen supports the lungs, etc.

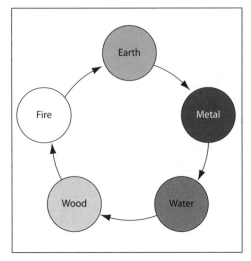

Figure 6.3 Generating cycle.

- The *ke* cycle implies a degree of control, as when water 'controls' fire. When an organ is weak it is unable to exert the control necessary to assist other organs. Thus, if the lungs are weak the liver may become too strong, leading to headaches or hypertension.

- The cosmological cycle (or sequence) considers water to be the most important element. As water corresponds to the kidney it reflects the importance that Chinese prescribers place on this organ. It is viewed as the centre of all yin and yang energy in the body and its health is therefore vital.

The five phases are in a complex relationship with other important elements of TCM as shown in Table 6.1.

Table 6.1 Relationships of the five phases

	Wood	Fire	Earth	Metal	Water
Seasons	Spring	Summer	Late summer	Autumn	Winter
Environment	Wind	Heat	Damp	Dry	Cold
Zang organs (yin)	Liver	Heart	Spleen	Lung	Kidney
Fu organs (yang)	Gallbladder	Small intestine	Stomach	Large intestine	Bladder
Directions	East	South	Middle	West	North
Tastes	Sour	Bitter	Sweet	Pungent	Salty
Senses	Eye	Tongue	Mouth	Nose	Ear
Tissues	Tendon	Vessel	Muscle	Skin, hair	Bone
Emotions	Anger	Joy	Worry	Grief	Fear

The five substances

In TCM five substances encompass both tangible and intangible elements within the body. They are summarised in Table 6.2

The first three substances, *qi*, *jing* and *shen*, are known as the 'three treasures' and are believed to be the essential components of an individual's life. They include such qualities as energy and spirit.

The other elements, blood and body fluids, are rather easier to understand, although these also have essential intangible properties.

Qi (chee)

Qi is usually translated as simply 'energy' but there is no one English word that conveys its true meaning. It is considered to be a vital or life force and is carried round the body through the meridians (see below)

Qi is responsible for the following day-to-day body functions:[11]

- Movement, both conscious (voluntary) and unconscious (involuntary)
- Transforming food and drink into blood, body fluids and energy
- Containment of organs, blood vessels and body tissues in their proper places
- Protection from external environmental factors including heat, cold and dampness
- Maintenance of body heat.

A number of *qi* disharmonies may be identified:

- A deficiency in *qi* will lead to debilitation, protracted recovery from illness, chronic colds, lethargy and other signs of weakness.
- Sinking *qi* is when *qi* can no longer perform its holding function and this is reflected in an organ prolapse.

Table 6.2 Summary of the five substances

Basic substance	Main responsibility	Possible symptoms of disharmony (deficiency or excess)
Qi Jing	Day-to-day functions	Debilitation, chronic colds, gastrointestinal problems
Shen	Development	Learning difficulties, kidney problems, ageing, weak constitution
Blood	Consciousness	Anxiety, insomnia, psychiatric problems Paleness, stabbing pains, fever
Body fluids	Nourishes, moistens	Dryness of skin, dry cough; weeping rashes, productive cough (phlegm)

- Stagnation of *qi* is caused by an irregular energy flow or blockage; this may be the result of physical injury or emotional stress and its symptoms include indigestion and irritability or swelling and inflammation following a knock.
- Rebellious *qi* is when *qi* flow is in the wrong direction – e.g. in the stomach *qi* is considered to flow downwards; a reverse flow might cause nausea and vomiting.

An excess of *qi* is not considered to be detrimental unless it is blocked or it is over-acting on another organ system, e.g. in the case of a migraine headache, where the *qi* of the liver is blocked and, in excess, it invades the stomach and causes vomiting; with this release of energy the intensity of migraine symptoms is often reduced.

Feng shui is an ancient Chinese practice believed to use the laws of both heaven (astronomy) and Earth (geography), to help one improve life by receiving positive *qi*. Most of today's feng shui schools teach that it is the practice of choosing a place to live or work, arranging objects and using colour to achieve harmony with one's environment.

Jing (*essence*)

The concept of *jing*, similar to *qi*, is difficult to convey in a single English word. It may be translated as 'essence' and underpins all aspects of organic life. If *jing* is plentiful life itself is good, full of harmony and vitality. If *jing* is lacking then *qi* will be weak, life will be dull and the person will be susceptible to contracting disease. *Jing* differs from *qi* in that the former is responsible for the developmental changes associated with growth throughout life, whereas the latter is associated with day-to-day bodily functions. *Jing* governs fertility, sexuality and growth, and is believed to have 7-year cycles in men or 8-year cycles in women, during which development and ageing take place.

Jing is responsible for:

- governing growth, reproduction and development
- production of bone marrow
- promotion of kidney *qi*
- determining the basic constitutional strength.

Deficiency of *jing* is the only disharmony and is said to be more prevalent in men than in women. The following symptoms may be identified:

- Developmental disorders, including physical, mental and learning problems – as *jing* deteriorates with age, so symptoms of baldness, deafness, brittle bones and senility may result

- Kidney-related disorders
- Poor memory and concentration
- Constitutional weakness
- Low libido.

Shen

Shen is both mind and spirit. It is based in the heart and governs spiritual, mental and emotional health. It has been described as responsible for 'the sparkle in one's eyes'.

If there is a *shen* disharmony human thought may be disturbed and the eyes may be cloudy with insomnia, forgetfulness and, in the worse case, incoherent speech. With extreme *shen* disharmony the condition may lead to unconsciousness.

Blood

In TCM blood is much more than simply a physical transport system, as in western medicine. It is closely linked to *qi* and is considered to have the following important functions:

- It nourishes the body by carrying nutrients to all tissues and structures and in so doing it helps to fulfil the nutritive functions of *qi*.
- It has a moistening and lubricating action. It aids clear and stable thought processes.

Disharmony may arise from three imbalances:

- Deficiency shows in pale face, dry skin, light-headedness and emaciation.
- Stagnation produces stabbing pains, and purple lips and tongue.
- Excessive heat in the blood can cause bleeding, skin conditions and fever.

Body fluids (jin ye)

Body fluids include external light and watery fluids, such as saliva and tears (known as *jin*), and the dense thicker fluids that circulate inside the body, e.g. gastric juices and joint fluids (known as *ye*). The function of all the body fluids is to nourish and lubricate the body. They are essential for the maintenance of healthy *qi*.

Disharmony due to deficient body fluids results in dryness of the eyes, lips and hair, a dry cough and excessive thirst. Excess body fluids can lead to problems known as dampness and phlegm, characterised by productive coughs, weeping skin rashes and vaginal discharge.

The five substances are summarised in Table 6.2.

The organs (zang fu)

The organs detailed below have a special status in TCM, being the creators and storers of the five substances. They are considered to be closely related to specific emotions and virtues and, if their essential requirements are not fulfilled, ill-health will result. Two types of organs are recognised:

1 The solid organs
2 The hollow organs.

The solid organs (*zang*) are associated with yin and include the following:

- The heart is the centre of *shen* and also governs the circulatory system. It is positively associated with compassion, love and affection, and negatively with overexcitement. Symptoms of ill-health include insomnia and hyperactivity.
- The lungs relate to *qi* and require confidence to function effectively. They are positively associated with conscientiousness and negatively with sadness. Symptoms of ill-health include irregular breathing, coughs and susceptibility to colds.
- The liver ensures that *qi* flows smoothly. When the liver is in harmony, a person will feel relaxed and optimistic but, when out of balance, the person will feel irritable and unable to move forward positively. Symptoms of ill-health may be irregular periods, premenstrual syndrome (or tension), headaches, irritable bowel syndrome and a bad temper.
- The spleen creates *qi*. Its health depends on a good diet and a non-stressful lifestyle. It is positively associated with empathy and negatively with obsession. Symptoms of ill-health include poor appetite and diarrhoea.
- The kidneys store *jing* and are associated with long-term growth. Their positive emotion is courage and their negative emotion is fear. Symptoms of ill-health include lethargy, diarrhoea, infertility and oedema.

The hollow organs (*fu*) are associated with yang, and include:

- the gallbladder
- the large and small intestines
- the bladder
- the stomach
- the *san jiao*, also known as the 'triple burner' or 'triple heater'. *San jiao* has no equivalent anatomical structure in western medicine,

although it roughly corresponds to the thoracic, abdominal and pelvic regions, including all the organs within. It coordinates transformation and transportation of fluids in the body. *San jiao* also helps move *qi* and maintains the ambient temperature in the body, a function from which the name 'triple burner' derives.

The meridians or channels

The word 'meridian' as used in TCM entered the English language through a French translation of the Chinese term *jing-luo*. *Jing* means 'to go through' and *luo* means 'something that connects'. Meridians are the channels that carry *qi* and blood throughout the body. They form an invisible network close to the surface of the body, which links together all the fundamental textures and organs. Kaptchuk mentions 14 meridians in his book;[12] other writers refer to different numbers ranging from 11 to 20. As the meridians unify all parts of the body and energy (*qi*) can pass along the channels, they are essential for the maintenance of harmonious balance. Set along the meridians are a number of points used by acupuncturists (see below).

The meridians are named for the organs or functions to which they are attached. Fulder explains the function of the meridians thus:[13]

> The meridian of the colon runs from a point on the nail of the index finger along the arm and over the shoulder and neck to the nose from whence it follows a deep pathway down to the colon. Because the meridian system connects the exterior of the body by pathways to the viscera, external factors can penetrate and produce symptoms such as abdominal pain, migraine, etc. Conversely, diseases of the internal organs will produce superficial symptoms that may appear along the lines of the meridians. Thus, kidney disease can induce back pain, while disease of the gall bladder can bring pain to the shoulder, these being areas through which the respective meridians pass.

Practice of TCM

Diagnosis

A diagnosis is achieved using four traditional methods:[14]

1 Listening carefully to the sound and quality of the patient's voice (auscultation) and evaluating any breath or body odours (olfaction).
2 Asking questions to ascertain the features of the illness (enquiry).
3 Observing the patient's general demeanour, emotional state and *shen*, and assessing the quality and texture of the skin and the shape, colour and coating of the tongue (inspection).
4 Palpation of the pulses and body.

After taking a full history, pulses are read (Figure 6.4). Chinese medicine recognises up to 28 pulses, which are palpable on the right and left wrists. The right-hand pulses represent conditions of the lung, spleen and kidney yang, whereas the left-hand pulses represent conditions of the heart, liver and kidney yin. The pulse is assessed in seven criteria: depth, fluency, rhythm, size/shape, speed, strength and tension. The experienced practitioner can deduce much information on the patient's past and present health status from reading the pulses and palpating the body.

The aim is to determine which organ(s) might be out of balance by considering all the elements outlined above, and to take appropriate action to rectify the problem according to the various principles outlined above. It appears to be a daunting task to the western healthcare professional, who is more used to making a decision on appropriate medication based on symptoms determined within a 3- to 5-min consultation.

Treatment

Treatment is by a range of different therapies; each is described below under the appropriate section headings.

Evidence

Many randomised controlled trials have been conducted in China to evaluate the effectiveness of TCM, but much of the information is either inaccessible to Western practitioners and/or may be flawed.

Tang et al. identified 2938 RCTs in 28 journals randomly selected from a total of 100 Chinese journals of TCM (4 national, 10 university, 10

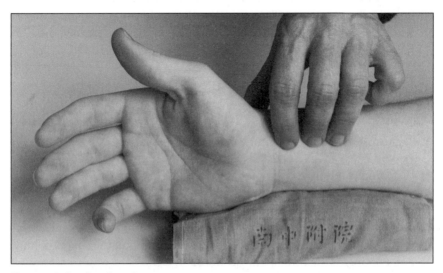

Figure 6.4 Reading the pulse.

provincial or regional, and 4 specialist).[15] The first trials were published in the early 1980s. The number of trials had doubled every 2–3 years over the past 15 years. The number of RCTs published in all 100 journals by the end of 1996 was estimated to be around 7500. Comparison of trials searched for by hand with trials of TCM found in electronic databases (which hold journals of conventional medicine as well) shows that journals of conventional medicine in China published about a quarter of the number of RCTs published in journals of traditional Chinese medicine. Thus, almost 10 000 RCTs were published in China before 1997. Over 90% of the trials in non-specialist journals evaluated herbal treatments that were mostly proprietary Chinese medicines. The 10 most common diseases in the trials were ischaemic heart disease, stroke, chronic viral hepatitis, peptic ulcer, childhood diarrhoea, hyperlipidaemia, primary hypertension, upper digestive tract bleeding, diabetes mellitus and pneumonia. They accounted for a fifth of the trials.

Unfortunately much of the early research was considered to be inadmissible because of problems associated with:[16]

- poor translation of studies
- the quality and design of the research not being up to western standards
- the use of unvalidated methods
- methodological difficulties of establishing control groups and sham procedures for the placebo arm of trials (e.g. it is impossible to 'blind' an acupuncturist)
- variations in what is understood by different terms.

From an initial sample of 37 313 articles identified in the China National Knowledge Infrastructure electronic database a study led by Wu of the Chinese Cochrane Centre at Sichuan University, found 3137 apparent randomized controlled trials on 20 common diseases published between 1994 and 2005.[17] Of these, 1452 were studies of conventional medicine (published in 411 journals) and 1685 were studies of traditional Chinese medicine (published in 352 journals). Interviews with the authors of 2235 of these reports revealed that only 207 studies adhered to accepted methodology for randomisation and could on those grounds be deemed authentic randomised controlled. The reviewers considered that a randomisation sequence generated from a random number table, calculator, or computerised random number generator was authentic but that tossing a coin, drawing straws, or allocating a participant according to date of birth or hospital record number was not.

It is vital that correct plant species are used when researching traditional herbal medicine and that tests are carried out on material prepared according to ethnic methods.[18] The choice of test system might also be difficult because, particularly with traditional Chinese or Indian ayurvedic medicine, where the aim may be to correct imbalances in health, there is no outcome to measure in the same way that western medicine allows. For the same reason animal models are unlikely to provide applicable results. Practitioners frequently use mixtures of ingredients and testing standardised individual elements may not be appropriate. Another significant factor with ethnic medicine is the charisma and seniority of the practitioner, which introduces a significant element of placebo response that cannot be quantified.

The number of RCTs of TCM has increased in recent years. However, there have been few systematic assessments of the quality of reporting of these trials. Wang et al. concluded from an assessment of 7422 RCTs, published in mainland China from 1999 to 2004, that, although the quality of reporting of RCTs of TCM was improving, it still remained poor.[19]

Modern Chinese medicine

Since the 1950s, the Chinese government and the government of the Republic of Chinese Taiwan have put great efforts into promoting the modernisation of Chinese medicine. This has been in response to national planning needs to provide comprehensive healthcare services. Previously, TCM had been viewed as part of an imperial legacy, to be replaced by a secular healthcare system. Integration was guided by health officials trained in modern medicine; harmonisation with modern medicine was the goal. This was accomplished by a science-based approach to the education of TCM and an emphasis on research. There are now Chinese professionals trained in both TCM and modern western medicine, who conduct research on the development of Chinese medicine. Western science methodologies have been employed to analyse the effectiveness of herbs and treatment on various individuals. Many of the differences between TCM and western scientific practices are now being studied for their synergistic potential.

Tang has asked whether the current western model of research – trying out unknown treatments in animals – is suitable for studying treatments that have long been used in humans.[20] Evidence-based medicine focuses on clinical research in humans. However, research in TCM has had a mechanism-centred approach. Despite occasional successes, such as in acupuncture,[21] most questions, e.g. the nature of disease in TCM, have not been satisfactorily answered.

TCM research has been accused of being in disarray.[22] A long history of use, traditions, faith, popularity and anecdotes is widely taken as evidence for the efficacy of traditional Chinese medicines. Some traditional therapies are undoubtedly effective but this does not mean that all are. These medicines have been used for thousands of years. Whether tested or not, they will continue to be used in places where TCM is officially recognised. Tang suggests that there is a much greater need to determine whether Chinese medicinal herbs *do* work rather than *how* they might work.[20] As traditional Chinese medicines are already in use, it would be better when studying them to start with showing efficacy in humans by RCTs.

Joint research projects have been undertaken in the USA[23] involving research institutes such as Stanford University, the College of Physicians and Surgeons of Columbia University and the National Cancer Institute to evaluate the effectiveness of Chinese medicine and improve the classification and selection/prescription of formulae.

In 2008 the Department of Health and Human Services (HHS) of the USA and the Ministry of Health (MOH) of China concluded a Memorandum of Understanding on Collaboration in Integrative and Traditional Chinese Medicine research. (Full text available online at http://tinyurl.com/5tm79l – accessed 31 August 2009.)

However, the process of integration has resulted in the loss of important aspects of traditional theory and practice. Fewer acupuncture points are taught than in the classic system, and aspects of the theory of TCM have been de-emphasised.

Hospitals practising TCM still treat 200 million outpatients and almost 3 million inpatients annually. Overall, 95% of general hospitals in China have traditional medicine departments, which treat about 20% of outpatients daily.[24]

Acupuncture

Acupuncture is a technique involving the insertion of fine needles into the skin at selected points over the body. Practitioners of acupuncture generally follow one of two broad approaches to the discipline, using either TCM with all its many ramifications for maintaining health, or the simpler symptom-oriented western acupuncture. This section gives an outline of both.

Acupuncture is used widely in western Asia, Australia, Canada and parts of Europe (Figure 6.5).

History

The theory that surrounds the practice of traditional acupuncture probably dates back as many as 4000–5000 years, although there are no reliable references in Chinese literature before the first century BC. Ancient works were generally written on bamboo strips and silk, and have not survived. The earliest physician reputed to be proficient in acupuncture techniques was Bian Que in around 500 BC.

The names and reputed functions of all the acupuncture points were established by about AD 259 when *The Classic of Acupuncture (Zhen Jiu Jia*

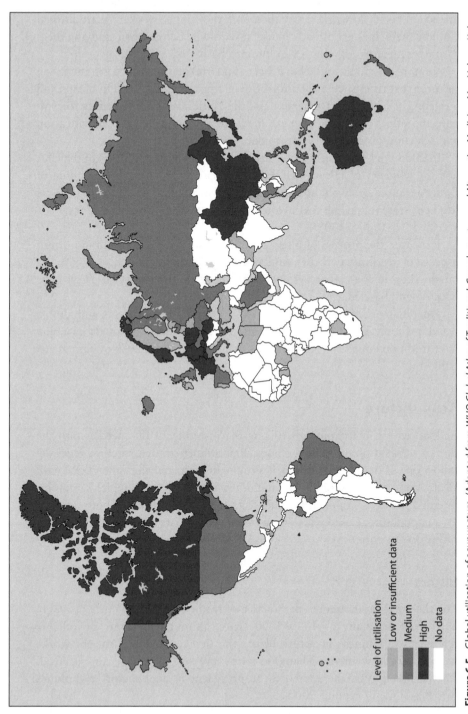

Figure 6.5 Global utilisation of acupuncture. (Adapted from *WHO Global Atlas of Traditional, Complementary and Alternative Medicine, Map Volume Kobe, Japan: WHO Centre for Health Development, 2005: 50.)

Jing) was published. Acupuncture flourished in China throughout the Ming period (1368–1644). Subsequently, it went into gradual decline until 1822, when it was finally banned by Emperor Dao Guang, who disapproved of its practices. In the early part of the twentieth century acupuncture became part of the ongoing debate as to whether Chinese culture should be overtaken by western influences or maintain its own traditions. With the arrival of western medicine, acupuncture was increasingly relegated to rural and remote backwaters.

In the 1950s the discipline was reintroduced by the communist authorities, who saw TCM as a solution to the problem of providing healthcare to an ever-growing population. Acupuncture developed once again as people were quickly trained and pressed into service. Today it is practised alongside western medicine.

News of the success of acupuncture was brought to the west in 1683 by Dr Willen Ten Rhijn, a physician working for the Dutch East Indies Company in Japan. Dr Rhijn's report was not the first, but it was the most reliable. Usage of the English word 'acupuncture' is attributed to him.

Acupuncture was widely practised in France in the late eighteenth century with Dr Berlioz, a Parisian doctor, becoming the first western practitioner of acupuncture in the early nineteenth century. John Churchill, the first British acupuncturist, used the technique in the treatment of rheumatism in 1821. Acupuncture was even mentioned in the first edition of *The Lancet* in 1823 as being chiefly used in 'diseases of the head and lower belly'.[25]

When China opened up to visitors shortly after President Nixon went to the country in 1971, physicians and others from the west made visits to witness how acupuncture was being used.[26] Indeed in 1972 one of the authors of this chapter (SK) visited Nanjing and saw a surgeon directing her own abdominal operation, and observed several other minor operations and the delivery of a baby; all the procedures were performed with the aid of acupuncture needles to control the pain.

Acupuncture is now among the best-known complementary therapies in the UK. In Scotland, a random survey found that an impressive 94% of respondents in a random survey knew something about acupuncture and 25% said that they would consider using it, although in practice only about 6% had actually done so.[27] It would be interesting to know why there was such a large discrepancy between the two figures.

Principles of acupuncture

In addition to the classic principles of Chinese medicine outlined above, there is one key aspect of practice still to consider. This is the theory of acupuncture points that are stimulated usually by the superficial insertion of needles into the skin. Other methods of stimulation include the application of pressure and the passing of a weak electrical current (see below).

A basic 365 mapped acupuncture points are situated along the meridians. A further 1000 extra points and special use points may also be identified on the hands, ears and scalp. It is not known how these points were discovered – probably it was by observation over hundreds if not thousands of years – nor is it known exactly how many points were first identified. Pain points can be located anywhere on the body where there is a pain locus. Figure 6.6 shows an acupuncture doll with acupoints on the head and neck marked.

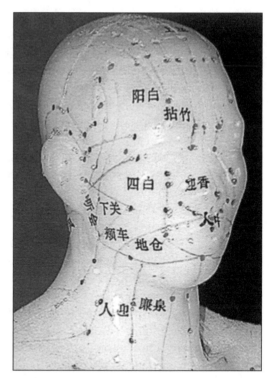

Figure 6.6 Acupuncture points on head and neck.

Acupoints cannot be identified by their appearance and no consistent features of their anatomy have been found that distinguish them from other tissues. It has been suggested that the points may be sites of tenderness.[28] The methodology for investigating the tenderness of acupuncture points has been explored.[29] The study of the acupoint known as spleen 6 found that there was no strong evidence to support the hypothesis that acupuncture points were more tender than control points.

Practice of acupuncture

There is archaeological evidence that shows that the earliest acupuncture needles date back to the Stone Age, when instruments called bian were thought to have been used in China.[30] By the Bronze Age acupuncture was already well developed and needles were made of bronze. Needles were subsequently made of many different metals: gold, silver, copper, etc. Modern acupuncturists use solid sterile disposable needles of narrow bore, about 3 cm long (although longer needles may be used at different sites). Recently two novel acupuncture techniques have been reported. In the first

Wang et al. described the use of a needle that looks rather like a scalpel for the treatment of myofascial pain.[31] The second is a new form of sustained stimulation by a plastic tube; this is introduced subcutaneously by a needle and left *in situ* for 24 hours before removal.[32]

The patient is usually treated lying down to minimise any tendency to faint. As many as 15–20 needles may be inserted superficially at the appropriate point(s). The practitioner then gently introduces the needles a little more deeply into the muscle, rotating them between finger and thumb. *Qi* and blood flow throughout the meridians and this is where manipulation of the needle is critical in properly moving this flow. The arrival of *qi* called *deqi* is signified by a dull ache or tingling sensation and slight inflammation. Some practitioners may use electrical stimulation, connecting the needles to a small piece of equipment powered by batteries. Needles are left in place for up to 20 min: the patient is invited to lie back and relax. Occasionally a needle may be left in place for several days, normally situated in the ear; these so-called indwelling needles should not be used in patients with heart valve disease or who are immunocompromised.

A single course of treatment usually comprises 10–12 sessions. Two or three courses may be required for the treatment of chronic conditions. Acupuncture point selection may vary at each treatment, depending on the patient's response. If significant improvement is achieved, the patient will be discharged at the end of the treatment but will normally be instructed to continue with other elements of TCM, e.g. dietary control and perhaps exercises.

Evidence

The reader is referred to the comments made in the section on TCM above. Evidence of effectiveness is largely restricted to case studies, although RCTs are available for western acupuncture (see below). The findings of many of these randomised trials have caused much debate. Positive trials have been criticised because of inadequate blinding, and negative trials because the intervention was not administered by properly trained practitioners or control interventions may have had analgesic effects.[33]

Cautious approval of some applications of acupuncture was given by the US National Institutes of Health consensus development meeting in 1997.[34] The 12-member panel was asked to evaluate current evidence for the efficacy of acupuncture and concluded that there is 'clear evidence' of efficacy in the control of nausea and vomiting occurring in some patients postoperatively and in association with chemotherapy, and for the relief of post-operative dental pain. The panel said that acupuncture was 'probably' also effective in the control of nausea in early pregnancy. The British Medical Association reached a similar conclusion in their report on acupuncture.[35] A number of correspondents to the *British Medical Journal* criticised this support, claiming that the evidence was not sufficient to reach a positive conclusion.[36]

There are problems with designing trials for acupuncture associated with the control arm of an RCT.[37] The most usual placebo method is sham acupuncture, when needles are inserted outside acupuncture points with minimum interaction between practitioner and patient.[38] It is argued that this is an incorrect method because it leads to a study of the importance of the acupuncture point rather than of acupuncture itself.[39] Furthermore, as stated above, there are doubts about whether acupuncture points and non-acupuncture points can be identified. Even if they can, there is evidence that acupuncture at non-classic points, the so-called trigger points, may have analgesic effects.

Kaptchk et al. investigated whether a validated sham acupuncture device had a greater placebo effect than an inert pill in people with persistent upper extremity pain due to repetitive strain injury.[40] During the placebo run-in, participants assigned to the acupuncture group received two treatments a week with a sham acupuncture device that looked exactly like a real acupuncture needle but had a blunt tip and retracted into a hollow shaft handle. When the needle was 'inserted into the skin' participants saw and felt the needle penetration. Both sham and genuine needles were held in place with a plastic ring and surgical tape so the procedure looked identical. After the run-in period, the acupuncturists followed identical protocols for administering real or continued sham acupuncture. Participants in the pill group were instructed to take one capsule each evening to minimise daytime drowsiness. The placebo capsule contained cornstarch, and the amitripty-line capsule contained cornstarch plus 25 mg amitriptyline. The primary outcome was self-reported intensity of pain in the most severely affected arm during the preceding week measured on a 10-point numerical rating scale ranging from no pain (1) to the most severe pain imaginable (10). The sham device had greater effects than the placebo pill on self-reported pain and severity of symptoms over the entire course of treatment, but not during the 2-week placebo run-in. It was concluded that placebo effects seem to depend on the behaviours embedded in medical rituals.

Notwithstanding the difficulties highlighted above, a number of RCTs have been conducted, providing results that, with a few notable exceptions, are not conclusive.[41]

Various methods of assessing clinically meaningful change associated with a course of acupuncture treatment have been studied.[42] The most effective was the Measure Your Own Outcome Profile (MYMOP), in which patients were initially invited to rank up to three symptoms for which they were most interested in seeking treatment with acupuncture. This helped the acupuncturists formulate a treatment plan for each patient. Subsequently they were asked to rate how much their clinical condition had improved or worsened over a specified period of time.

The BMJ Group has taken over the publishing of *Acupuncture in Medicine*, a quarterly title medical journal on acupuncture from 2009. This will be the first complementary medicine title that the BMJ Group has published and aims to build the evidence base for acupuncture.

Safety

A study that investigated the incidence and severity of acupuncture reactions has been carried out in Japan.[43] In 1441 treatment sessions involving 30 338 insertions in 391 patients, 9 episodes of failure to remove the needle were reported and classified as negligence rather than an adverse reaction. The most common systemic reactions were tiredness and drowsiness (11%), aggravation of symptoms (2.8%), irritation (1%), vertigo (0.8%) and fainting (0.8%). The most common local effects were bleeding (2.6%) and pain (0.7%). The authors concluded that there were some adverse reactions associated with acupuncture, but that they were generally transient and mild. However, serious complications have been reported.[44]

There is some evidence from a lack of recent cases in the literature that the situation is improving, i.e. the incidence of adverse reactions is decreasing, particularly in the west.

As fainting and drowsiness are commonly reported,[45] patients should be advised not to drive immediately after treatment if affected, and to exercise particular care if any prescribed or over-the-counter (OTC) medication is being taken that might enhance these effects. It has been suggested that a fall in blood sugar could be involved[46] and this might be a problem for patients with diabetes using insulin or oral hyperglycaemic drugs. Advice from a pharmacist on the rescheduling of administration would be appropriate.

The adverse effects that may be attributed to acupuncture have also been catalogued.[47,48] Examples of potential dangers identified in the reviews include infection during needling and trauma.

Infection during needling

Hepatitis
Re-using needles with inadequate sterilisation has been the source of hepatitis in a number of patients, although the literature refers mainly, but not exclusively, to the 1980s and earlier.[49-51]

HIV
Human immunodeficiency virus (HIV) infection has been linked to acupuncture. In one case a patient became HIV positive after a 6-week

course of acupuncture.[52] In another case two acquired immune deficiency syndrome (AIDS) patients were strongly suspected of contracting their condition as a result of acupuncture.[53] It must be stressed that due to lack of information a direct causal link in this case could not be established. There may also be some risk to the acupuncturist from treating a patient who already has HIV.

Other infections

Other infections reported include those due to *Pseudomonas* spp. and *Staphylococcus aureus*.[54]

A recent report describes an outbreak of post-acupuncture cutaneous infection due to *Mycobacterium abcessus* in Seoul, South Korea. The report details a large outbreak of rapidly growing mycobacterial infection among patients who received acupuncture at a single clinic and concludes that physicians should suspect mycobacterial infections in patients with persistent cutaneous infections after acupuncture, and infection control education should be emphasised for acupuncture practitioners.[55]

Since the adoption of disposable needles and avoidance of touching the needle shaft before insertion, the incidence of infection during needling is likely to fall even more. It is no longer considered appropriate to use autoclaves to sterilise acupuncture needles due to the validation problems associated with bench-top autoclaves. The British Acupuncture Council (BAcC) has a comprehensive code of safe practice that, among other things, gives direction on clean needle technique.

Trauma

A number of cases of damage due to acupuncture needling, including pneumothorax, cardiac tamponade and spinal cord damage, have been reviewed.[47,48] Five fatalities have been reported, although the evidence that acupuncture was solely to blame is compelling in only one of these cases, involving a 40-year-old Norwegian woman whose heart was pierced by a needle.[56] A case of spinal cord injury from a broken, small needle-knife (known as *Xiaozendao* in Chinese) insertion into the spinal cord with delayed onset of neurological symptoms has also been reported.[57]

Local traumatic damage to blood vessels may produce a haematoma.

Other adverse effects

Other possible adverse reactions to acupuncture include cardiac arrhythmias,[58] the triggering of asthma[59] and the exacerbation of symptoms.[59] Allergic reactions caused by the metal of the needles, particularly chrome and nickel, are possible.[61–63] There is some evidence that it might be inappropriate to use electro-acupuncture on patients with pacemakers.[64] Some concerns have been expressed about the safety issues involved with electrostimulation and the possibility of tissue damage.[65]

Accidental burns from moxibustion procedures (see below)[66] or excessively warm acupuncture needles[67] have been reported. Clinical misjudgement may give some cause for concern.

A summary of some of the complications of acupuncture is set out in Table 6.3, which gives a simple summation of the cases of each episode computed from a literature search. The results cannot be used to make deductions of the frequency of such events.

Contraindications

Acupuncture is contraindicated or must be used with extreme care in patients who:

- are unwilling to be needled; they should not be pressurised to undergo treatment
- have a tendency to bleed excessively
- have a pacemaker; it might be affected by the electrical stimulation of acupuncture needles.

Table 6.3 Complications of acupuncture

Event documented	Number of cases in the literature
Drowsiness, fainting	1429
Increased pain	1129
Nausea, vomiting	540
Infections	228
Pneumothorax	129
Hepatitis	127
Psychiatric complications	112
Convulsions	80
Cardiac trauma	7

Precautions

A number of precautions may be suggested when practising acupuncture:

- Patients should lie down during treatment.
- Disposable sterile needles should be used.
- Needles should be counted before and after treatment so that all may be accounted for.
- Patients should be carefully observed for excessive bleeding.

Western acupuncture[68]

Some general practitioners (GPs) and physiotherapists with orthodox backgrounds find it difficult to accept the intangible nature of traditional acupuncture, which relates to the flow of *qi*. Many dispute the existence of meridians or acupuncture points,[69] preferring to link their practice to trigger points instead.[70,71] Trigger points are small areas in muscle that have been strained or injured and have not healed. They may remain sensitive for many years, causing pain that may be experienced some distance away from the trigger point. Interestingly, the trigger points and pain referral sites appear to be similar in all people and, furthermore, many of the trigger points are identical to acupuncture points.

It is suggested that acupuncture works by stimulating the nervous system, leading to the release of opioid peptides (endorphins), compounds that are closely involved with the mechanisms by which the body controls its perception of pain. Thus, acupuncture is used in the treatment of intractable pain without the attendant traditional Chinese theory. This variant, which involves very brief needling lasting no more than a few seconds at trigger points, has been termed 'minimal acupuncture'.[72] Exponents of minimal acupuncture commonly treat musculoskeletal pain, arthritis and symptoms of stress, including tension headaches, gastrointestinal problems and nausea.

Applications of acupuncture

Therapeutic areas in which acupuncture has been used include the following.

Pain

Back pain

Many systematic reviews for back pain include trials that use different techniques and control procedures.[73] However, the balance of evidence appears to suggest that acupuncture can be useful in the treatment of back pain when compared with placebo.[74,75] A pilot study for an RCT of acupuncture in low back pain concluded that the results were 'promising' and worthy of further research.[76]

A study was conducted as part of a major acupuncture research initiative by health insurance companies in Germany: 2807 patients with chronic back pain who attended over 1000 study centres were randomised to receive either acupuncture or no acupuncture in addition to whatever conventional care they chose to have. After 3 months of treatment, patients who received the acupuncture showed significantly greater improvements in back function and quality-of-life scores.[77]

A short course of traditional acupuncture for persistent non-specific low back pain in primary care has been shown to provide a modest health benefit for minor extra cost to the UK NHS compared with usual care.[78] Acupuncture care for low back pain appeared to be cost-effective in the longer term.

Dental pain
Most of the studies included in a systematic review of 16 trials of dental pain suggested that acupuncture does have a greater effect than placebo.[79]

Headache and migraine
Four hundred and one patients with chronic headache were recruited from general medical practices in England and Wales and were randomly assigned to receive either standard care or acupuncture (12 treatments over 3 months). At 12 months after the onset of treatment headache scores in the acupuncture group fell by 34% (compared with 16% in the control group), with 22 fewer days of headache per year. They took 15% less medication, made 25% fewer doctor visits and took 15% fewer days off work. The greatest improvements were found in patients with migraine.[80]

A study investigated the effectiveness of acupuncture compared with minimal acupuncture and no acupuncture in patients with tension-type headache.[81] The end-point was the difference in numbers of days with headache between 4 weeks before randomisation and 9–12 weeks after randomisation, as recorded by participants in headache diaries. The acupuncture intervention investigated in this trial was more effective than no treatment, but not significantly more effective than minimal acupuncture for the treatment of tension-type headache.

Vickers et al. determined the effects of a policy of 'use acupuncture' on headache, health status, days off sick and use of resources in patients with chronic headache compared with a policy of 'avoid acupuncture'.[82] Headache score at 12 months, the primary end-point, was lower in the acupuncture group (16.2, standard deviation [SD] 13.7, $n = 161$, 34% reduction from baseline) than in controls (22.3, SD 17.0, $n = 140$, 16% reduction from baseline). It was concluded that acupuncture leads to persistent, clinically relevant benefits for primary care patients with chronic headache, particularly migraine and that expansion of NHS acupuncture services should be considered.

Knee pain

Patellofemoral pain syndrome is the leading cause of chronic knee pain in young adults and may affect up to 15% of young men in the US military service.[83] The results of a controlled trial, which included a total of 75 patients with patellofemoral pain, led the authors to conclude that acupuncture may be beneficial as a treatment for the condition.[84] A systematic review of high-quality RCTs also suggested that acupuncture can reduce pain and disability in people with chronic knee pain.[85] Despite this evidence the role of acupuncture in the management of chronic knee pain is still unclear.

Neck pain

There is some evidence that acupuncture may be effective when it is used for neck pain,[86,87] although a systematic review of 14 RCTs of this application concluded that existing data were insufficient to make a firm judgement.[88]

Pelvic girdle pain

A randomised, single-blind trial at a hospital, and at 27 maternity care centres in Gothenburg from 2000 to 2002, showed that acupuncture and stabilising exercises were both efficient complements to standard treatment for the management of pelvic girdle pain during pregnancy, with acupuncture being superior.[89]

Pain after surgery

A randomised trial of auricular acupuncture given for pain relief after arthroscopic knee surgery performed under general anaesthesia found that acupuncture reduced the need for ibuprofen after surgery more than an invasive needle control procedure.[90] Interestingly, most patients in both groups believed that they had received true acupuncture and wanted to repeat it in future.

Drug dependence

In a randomised, sham-controlled open trial with one active and two control arms the use of acupuncture in cocaine dependence was investigated.[91] The primary outcome was cocaine use assessed by three times weekly urine analysis. A total of 52 patients completed the study. Patients who completed a course of auricular acupuncture appeared to be more likely to abstain from using cocaine than either of the other two control groups. Another study showed that acupuncture could be of use in cocaine abusers stabilised on buprenorphine as a substitute.[92] To combat the severe drug problem, the Chinese government has adopted the methadone maintenance treatment programme, a multi-faceted therapeutic approach that aims to reduce the health and social problems induced by drug epidemics. In addition, TCM, including acupuncture and herbal therapy, is found both to be effective in the prevention of relapse and to cause few side effects, making it useful for the treatment of opiate addiction.[93]

Gastrointestinal disorders

Acupuncture has a long history of use for gastrointestinal disorders, including dyspepsia, ulcers and inflammatory bowel disease.[94]

HIV

Preliminary data from small numbers of participants in a pilot study using acupuncture for symptomatic relief have shown trends towards improvement in symptoms and quality of life.[95]

Insomnia

A systematic review of auricular acupuncture treatment for insomnia found 6 trials involving a total of 402 patients that met the authors' inclusion criteria.[96] Auricular acupuncture appeared to be effective for treating insomnia. However, as the trials were adjudged to be of low quality, it was concluded that further work involving better design, longer duration of treatment and longer follow-up should be undertaken.

Nausea and vomiting

For nausea and vomiting the P6 acupoint on the inner wrist is usually used. In a review of 29 trials in the literature that referred to nausea and vomiting from all causes, 27 gave positive results.[97]

Osteoarthritis

In a review of acupuncture in osteoarthritis, 13 studies were identified, of which 7 reported a positive and 6 a negative result.[98] However, most of the positive trials were not placebo controlled so no conclusions could be reliably drawn. In a trial involving 352 adults aged 50 or more with a clinical diagnosis of knee osteoarthritis the addition of acupuncture to a course of advice and exercise delivered by physiotherapists provided no additional improvement in pain scores (measured on the Western Ontario and McMaster Universities osteoarthritis index [WOMAC] subscale).[99] This finding agreed with an earlier trial that compared acupuncture with sham acupuncture given in addition to exercise in people with knee osteoarthritis.[100] Small benefits in pain intensity and unpleasantness were observed in both acupuncture groups, making it unlikely that this was due to acupuncture needling effects.

Vas et al. analysed the efficacy of acupuncture as a complementary therapy to the pharmacological treatment of osteoarthritis of the knee, with respect to: pain relief, reduction of stiffness and increased physical function during treatment; modifications in the consumption of diclofenac during treatment; and changes in the patient's quality of life.[101] Acupuncture plus diclofenac was found to be more effective than placebo acupuncture plus diclofenac for the symptomatic treatment of osteoarthritis of the knee.

A systematic review by Minns Lowe and colleagues assessed the effects of physiotherapy exercise programmes given after total knee replacement surgery in people with osteoarthritis.[102] The review found a small-to-moderate effect of functional exercise on joint motion and quality of life at 3–4 months after surgery, but the effect was not sustained at one year.

Pregnancy

Among women in labour[103,104] and women at various stages of pregnancy,[105–107] systematic reviews and randomised trials have shown acupuncture to be safe, although limited sample sizes preclude definitive conclusions.

One hundred healthy women with singleton pregnancies took part in an RCT.[108] The researchers were most interested in the impact of acupuncture on the speed of delivery, the length of the active phase of labour, the need for induction and the need for augmentation of labour with intravenous oxytocin. This small and preliminary study suggests that acupuncture has detectable beneficial effects on labour among women with spontaneous rupture of membranes at term. But as there was no active control (such as sham acupuncture), it is hard to say whether the benefits were due to the acupuncture itself or to the 20 minutes of personal attention received during treatment.

About 90% of all assisted reproductive treatment cycles result in the transfer of at least one embryo, but only about 25% of all cycles end in implantation of the embryo and live birth.[109] Some preliminary evidence suggests that acupuncture given with embryo transfer may increase the odds of clinical pregnancy compared with control groups,[110] although there is other evidence to the contrary: Wang et al. carried our a trial to determine if acupuncture performed during the follicular phase and luteal phase, but not on the day of embryo transfer, could improve the outcome following in vitro fertilisation pre-embryo transfer (VF-ET) compared with controls. The pregnancy rate was not improved.[111]

Shoulder injury

Trials investigating the effect of treating shoulder injuries with acupuncture have yielded encouraging results.[112,113]

Smoking cessation

A Cochrane review for smoking cessation included 18 reports, with 20 trials, that compared acupuncture with various other interventions.[114] Acupuncture did not show any advantage over sham acupuncture.

Stroke

Systematic reviews and one RCT would appear to indicate that there is some effect of acupuncture on the rate of recovery of stroke patients.[115–117]

Temporomandibular joint dysfunction

A small systematic review of three RCTs of acupuncture for temporomandibular joint dysfunction suggested that the treatment provided some symptomatic relief comparable with that provided by orthodox measures.[118] A caveat of 'more rigorous investigation needed' was expressed by the authors.

Weight loss

Contrary to popular opinion, there is no firm evidence that acupuncture is effective in promoting weight loss.

The effects of pressing ear points at ear meridian points on obesity-related parameters including body weight, body fat, body mass index and waist:hip circumference was studied in two groups of non-obese healthy and obese volunteers.[119] The authors concluded that further studies were needed with larger sample sizes and RCTs with both healthy and obese volunteers.

Other conditions

Conditions for which acupuncture has been used but for which there is no robust evidence include glaucoma[120] and Bell's palsy.[121]

It would appear that acupuncture can be shown to be effective in the treatment of various forms of pain, and nausea and vomiting. Evidence for other applications is sparse and the Scottish verdict of 'not proven' would seem to be the most appropriate in these circumstances.

Availability of acupuncture

UK NHS

Medical opinion

A questionnaire was sent to a random sample of 650 UK GPs selected from the BMA database and representing 1.6% of the country's GP population.[122]

A number of questions relating to the provision of complementary and alternative medicine were asked in the survey. The response rate was 56%. The most popular therapy arranged for patients was acupuncture (47% of respondents). In almost half these cases the service was provided within an orthodox setting such as the GP's own surgery. Pain relief and musculoskeletal disorders were the most frequently cited conditions treated; other applications included smoking cessation, stress and morning sickness.

When asked whom they thought should provide acupuncture, the GPs replied strongly in favour of registered medical practitioners, followed by physiotherapists and dentists. Less than half the respondents thought that TCM practitioners should be involved.

Reasons for not offering acupuncture were lack of demand (63%), lack of knowledge of the services available (63%) and lack of guidelines on how to assess the competence of practitioners.

The percentage of physicians who practise acupuncture in the UK has varied widely over the last 20 years, with estimates of 1% in Scotland,[123] from 3%[124] to 21%[125] in England, and from 4%[126] to 5%[127] in the country as a whole. This compares with the USA (1%)[128] and New Zealand (Wellington 18%[129] and Auckland 21%[130]). In Australia the use of acupuncture by doctors has increased greatly since the 1984 introduction of a Medicare rebate for acupuncture. In 1996, 15.1% of Australian doctors claimed for acupuncture, with almost one million insurance claims being made.[131]

In the UK the practice of acupuncture is not legally restricted to medically qualified doctors as it is in many other European countries (e.g. France, Hungary, Italy, Poland and Portugal), so the market may be partially satisfied by professional or non-medically qualified practitioners (NMQPs). There are more than 5500 acupuncturists in the UK, of whom 3500 are statutorily registered health professionals.

There are 3000 traditional acupuncturists in British Acupuncture Council, 5000 physiotherapists, 2500 GPs and about 3000 in other associations.

Cost-effectiveness studies of acupuncture

Cost-effectiveness studies of acupuncture have been mainly restricted to the treatment of pain. Wonderling et al. evaluated the cost-effectiveness of acupuncture in the management of chronic headache.[132] The main outcome measure was incremental cost per quality-adjusted life-year (QALY) gained. Total costs during the 1-year period of the study were on average higher for the acupuncture group £403 (€460, US$663) than for controls £217 (€248, US$357) because of the acupuncture practitioners' costs. The mean health gain from acupuncture during the 1-year trial was 0.021 QALYs, leading to a base case estimate of £9180 (€10,500, US$15,240) per QALY gained. This result was robust to sensitivity analysis. Cost per QALY dropped substantially when the analysis incorporated probable QALY differences for the years after the trial. It was concluded that acupuncture for chronic headache improves health-related quality of life at a small additional cost; it is relatively cost-effective compared with a number of other interventions provided by the NHS.

Canter et al. systematically searched seven electronic databases, and included all prospective controlled studies carried out in the UK before April 2005, for rigorous cost-effectiveness studies of complementary treatments.[133] Five studies, all randomised, met the criteria set and were included, one of acupuncture for chronic headache and four of spinal manipulation for different types of spinal pain. The provision of the treatments represents an additional healthcare cost in four out of the five studies considered. Estimates of cost per QALY from three studies compared favourably with other treatments approved for use in the NHS, but for spinal manipulation the health benefits were small to moderate and of questionable clinical significance. The authors acknowledged that estimates of cost-effectiveness may be less favourable in situations for which the complementary treatment is offered routinely rather than in the novel situation of a clinical trial.

Ratcliffe et al. have assessed the cost-effectiveness of acupuncture in the management of persistent non-specific low back pain.[134] Lower back pain is a common ailment that places a considerable burden on society in terms of reduced quality of life and lost productivity.[135] The study was based on a well-conducted pragmatic RCT, which found weak evidence of an effect of acupuncture on persistent non-specific low back pain at 12 months, but stronger evidence of a small benefit at 24 months.[136]

Availability of acupuncture in the USA

Acupuncture has been increasingly embraced by practitioners and patients in the USA since the appearance of an article describing successful postappendectomy pain management using acupuncture needles.[137] California became the first state to license acupuncture as an independent healthcare profession in 1976.[138] Since then, 40 states and the District of Columbia have adopted similar laws. Most states (27) allow herbal medicine within the scope of acupuncture practice; only a few states (10) require the supervision of a physician for the almost 11 000 practising non-physician acupuncturists. The number of acupuncturists is rapidly growing and is projected to quadruple by 2015.[139] A National Health Interview Survey carried out in the USA revealed that 4.1% of the respondents reported lifetime use of acupuncture and 1.1% reported recent use.[140] This utilisation of acupuncture was somewhat lower than expected given its significant national and international recognition and its visibility in the media, This may in part be a function of provider availability.

Variants of acupuncture

Acupressure

Acupressure is a form of acupuncture in which fingers, thumbs and elbows are used to stimulate the body's acupuncture points. Acupressure relieves muscular tension, facilitating blood flow and therefore distributing more nutrients and oxygen throughout the body, as well as removing waste products. This helps to promote both physical calmness and mental alertness. The technique involves repeatedly pressing the acupuncture points for 3–5 seconds and then releasing the pressure. It is believed that the practitioner's *qi* helps to strengthen the weakened *qi* of the patient. Thus it is important that the practitioner maintains a healthy body so that his or her *qi* is stronger than that of the recipient.[141] As a result of these *qi* differentials, self-acupressure is not considered to be as effective as having a practitioner do it for you.

Acupressure has been used to relieve mental tension, for tired and strained eyes, headaches, menstrual cramps and arthritis, as well as to promote general healthcare.[142] A trial to minimise motion sickness by intermittent pressure on the wrist point P6 with wrist bands found no reduction in symptoms.[143] However, in a later study regular pressure was applied and, under these circumstances, a clear positive outcome resulted.[144] Acupressure in sickness during pregnancy may also be helpful,[145] although the use of the P6 point with wristbands as outlined above has not been successful in this context.[146] A study to evaluate the effectiveness of acupressure in terms of disability, pain scores and functional status found that it was effective in reducing low back pain and that benefit was sustained for 6 months.[147]

Acupressure should not be applied to an open wound, or to a place where there is inflammation or swelling. Areas of scar tissue, boils, blisters, rashes and varicose veins should also be avoided. Certain pressure points should be avoided during pregnancy and in patients with hyper- or hypotension.

Shiatsu

This is a deeply relaxing therapy originating in Japan that provides stimulation by using the fingers and palm of the hand to apply pressure and gentle stretches to the meridians. It consists of a whole body treatment, as it is believed that a disorder in one area can have effects elsewhere on the body. There are two main Shiatsu schools – one based on western anatomical and physiological theory and the other based on TCM (see Chapter 8).

Moxibustion

The tradition of moxibustion was originally developed in Mongolia and later incorporated into TCM and Tibetan medicine. It is similar to both acupuncture and acupressure in its effects but uses a glowing wick instead of needles or fingertips as the source of stimulation for the acupoints. Traditionally moxa is the dried leaves of *Artemisia vulgaris* and *Artemesia argyi* and other species of mugwort, made into various forms including:

- punk – loose moxa, rather like green cotton-wool
- moxa rolls – similar to cigars in appearance
- moxa cones.

When lit, the moxa smoulders slowly. The glowing moxa rolls are held about 2 cm from the acupoint. Another method is for a small moxa cone to be placed on the blunt end of an acupuncture needle while it is in place. It is lit, transmitting the heat down the needle into the acupuncture point. A cone may also be placed directly on the skin over a slice of ginger. It is lit at its apex and burnt down until the patient is able to feel the heat; it is then removed. Cauterising moxibustion involves the burning of loose punk directly on the skin until blisters form; however, this technique is unlikely to be used in the UK.

Moxibustion tones, stimulates and supplements energy in the meridians. It is claimed to be an effective treatment for arthritis and menstrual problems.

Chinese herbal medicine

In the west it is quite normal to equate the word 'herbal' with something that grows in the garden. Certainly most Chinese herbal remedies are made from plant material, but others are of mineral or animal origin, e.g. gypsum (*shi gao*) is a cooling mineral 'herb' commonly used to treat conditions characterised by much heat. Oyster shells (*mu li*) may be used for hypertension. The use of animal parts is a controversial issue in western communities and it is currently illegal in the UK to use anything other than plant material in herbal decoctions. In China and other Asian countries the practice is still widespread, but it has been largely discontinued elsewhere after action by regulatory authorities with enthusiasm that may occasionally be misplaced. The famous highly aromatic salve marketed around the world known as Tiger Balm was once the subject of a dawn raid of Chinese herbalists by police in Manchester. They thought that they had uncovered the illegal use of parts from a protected wild animal. There were a few red faces when it was realised that the title merely referred to the nickname of the brand owner!

History

China's greatest materia medica (*Pen Ts'ao*) was published by Li Shizhen in 1578.[148] The culmination of 26 years' work, it comprises 1892 species of drugs of animal, vegetable and mineral origin, and includes no fewer than 8160 prescriptions.

Secret recipes (also known as 'prepared medicines') were the equivalent of modern patent medicines. They were first produced during the Song dynasty (AD960–1234) and were dispensed by government agencies such as the Imperial Benevolence Pharmacy.[149] A variety of dose forms were available including pills, liquids and honey boluses. By the time of the Ming dynasty (1368–1644) more than 60 000 formulae had been recorded in the 1406 book entitled *Formulas of Universal Benefit* (*Pu Ji Fang*). In recent years many of these formulae have passed into public usage, but there may be as many as 5000 licensed patent medicines still circulating in China. The most famous factory is at the Tong Ren Tang pharmacy in Beijing, which has been operated by the same family since the late seventeenth century.

Availability of CHM

In the UK, Chinese herbalism is the most prevalent of the ancient herbal traditions currently being practised.[150] About 500 different herbal materials are imported into the UK and are worth several million pounds each year.[151] In addition an unquantified amount of material enters the country illegally by suitcase smuggling. There is ongoing concern about the lack of controls. In the USA legislation now allows the import of Chinese herbal materials, because the Food and Drug Administration (FDA) has lifted earlier restrictions that limited imports to ethnic groups. This has prompted the wider availability of prepared medicines.

There are now over 3000 clinics in the UK that prescribe Chinese herbal remedies for various disorders and the use of these remedies seems set to increase further, given the apparent success being reported,[152] despite a lack of firm evidence of effectiveness in many cases. In the USA a survey of 575 users of CHM also showed an extremely high level of satisfaction.[153]

Practice of CHM

Herbs are given to achieve eight general outcomes in TCM. These are:

- cooling
- diaphoresis
- elimination
- emesis
- mediation
- purging
- tonification
- warming.

Categorisation of Chinese herbs

Chinese herbs may be categorised according to:

- the four natures
- the five tastes
- the meridians.

The four natures

Similar to other TCM disciplines, CHM is based on the concepts of yin and yang and of *qi* energy. The herbs are ascribed qualities ranging from cold (extreme yin), cool, neutral to warm and hot (extreme yang), and are often used in combination according to the deficiencies or excesses of these qualities in the patient.

The five tastes

The five tastes are:

- Pungent: pungent herbs are often used to generate sweat and to direct and vitalise *qi* and the blood
- Sweet: sweet-tasting herbs are often used to tonify or harmonise bodily systems
- Sour: sour tasting herbs are most often used as astringents
- Bitter: bitter tasting herbs are used to dispel heat and purge the bowels
- Salty: salty tasting herbs are used to soften hard masses as well as purge and open the bowels.

The meridians

The meridians refer to which organs the herb acts upon, e.g. menthol is pungent, cool and linked to the lungs and the liver.

Formulation of Chinese herbal medicines

The unique characteristic of CHM is the degree to which it is formulated. In other forms of herbal medicine, especially western herbal medicine, herbs are often delivered singly or combined into very small formulae of herbs with the same function. In contrast, Chinese herbalists rarely prescribe a single herb to treat a condition. They create formulae instead. A formula usually contains from 4 to 20 herbs. They may also be combined with animal or mineral materials.

Examples of herbs from vegetable and animal origin are shown in Figure 6.7.

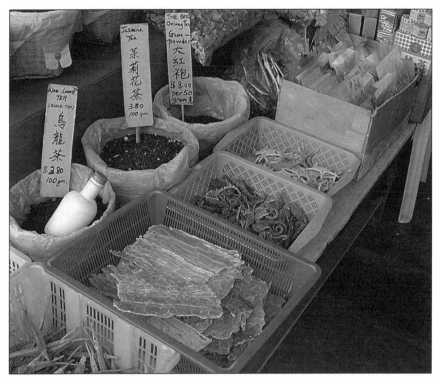

Figure 6.7 Loose herb display.

Medicinal substances are combined to:

- increase therapeutic effectiveness by synergy
- reduce toxicity or adverse reactions
- accommodate complex clinical situations
- alter the actions of the substances.

A typical Chinese herbal formula usually comprises the following components:[154]

- The main ingredient, which treats the main disease
- The associate ingredient, which assists the main ingredient
- The adjuvant, which acts as an enhancer of the main ingredient, and moderates or eliminates the toxicity of other ingredients; it may also have an opposite effect to the main ingredient to produce supplementary benefits
- The guide ingredient (or envoy), which focuses the actions of the formula on certain meridians or areas of the body, or harmonises and integrates the actions of the other ingredients.

Presentation

When herbs are prescribed for individual patients the practitioner weighs out a day's dosage of each herb and combines them in a bag. The patient is given a bag for each day that the herbal formula will be taken. The herbs are then boiled in water by the patient at home. The boiling process takes from 30 minutes to 60 minutes, and portions of the resulting decoction are consumed several times during the day.

A Chinese herbal dispensary and dispensing area are shown in Figures 6.8 and 6.9.

Another modern way of delivering herbs is through granulated herbs, which are highly concentrated powdered extracts. These powders are made by first preparing the herbs as a traditional decoction, after which the decoction is dehydrated to leave a powder residue. Practitioners can mix these powders together for each patient into a custom formula. The powder is then placed in hot water to recreate the decoction, which eliminates the need to prepare the herbs at home, but still retains much of the original decoction's potency.

Example of a prescription

An example of the ingredients for a dried herb prescription is shown in Figure 6.10.

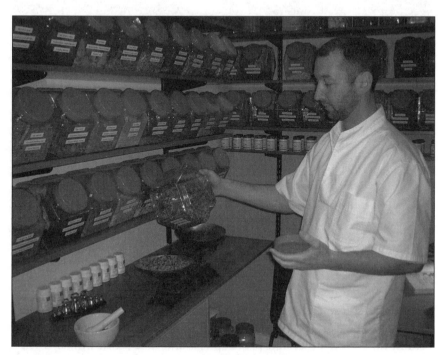

Figure 6.8 Dispensing area in Chinese herbal medicine pharmacy.

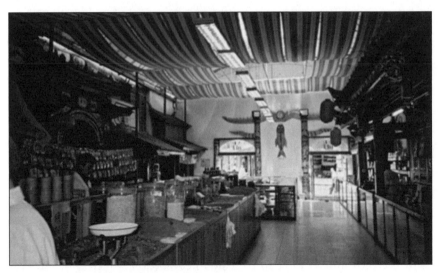

Figure 6.9 Herbal dispensary, Yunan, China.

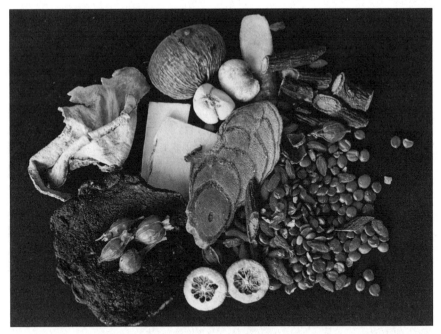

Figure 6.10 The ingredients of a CHM prescription.

Chinese patent medicines

Pre-made formulae are available as pills, tablets, capsules, powders, alcohol extracts, water extracts, etc. Most of these formulae are very convenient because they do not necessitate patient preparation and are easy to take. These products are usually not as potent as the traditional extemporaneous preparation of decoction described above. They are not 'patented' in the western sense of the word because there are no exclusive rights to the formula. Instead, 'patent' implies standardisation of the formula. All Chinese patent medicines of the same name have the same proportions of ingredients.

A medicine known as 'four gentleman decoction' (*si jun zi tang*) is an example of such a product.[155] It is used for fatigue, reduced appetite, loose stools, pale tongue and weak pulse, which occur because of the deficiency of spleen and stomach *qi* and dampness in the digestive system. The formula comprises:

- Main herb: *Radix panax ginseng* (ren *shen*), to enhance spleen *qi*
- Associate: *Rhizoma atractylodis macrocephalae* (*bai zhu*), to strengthen the spleen and dry off the 'dampness'
- Adjuvant: *Sclerotium poriae coco*s (*fu ling*), to assist the main and associate herbs
- Guide: *Radix glycyrrhizae uralensis* (*zhi gan cao*), to harmonise the other three herbs and regulate spleen *qi*.

The use of this formula is an example of tonification.

Regulatory affairs

Licensing of CHMs in China
Remedies used in TCM are subject to rigorous licensing procedures.[156] The pharmacological, toxicological and clinical studies required by the regulatory authorities depend on the class of TCM product being licensed. Nine classes of medicines are recognised

- Single compound isolated from natural material(s)
- Newly discovered medicinal plants
- Medicines containing a substitute for a TCM raw material
- Medicines made from a medicinal plant part different to (and combined with) a plant part traditionally – used in TCM raw material
- Medicines containing effective fraction(s) isolated from natural material(s)
- A multi-ingredient TCM preparation
- Medicines involving a change in the route of administration
- Medicines involving a change in dose form
- Generic drug.

Under the Drug Administration Act 2001 post-marketing surveillance of adverse drug reactions is mandatory in China. Whenever an adverse reaction event occurs, the manufacturer, the medical institutions and the seller are obliged to report it.

Some examples of licensed Chinese herbal medicines are shown in Figure 6.11.

Licensing of CHMs in Europe

Most herbal medicines on the UK market are sold and supplied as unlicensed herbal remedies under the provisions of the 1968 Medicines Act (http://tinyurl.com/ 3yhq9p). The main legislation requires that medicines placed on the market must have a licence, which requires meeting standards of safety, quality and efficacy. These licensing conditions pose inappropriate demands on most herbal medicines, because plants are chemically complex and variable, active constituents are not always known and the huge costs cannot be recouped through patenting. Hence, there are very few licensed herbal medicines on the UK market.

Under the 1968 Act, herbal remedies are exempt from the licensing requirement if *either* the herbal remedy is made up on the premises from which it is supplied, after a one-to-one consultation (Section 6.1 of the Act), *or* it is an over-the-counter (pre-prepared) remedy, in which case no therapeutic claims can be made for it (Section 6.2 of the Act). These exemptions only apply to plant remedies, so medicines containing non-plant ingredients require a medicine licence.

In recent years these provisions, which provide no specific regulation for herbal medicines, have been considered inadequate to ensure their safety and quality. There are a number of reasons including: adverse effects from some herbal ingredients (natural does not mean safe); misidentification of some

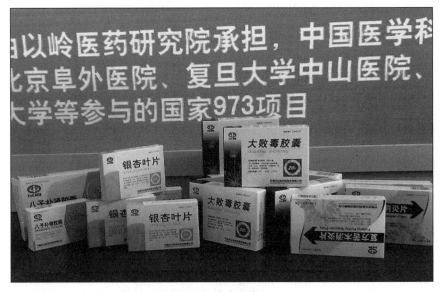

Figure 6.11 Examples of licensed Chinese Herbal Medicines.

herbs and occasional substitution of toxic for safe species; illegal inclusion of prescription-only drugs or heavy metals in some 'herbal' medicines; microbial contamination; and discovery of problematic herb–drug interactions. However, this situation is about to change.

For these various reasons a reform of the 1968 herbal provisions was undertaken. The UK law relating to the sale and supply of over-the-counter herbal remedies (Section 6.2 of the Act) has now been replaced by the European Directive on Traditional Herbal Medicinal Products of the European Parliament (2004/24/EC) and of the Council of 31 March 2004 amendment (available at http://tinyurl.com/2w9nfw). This establishes a registration scheme for industrially produced over-the-counter herbal medicines, under which manufacturers have to demonstrate safety and quality, but not efficacy. Quality is guided by European good manufacturing practice, and safety is protected by requiring evidence of at least 30 years of safe use, of which at least 15 years must be within the European Community. There is a lead-in time to allow manufacturers and suppliers to make the necessary adjustments, but after 2011 any over-the-counter herbal product that is not registered under this scheme will be illegal. This lead time is, however, only for products that were on the market before April 2004. All new herbal medicinal products must have a traditional use registration before being placed on the UK market. Further advice on the Traditional Herbal Medicines Registration Scheme is available at the UK Medicines and Healthcare products Regulatory Agency (MHRA) site at http://tinyurl.com/2ls8wm. By 3rd September 2009 a total of 88 THMR applications had been received by the MHRA of which 45 had been granted.

The European Directive leaves intact the UK exemption for herbal remedies made up by practitioners after a personal consultation, i.e. the exemption created by Section 6.1 of the 1968 Act. Such medicines will not have to be licensed and, because they are not industrially produced, will not have to be registered under the European Directive. There are, however, concerns about the quality and safety of herbal medicines supplied by this route. This is the context of the proposals for reform of Section 6.1 of the 1968 Act, published as a consultation document by the MHRA in March 2004, known as MLX 299 (available at http://tinyurl.com/3ctap2).

The issue is how to strengthen the public's protection while preserving their access to herbal medicines. This consultation document looked at a number of possible changes, including those discussed below:

- The statutory regulation (SR) of the herbal medicine profession provides the main mechanism, in a number of ways. First, members of the statutory register can be tied, through a codes of practice, to suppliers that have been audited and demonstrated satisfactory standards of quality assurance. The Register of Chinese Herbal

Medicine has provided a good model for such an arrangement through its Approved Suppliers scheme. Under SR an arrangement of this kind can be extended to all registered practitioners. As it will be illegal to practise under the title of herbalist or Chinese medicine practitioner without membership of the register, the public will have stronger assurance about the quality of Section 6.1 products than at present. Second, some more potent items in the materia medica can be restricted to use by registered practitioners. Third, SR provides a possible route for preserving access to so-called patent medicines (see below).

- At present practitioners have access to a wide range of Chinese medicine 'patents'. These are unlicensed medicines that would be considered industrially produced and thus, once the European directive is in force, would have to be registered under that scheme in order to remain legal. However, it seems likely that most of these patents would be considered unsuitable for registration under the European directive, because even if they met the tough quality assurance standards, most would not be suitable for over-the-counter use. On the other hand, they are industrially produced, so they could not be supplied under the normal Section 6.1 conditions. One way in which access might be preserved is through the so-called 'Specials' regimen, a provision in European medicines law that allows *authorised health professionals* to commission a third party (who would have to possess a manufacturer's license) to make up medicines according to a particular specification. As registered herbalists would be authorised health professionals, it would in principle be possible for herbalists to commission a range of products for the exclusive use of practitioners on the statutory register. This possibility was put forward by the MHRA.

- For acupuncturists to be able to commission specials they would also need to be designated 'authorised healthcare professionals' and able to demonstrate that they operate on a comparable level to herbalists in terms of the public's protection. Under the new specials regimen, it is the practitioner who would be responsible for the formulation of any herbal patent medicine. Suppliers would not be able to advertise their products but would be able to advertise that they are able to provide a service.

- The current licensing exemptions apply only to plant remedies. The 1968 legislation was brought in when very little non-European herbal medicine was practised in the UK, and the question of non-plant ingredients did not arise. However, the use of CHM, in which mineral and animal ingredients play an important role, has grown rapidly in the UK since then. Although there have been no prosecutions to date arising specifically from the use of non-plant ingredients – hence the law has never been tested in the courts – the wider concerns about the lack of regulation of herbal medicines have put this issue in the spotlight and it is clearly desirable to put this part of the materia medica onto a secure legal footing. The herbal community is therefore pressing for an extension of the licensing exemptions to non-plant medicines.

Licensing of TCMs in Australia

Chinese herbal products in Australia are regulated by the Therapeutic Goods Administration (TGA) and need to meet quality and safety standards.

Evidence

There is research that has demonstrated the usefulness of CHM in many disorders[156] and supports its provision in state hospitals throughout China, alongside conventional medicine. It is suggested that, although the research is of variable quality, it should not be ignored.[157] Some promising trials have been carried out in the west.[158,159] Standardised oral herbal preparations that are monitored in a conventional western manner have been shown to be beneficial in eczema.[160] CHM may also be effective in the treatment of primary dysmenorrhoea.[164]

Other applications that have been studied include atopic dermatitis and the treatment of side effects associated with chemotherapy treatment.

Atopic dermatitis

A twice-daily concoction of an ancestral formula containing five herbs (CHM) was assessed as a treatment for atopic dermatitis (AD).[161] After a 2-week run-in period, children with long-standing, moderate-to-severe AD were randomised to receive a 12-week treatment with twice-daily dosing of three capsules of either traditional CHM or placebo. The SCORing of Atopic Dermatitis (SCORAD) score, Children's Dermatology Life Quality Index (CDLQI), allergic rhinitis score, and requirement for topical corticosteroid and oral antihistamine were assessed before and at weeks 4, 8, 12 and 16 after treatment. Adverse events, tolerability, and haematological and biochemical parameters were monitored during the study. The CHM concoction was found to be efficacious in improving quality of life and reducing topical corticosteroid use in children with moderate-to-severe AD. The formulation was palatable and well tolerated.

Treatment of side effects associated with chemotherapy treatment

Short-term side effects of chemotherapy include fatigue, nausea, vomiting, mucositis, and myelosuppression or neutropenia. These occur during the course of treatment and generally resolve within months of completion of chemotherapy. A variety of Chinese medicinal herbs has been used for managing these side effects. A review by Zhang et al. has provided limited evidence concerning the effectiveness of Chinese herbs in alleviating chemotherapy-induced short-term side effects.[162]

Wei et al. assessed the efficacy and possible adverse effects of the addition of two Chinese medicinal herbs to treatment with radiotherapy or chemotherapy for oesophageal cancer.[163] Only two studies of limited quality were included in their review and the results were inconclusive. CHM has been shown to have a significant impact on control of nausea experienced by patients with early stage breast or colon cancer who required postoperative adjuvant chemotherapy.[164]

Safety

Competence of practitioners

The use of CHM is increasing in the UK and fewer patients are now Chinese. This has led to problems, because most of those who seek treatment are unable to distinguish between adequately and inadequately trained practitioners.

Practitioners fall into three broad categories:

- Those who have had a full training in the discipline This may be practitioners who have trained in China, normally for 5 years. or have graduated from a UK college or university, once again after a 4- or 5-year training to BSc or MSc level.
- Those who have received limited training in the UK or China.
- Those who have no training.

There are no data on exactly how many practitioners now offer Chinese herbal treatment in the UK, and only some of them will belong to a professional body. The main body is the Register of Chinese Herbal Medicine (RCHM), which maintains minimum standards of training and practice. Another organisation, the Association of Traditional Chinese Medicine (ATCM), also exists to represent mainly ethnic Chinese practitioners of both acupuncture and CHM. The RCHM and ATCM work in close collaboration in many areas and hold regular joint seminars and continuous professional development days in order to promote increased integration between the two groups.

Fully trained practitioners have training similar to that given to orthodox doctors in the west. They receive some training in western medicine and can distinguish those conditions that would be best treated by western medicine.

Intrinsic toxicity of herbs

Some CHMs have already caused serious health problems in the UK and other developed countries and, despite initiatives from both the MHRA and some representatives from the Chinese herbal medicine sector, problems with the quality of CHMs continue to arise.[166]

Large amounts of traditional medicines are imported into the UK, legally and illegally, and use of such medicines is frequently not admitted on occasions when serious illness forces patients to consult western medical practitioners. These medicines carry with them a risk of adverse reactions; the risk needs to be quantified and as far as possible minimised. A correspondent to the *Pharmaceutical Journal* has expressed concern that the availability of traditional CHMs in the western world will, at some time in the future, pose serious problems.[167]

A warning that there can be no guarantee of the safety or quality of traditional CHMs was issued by the MHRA in 2004 (http://tinyurl.com/2olbvg), following a similar warning 3 years before. The warning was circulated again in the light of clear evidence that problems with traditional CHMs containing toxic, and often illegal, ingredients persist, with the ingredients not always being declared on labels.

The MHRA said:

> There is no reliable way for the public to identify those CHMs which could be unsafe. In the light of this evidence we are unable to give the public any general assurances as to the safety of CHMs on the UK market. When buying TCMs people should always be aware of the possibility of low quality or illegal products. They should not take them if they are not labelled and [do not] include a list of ingredients in English. Even then, clear labelling is not in itself a guarantee of good quality standards.

Other general and specific safety warnings associated with the use of CHMs may be found at http://tinyurl.com/2p6rp4.

The herbs prescribed by practitioners of TCM in the UK are generally purchased from wholesale companies that specialise in this trade. These companies import herbs from the People's Republic of China either directly or through dealers in Hong Kong. The quality of imported herbs varies considerably, and great skill is needed to ensure that the correct herbs are provided to the practitioner. Some substitution of herbs is acceptable in China but can lead to problems if the wholesaler or practitioner is unaware of the substitution (see below). Confusion may arise over the precise identity of the herb being ordered; no standardised nomenclature exists for herbs. Fortunately, the best wholesalers and properly trained practitioners are able to make fairly reliable checks, at least visually. Unrecognised contamination by other herbs, drugs and various chemicals (including heavy metals or insecticides) is another possible hazard.

In an effort to improve the provenance of Chinese medicinal herbs a field cultivation project has been set up in Germany.[167] Herbs are grown under controlled and documented conditions, improving drug safety and material quality.

CHM has frequently been used as an alternative to orthodox therapies, especially where the latter have been considered to be ineffectual or have unacceptable side effects. One of the most popular uses of CHM in the UK is in the treatment of atopic eczema, particularly in cases resistant to orthodox therapy. As the herbal medicines are of natural origin, they are often perceived as being totally safe by consumers, but unfortunately many TCM remedies are potentially toxic when used in large doses and/or over extended time periods. Some examples of potentially toxic herbs are given in the following sections.[168]

Examples of toxic herbs

It is estimated that there are 7000 species of medicinal plants in China and, of the 150 species most frequently used, 10 are toxic.[169] In Hong Kong most cases of serious poisoning are related to the use of the roots of *cao wu* (*Aconitum kusnezoffiii*), *fu zi* and *chuan wu* (*Aconitum carmichaeli*). These herbs contain variable amounts of highly toxic alkaloids, including aconitine, which activates sodium channels and causes widespread excitation of cellular membranes. Several other herbal preparations containing aconitine alkaloids, e.g. monkshood (*Aconitum* spp.), are commonly used in Chinese medicine to treat arthritic, rheumatic and musculoskeletal pain. The alkaloids have analgesic, antipyretic and local anaesthetic properties but they are potentially toxic. The toxic effects include severe cardiac arrhythmias, nausea, vomiting and general debility. Unfortunately there is only a small margin between therapeutic and toxic doses. Aconite species are currently classified as a prescription-only medicine (POM) in the UK for internal use, although they are allowed for use externally by herbalists.

Anticholinergic poisoning due to the flowers of *yang jin hua* (*Datura metel* L.) and *nao yang hua* (*Flos rhododendri mollis*) has been reported. These herbs, which are used to treat asthma, bronchitis and toothache, may contain hyoscine, hyoscyamine and atropine, and can cause flushed skin, dilated pupils, confusion and coma.

Ba jiao lian (*Dysosma pleianthum* [syn. *Podophyllum pleianthum*]) is a species of the May apple that is used for the treatment of weakness and snake bites. The resin is extracted from the plant rhizome and is thought to contain a toxin that can cause nausea, vomiting, diarrhoea and abdominal pain.[170]

There are two species of senecio plants: *Senecio scandens* (grown in China) and *Senecio vulgaris* (grown in Europe). *Senecio scandens*, used in TCM, contains eight times less pyrrolizidine alkaloids than *Senecio vulgaris* and has little toxicity to the liver, whereas *Senecio vulgaris* exhibits significant toxicity.

Hepatotoxicity is a feature of various Chinese herbal preparations. Between November 2003 and June 2004 four patients developed severe acute liver injury within 2 months of starting to take a slimming aid (*Shubao*), widely available in the West Midlands of England.[171] Three patients fully recovered on discontinuing the agent; one patient progressed to fulminant hepatic failure, requiring liver transplantation. Laboratory analysis showed adulteration with N-nitrosofenfluramine, a recognised hepatotoxin. Warnings about taking slimming products have been issued by the MHRA (see below).

Administration during pregnancy

A number of herbs, e.g. pennyroyal (*Mentha pulegium, Hedeoma pulegoides*) and valerian (*Valerian wallichi*) have abortifacient properties and should be avoided during pregnancy.[172] Their action is thought to be due to the presence of volatile oils, which can induce uterine contractions.

Administration to children

Infants are at greater risk of possible poisoning from CHM than adults because of their inadequate biotransformation processes. Chinese infants are frequently given *huang lian* (*Coptis chinensis*) by their mothers to clear up 'products of pregnancy'.[173] The main alkaloid of this herb is berberine and it can displace bilirubin from its serum-binding proteins, causing a rise in free bilirubin concentration and a risk of brain damage. *Yin-chen hao* (*Artemisia scoparia*) is used for the treatment of neonatal jaundice and has a similar effect although it does not contain berberine.

Concurrent use with orthodox medicines

There are two problems here: an enhanced activity from the herbal medicine or the orthodox medicine, or both, and an intrinsic toxicity, real or threatened, from the allopathic ingredient.

Aristolochia is an example of a herb that not only is toxic in its own right but also its administration concurrently with allopathic drugs in Chinese herbal preparations (albeit inadvertently) may potentiate its action, causing severe adverse reactions (see below).

There are several examples of the inclusion of illegal ingredients in Chinese medicines over many years and pharmacists should be aware of this possibility. In 1975, a herbal-based preparation called Toukuwan was manufactured in Hong Kong and widely promoted in the USA for rheumatism and arthritis. It was discovered that the product contained four orthodox medicines, including the prescription drug diazepam, and its continued import was swiftly banned by the FDA. More recently, the New Zealand Director General of Health advised consumers against taking a Chinese product known as *cheng kum* because it contained a pharmacy-only antihistamine that could cause drowsiness.[174] The capsules have now been withdrawn from sale. They were advertised for use in the treatment of various conditions, including the promotion of joint mobility, healthy skin, as a support during menopause and of benefit while consuming alcoholic drinks. The Ministry of Health made the ruling following complaints from doctors about the product.

Another example is the intentional inclusion of steroids in oral[175] and topical preparations[176] used for the treatment of dermatological conditions. Following reports of positive clinical effects in the treatment of eczema, 11 Chinese herbal creams were analysed. Eight were found to contain dexamethasone in varying amounts.[177] The mean value approximated to a proprietary brand of 0.05% betamethasone valerate, a commonly prescribed steroid ointment in the UK. None of the patients was aware that the creams contained a steroid. The authors concluded that the risk of adverse reactions with such potent steroids is increased by their inappropriate use and application to areas of thin skin and on the face.

It has been suggested that exported herbal remedies have been adulterated with synthetic drugs to improve their activity, and their popularity, in western countries. A dangerous evolution in the formulation of a Chinese herbal arthritis cure, *Chuifong Toukuwan*, manufactured by a laboratory in Hong Kong, has been dsecribed.[178] The undeclared presence of phenylbutazone, indometacin, hydrochlorothiazide, chlordiazepoxide, diazepam and corticosteroids was reported in the product, a mixture of 23 herbs.

Dangerously high levels of undeclared pharmaceuticals have been discovered in a supposed 'herbal Viagra' being sold in many TCM stores in the UK.[179] The product '*Jia Yi Jian*' was seized by the MHRA in 2009 and claimed to contain only herbal ingredients. However, laboratory analysis revealed the unlicensed product contained 68.1 mg sibutramine and 50.06 mg tadalafil, four times the level found in prescribed medicinal products licensed for the treatment of erectile dysfunction and obesity respectively.

Inclusion of adulterants

Major problems resulting from the presence of adulterants in CHM have been experienced. It is therefore extremely important that TCM products are monitored closely. The European Agency for the Evaluation of Medicinal Products in London has a working party on herbal medicinal products, with the remit to include pharmacovigilance and the introduction of safety measures throughout member states. The MHRA performs a similar task in the UK. Currently, Chinese herbal suppliers are engaged in agreeing guidelines to ensure that their medicines are of the highest quality and free from adulterants.

The RCHM introduced a system of approving suppliers in 2002, where companies are required to submit themselves to an independent audit by a trained pharmaceutical auditor.

The audit examines the quality system of the UK supplier and focuses on the five Ps of GMP: premises, personnel, products, procedures and processes. The company is then inspected at yearly intervals.

Although still in its infancy, this approved suppliers' scheme has provided a framework for future initiatives to increase confidence in the quality of Chinese herbs and herbal products.

The aristolochia story – a complex problem[180]

Severe concerns about the safety of the herb *Aristolochia* arose in early 1992, when two women presented with extensive interstitial renal fibrosis to doctors in a Belgian clinic that specialised in weight-loss regimens. The condition rapidly progressed to terminal renal failure.[181] The total number of patients exposed to the herb is not known exactly, but around 100 people with renal disease were eventually recorded, representing about 5% of those who took the slimming preparation.[182]

The diet regimen used by the clinic for many years without problems comprised a mixture of acetazolamide, fenfluramine, and various animal and vegetable extracts. In the mid-1990s the formula was supplemented by the addition of powdered extracts of Chinese herbs. A possible relationship between the renal disease and the herbs was suspected. Subsequently, it was established from an epidemiological survey that *Stephania tetrandra* was the only herb associated with all the cases of renal disease. Most unexpectedly, the alkaloid normally derived from *Stephania* – tetrandrine – could not be found in the capsules taken by the affected patients.[183] Instead, analysis revealed the presence of a series of substituted nitrophenanthrene carboxylic acids, known as aristolochic acids. These were considered to be the cause of the adverse reactions.[184,185] The acids form the main active principle of various species of another Chinese herb, namely *Aristolochia*.

It was finally concluded that the *Stephania tetrandra* (*han fang ji*) must have been inadvertently replaced by *Aristolochia fangchi* (*guang fang ji*) in the powdered extracts delivered to Belgian suppliers. Herbal ingredients are usually traded using their common Chinese names and this can lead to confusion during translation. About 185 kg of the substituted *han fang ji* was distributed to practitioners throughout Belgium but it was only one particular clinic that reported problems. The intrinsic nephrotoxic effects of the *Aristolochia* may have been potentiated in this case by the combination of orthodox drugs administered concurrently. The *British National Formulary*[186] states that the use of diuretics for weight loss is inappropriate; this would seem to question the wisdom of including acetazolamide in the product. The Belgian medical authorities have also warned doctors not to prescribe slimming products composed of appetite inhibitors and diuretics. The women may have been more vulnerable to adverse reactions due to a weakening of general health caused by the calorie-controlled diet that they were following.[187] In addition, the herbs were prescribed by untrained doctors and not in accordance with Chinese medical theories.

Since 1994 a total of seven cases of Chinese herb nephropathy have been reported in France. In 1998 a case of reversible acute hepatitis in a patient using a Chinese herbal tea was reported in the Netherlands.[188] *A. debilis* was identified in the tea mixture. Also around this time a case was reported in Spain of a patient with renal failure resulting from chronic intake of an infusion made with a mixture of herbs containing *A. pistolochia*. This species of the herb is native to Catalonia.[189]

The first two cases of a specific nephropathy caused by ingestion of an unlicensed Chinese herbal remedy in the UK were reported in 1999.[190] The first case was a 49-year-old woman who initially presented to her GP with headache and hypertension. Her only existing medication was a herbal preparation that she had been taking for about 2 years to treat her eczema. Renal function tests and a biopsy revealed substantial tubular atrophy and interstitial fibrosis in the cortex. The patient rapidly progressed to renal failure and dialysis was begun. Three years later she received a renal transplant.

The second patient was a 57-year-old woman who was admitted with renal failure and a 6-month history of anorexia, lethargy, nausea and weight loss. She had been taking Chinese herbal tea for eczema for 6 years. A renal biopsy showed evidence of deterioration, as in the case above. The patient was started on dialysis.

Subsequently, it was found that both patients had been exposed to aristolochic acids as a result of ingesting *A. manshuriensis* used as a substitute for *mu tong* in the herbal tea, in place of *Clematis* or *Akebia* spp.

An emergency ban was imposed on the import, sale and supply of *Aristolochia* by the UK Medicines Control Agency (MCA) in 1999. The ban was made permanent 2 years later.

Following the two cases in the UK the Australian Office of Complementary Medicine initiated a survey of products containing *Clematis* to determine whether inadvertent substitution with *Aristolochia* had occurred.[191] Their concern was prompted by a realisation that the Chinese name *mu tong* could be used to describe three different herbs: *Clematis* spp. (*chuan mu tong*), *Akebia* spp. (*bai mu tong*) and *Aristolochia manshuriensis* (*guan mu tong*). Of the 14 samples tested, a raw herbal material and a manufactured clematis product were found to contain *Aristolochia*. In TCM *Aristolochia* spp. are considered to be interchangeable with other commonly used herbal ingredients and substitution of one plant for another species is an established practice, when in fact this may not be the case (Table 6.4).

Pharmokinetic data for aristolochic acids 1 and 11 have been studied in rats, mice, guinea-pigs, dogs and humans after oral treatment.[192] The doses studied were in the range 0.6–85 mg/kg body weight. Most of the results relate to rats. After oral administration, aristolochic acid 1 was readily absorbed from the gastrointestinal tract. After oral administration of aristolochic acid 1 to rats, about 91% of the dose was recovered from the excreta, equally divided in the urine and faeces.

In vivo and in vitro studies have shown that aristolochic acids are both nephrotoxic and carcinogenic. Hence most European Union states have taken regulatory action to protect the public from unlicensed medicines that contain *Aristolochia*. In many member states (including the UK) *Stephania tetrandra, Akebia and Clematis* spp. are also being controlled because of the risk of substitution. Following the interim measures taken in July 1999, the UK MHRA introduced a permanent ban on the import, sale or supply of preparations containing plants of the genus *Aristolochia* and of *Akebia* and *Clematis* spp. used as *mu tong*. It is unfortunate that such action is necessary and some would say that this represents another example of the government restricting consumers' choice.

There is undoubtedly a substantial potential risk to health from *Aristolochia*. Effective control is vital to ensure that the herb is used under appropriate supervision and is of the highest quality. *Aristolochia* has been a POM since 1997 but exempt from control when used in herbal or homoeopathic medicine. Homoeopathic medicines were unaffected by the legislation, although it is possible that at a later date the potencies (strengths) available could be restricted to those above 9c, when the dilution is of such magnitude that no molecules of drug are considered to be present.

Table 6.4 Species of *Aristolochia*		
Species	**Part used**	**Indication**
A. fangchi	Root	Diuretic, antirheumatic
A. contorta, A. debilis	Fruit	Antitussive, antiasthmatic
A. contorta, A. debilis	Herb	Diuretic and anti-inflammatory
A. debilis	Root	Analgesic

Slimming aids

Despite the permanent ban on *Aristolochia*, the UK MHRA has continued to find evidence of the supply of TCMs containing the herb in the UK. The Agency has advised dieters to be cautious when using any TCM slimming aid to help weight loss, following the discovery of a number of potentially dangerous and illegal products (including *Xiao Pang Meion* and *Qian Er/Ma zin dol/Chaso/Onshido*) in the UK and international markets in addition to *Aristolochia*. The Agency has posted information on its website (http://tinyurl.com/yoly5t).

Heavy metals

Another reported concern with regard to CHMs is the presence of heavy metals. Much confusion has arisen regarding the presence of heavy metals probably due in part to the way news is reported in the press. There have been reports of herbal products contaminated with extremely high levels of heavy metals when in fact the heavy metals were an intended constituent of the formula. An example of this would be the formula *tian wang bu xin dan* or 'Emperor of Heavens Special Pill to Tonify the Heart'.

This formula contains *zhu sha* (cinnabaris or red mercuric sulphide) and is prescribed in China in small doses and for short periods of time to treat mental and emotional conditions. It is prescribed in small doses and used for short periods of time and is still used in China today. There are only a few Chinese herbal formulae that contain heavy metals and, when a case does occur citing heavy metal contamination with thousands of times the permitted level, it is almost certainly due to the use of one of these formulae, probably smuggled in from China.

The problem with heavy metals for mainstream CHM is a very different one. Here we see a situation where heavy metals may be found in low levels in formulae that do not traditionally contain any compounds that could be responsible. It is a contamination problem. At the moment China is undergoing its own industrial revolution, manufacturing industries are everywhere and the result of this frenetic manufacture is increased pollution into the rivers, many of which go on to irrigate farmland, including those that grow herbs. Testing programmes are in place to monitor heavy metal levels but a longer-term solution is needed.

Not all herbs are susceptible to heavy metal contamination and many herbs are grown in areas free from contamination. Many herbs are now cultivated rather than picked from the wild, not only protecting the environment, but also making it possible to control growing conditions. Good agricultural practice (GAP) has been introduced to herb farms across China and steadily a situation is developing where it is possible to trace herbs back to the field where they were grown. This is a far cry from the previous situation, where most herbs would be purchased from central markets dotted around the country.

Accidental contaminants may also include allergens, pollen, insect parts, moulds and mould spores. Mycotoxins are contaminants in a wide variety of natural products.[193]

Future measures to improve safety

The problems of TCM are not unlike those of orthodox medicine. There are both intrinsic adverse reactions resulting from the toxicity of the product and extrinsic adverse reactions arising from ancillary procedures, e.g. inappropriate diagnosis and prescribing. Both groups of problems need to be addressed. To minimise the chance of adverse reactions leading to a recurrence of the circumstances surrounding the use of *Aristolochia* with other herbs, the following measures should be instigated:

- Quality assurance and quality control should be put in place to ensure that unadulterated herbs are supplied to manufacturers and practitioners.
- Herbal practitioners should undergo a course of training to ensure that they provide a safe and effective service.
- Herbs with known potential to cause adverse reactions should not be mixed with orthodox drugs unless careful monitoring is carried out.
- Accurate records should be kept by all practitioners to monitor the incidence of adverse reactions. Regular audits should also be carried out. This is in any case a minimum requirement for the collection of the evidence of successful outcomes required by purchasing authorities. Effective use of the Yellow Card system by all disciplines of complementary medicine is long overdue. Non-medically qualified practitioners ('professional practitioners') should also be encouraged to take part. This would make sense because there are many more NMQPs than health professionals involved in TCM.

Yellow Card ADR reporting schemes

RCHM

The RCHM's Yellow Card scheme was established in order to gather safety data on CHMs, through identifying suspected adverse drug reactions (ADRs) to herbs. Although Chinese herbs have a long established history of use there is still relatively little present-day information on herbal safety. An example of the card used to record the reactions is provided in Figure 6.12.

Register of Chinese Herbal Medicine
Office 5, Ferndale Business Centre, 1 Exeter Street, Norwich
NR2 4QB.
Tel: 01603 623994
Fax: 01603 667557
Email: herbmed@rchm.co.uk
Website: www.rchm.co.uk

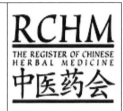

YELLOW CARD
for reporting suspected adverse events in confidence

Please fill in this form clearly in blue or black ink.
Please note that all information is completely confidential.

---

1) About you, the practitioner completing the Yellow Card report

Family name ....   First name ....

Address ....

....   Postcode ....

Telephone number ....   First name ....

---

2) About the patient who had the suspected adverse reaction

Family name ....   First name ....

Weight .... Height......................   Ethnic group ....

Date of birth ....   Male/Female ....   Pregnant? Yes/No

---

3) About the herbal medicine(s) that you think caused the adverse reaction

Type of prescription: Raw herbs/Concentrated Powder/Tincture/Pills/Cream/
(Delete as appropriate)

or other (please describe) ....

Prescription (please list all ingredients and brand name if applicable ....

....

....

....

....

What was the herbal medicine prescribed for (e.g. Asthma) ....

....

....

Supplier of the medicine ....

Dosage of the medicine ....

Date prescription was started ....   Date prescription was stopped (if stopped) ....

Figure 6.12 Example of Yellow Card used by the Register of Chinese Herbal Medicine (RCHM) to record adverse reactions.

RCHM YELLOW CARD continued

4) About the suspected adverse reaction

Did you consider the reaction to be serious? Yes/No

Please describe the suspected adverse reaction in your own words including any treatment

received for the reaction ....

....

....

....

How bad was the suspected adverse reaction? – please tick:

- Mild or slightly uncomfortable
- Uncomfortable, a nuisance or irritation, but able to carry on with everyday activities
- Bad enough to affect day to day activities, i.e. persistent or significant disability or incapacity
- Bad enough to be admitted to hospital
- Life-threatening
- Caused death
- Caused congenital abnormality

Date adverse reaction started ....

Has the adverse reaction stopped? Yes/No   If yes, what date did it stop? ....

How is the patient now? – please tick

- Recovered completely
- Getting better
- Still has reaction
- Recovered but with some lasting effects (please describe these below) ....

  ....

  ....

Was the patient rechallenged? Yes/No   If yes, at what dose ....

Did the adverse reaction re-occur? Yes/No

5) More information about the person who had the adverse reaction

Other medical conditions including known sensitivities ....

....

....

....

Figure 6.12   *Continued*

RCHM YELLOW CARD continued

6) Other medicines

Please list any other medicines (including your own previous prescriptions, prescribed medicines and other herbal remedies) used three months prior to the suspected adverse reaction including the name of the medicine, the dosage, what it was used for, when started, and when stopped.

Name of medicine including brand name if known and type of medicine e.g. pill, powder, cream	Type of medicine e.g. external cream, raw herbs, powder	Source	Used for?	Dosage	Date started	Date stopped
....	....	....	....	....	....	....
....	....	....	....	....	....	....
....	....	....	....	....	....	....
....	....	....	....	....	....	....

7) Additional information and comments

Was a doctor, pharmacist or other health professional told about the suspected adverse reaction? Yes/No/Don't know (please delete as appropriate)

If yes, did the health professional complete a Yellow Card report? Yes/No/Don't know (please delete as appropriate)

Please give any other information that you think might be relevant including test results, oriental medical diagnosis e.g. patient yang xu treating for wind heat attack, dietary information, your conclusions and suggestions. For congenital abnormalities please state all other drugs taken during pregnancy and the last menstrual period. Please continue on a separate sheet if necessary.

....

....

....

Are you happy for the MHRA to contact you in the future to discuss the suspected adverse reaction or ask for more information? Yes/No

8) Would you like your Yellow Card submission to be analysed by an expert?

The RCHM provides a service whereby the Yellow Card information that you have submitted, along with a full case history, can be analysed by an expert practitioner. This process is completely anonymous and confidential. If you wish for your Yellow Card report to be sent for analysis then please enclose a copy of your full case history notes and tick this box

9) Finally, please sign and date this Yellow Card submission, thank you.

Signed (practitioner signature) .... **Date** ....

Please return this form to: Yellow Card Report, Register of Chinese Herbal Medicine, Office 5, Ferndale Business Centre, 1 Exeter Street, Norwich, NR2 4OB.

Figure 6.12 *Continued*

The Yellow Card scheme for drug monitoring of orthodox drugs asks only for serious suspected reactions to established drugs and all suspected reactions to newer drugs. However, the RCHM's Yellow Card scheme asks for **any** suspected reaction, however minor. This does not include minor known side effects such as loose stools with the use of greasy yin tonics, or any other symptom that you might warn your patient about as a mild transient side effect.

Sometimes it is hard to tell whether a possible adverse reaction is due to herbs prescribed or something else. However, even if a practitioner is unsure as to whether a herbal medicine or a combination of herbal medicines and other medicines has caused a side effect, but has a suspicion, completion of a card would be appropriate. Actively using the Yellow Cards will further every practitioner's knowledge. Contact herbmed@rchm.co.uk.

MHRA

The Yellow Card scheme operated by the UK MHRA has been widened to encourage reporting of suspected ADRs in association with herbal medicines, including unlicensed products. Patients are now able to report suspected ADRs direct.

Endangered species

The conservation of rare medicinal plants is a worldwide problem affecting many cultures.[194] The issue of the usage of various endangered species, including bears and tigers, which are ingredients in the formulation of Chinese herbal patent formulae, was brought to the public eye in the USA by a World Wildlife Fund-supported report entitled *Prescription for Extinction: Endangered species and patented oriental medicines in trade.*[195] This report was released in 1994 and resulted in widespread media attention and subsequent public concern. Researchers at Bastyr University are studying the issue of endangered species usage in depth, along with the issues of excessive toxins, drugs, adulterants, and illegal and inaccurate labelling practices, which are prevalent in these formulae. Bastyr University is near Seattle, and integrates the pursuit of scientific knowledge with the wisdom of ancient healing methods and traditional cultures from around the world. Researchers plan to work with the manufacturers of Chinese herbal patent formulae toward establishing guidelines that may be implemented in the west and in Asia.

Modern developments in CHM

Over the last 20 years there have been initiatives in China to find new dosage forms that are more convenient than the traditional practice of boiling up loose herbs at home. This has resulted in the now widespread use of concentrated powder and granule extracts. These products are proving popular with both western patients and in Chinese cities where the pace of life has recently increased significantly. Although there is no doubt that these products make the process of taking herbal medicine much easier and therefore patient compliance has certainly improved, traditionalists argue that the effectiveness of these products is less than when using raw herbs. Until more comparable research is undertaken it will remain a matter of practitioner preference.

One of the major advantages of these products is in the microbiological quality. Traditionally made powders are produced from grinding the raw herb and can have very high microbial loads. As a result of the heating steps involved in the manufacture of concentrated extracts, the microbiological loading will be close to zero. These products can be stored for several years without microbial spoilage.

Western CHM

The use of CHM has been continued in the traditional manner by physicians and pharmacists serving Chinese communities around the world.

In many western cities the Chinatown districts support herb shops and practices with remedies imported directly from Asia, and practitioners trained by the old system of long apprenticeship. Increasingly, local western practitioners are training in their home countries to satisfy the growing interest for CHM. In particular, acupuncturists seem to be extending their practice. Many are taking a 2-year postgraduate course accredited by the European Herbal and Traditional Medicine Practitioners Association (EHTPA) and offered by many colleges and universities around the UK, which covers around 200 herbs and 100 classic formulae.[196]

Examples of Chinese herbs used in the UK

Examples of herbs used in TCM formulae in the UK are listed in Table 6.5.[195]

With the introduction of these new dosage forms modern manufacturing and testing facilities have developed. Since March 2005 factories in China must be GMP certified and companies who failed to reach the standard have been closed down.

As relations are further developed between Europe and China it is likely that UK inspectors will also travel to China in order to assess suitability for the European market. This will be a challenging and exciting development.

Table 6.5 Examples of common Chinese herbs[195]

Source material	Chinese name	Parts used	Main constituents	Clinical use
Agastache rugosa	Hua xiang	Herb	Essential oil	Digestive stimulant, antiemetic
Cinnamonium spp.	Rou gui	Bark	Essential oil, resin	Warms, circulatory stimulant
Clematis chinensis	Wei ling xian	Root	Anemoonin, saponins, sterols, phenols	Antirheumatic, stimulant, expels wind and damp
Glycyrrhiza uralensis	Gan cao	Root	Saponins, flavonoids	Expectorant, tonic, detoxifier
Lonicera japonica	Jin yin hua	Flowers	Luteolin, tannin	Cooling and disinfecting, antipyretic, detoxifier
Magnolia spp.	Xin yi hua	Bark	Essential oil, alkaloids	Digestive stimulant, expectorant
Panax ginseng	Ren shen	Root	Saponins, glycosides	Sedative, tonic
Phellodendron amurensei	Po-mu	Bark	Alkaloids, triterpenoids, sterols	Bitter digestive, diuretic, antipyretic
Taraxacum mongolicum	Pu gong ying	Whole plant	Bitters, sterol	Anti-infective, antipyretic

The Bristol Chinese Herb Garden

The Bristol Chinese Herb Garden (Figure 6.13) was started in 2000 as a partnership between the University of Bristol Botanic Garden and the RCHM. With the move of the University Botanic Garden in 2006, an opportunity was taken to greatly enlarge the size and scope of the Chinese Herb Garden.

The Chinese Herb Garden aims to provide a comprehensive living collection of plants used in Chinese medicine that can be used in the teaching of students of herbal medicine and for research by the University and the herbal profession into the cultivation and chemistry of the plants.

The garden is affiliated to several University and botanic gardens in China and is divided into several distinct areas, including a herbal teaching display where plants are divided into: 'use class' categories in line with Chinese medicine theory; a conservation bed highlighting some of the plants that are currently under threat from overuse or habitat loss; a research bed; a peony bed; and an area for ferns.

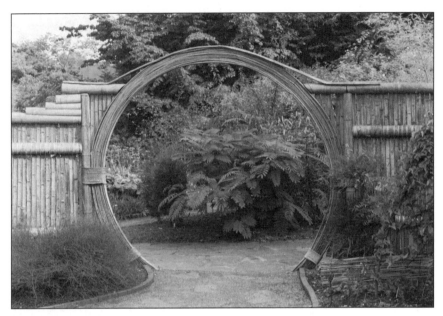

Figure 6.13 Bristol Chinese Herb Garden.

Over the next few years it is planned to further develop the facilities into an advanced teaching and research centre using the combined expertise of the University of Bristol and the herbal profession.

Other elements of TCM[196]

Chinese massage (tui na)

Massage has been an important element of TCM for at least 2000 years, featuring in the Yellow Emperor's famous text. The therapy uses hand manipulation, pushing, rolling and kneading, on specific points and parts of the body. It may be used to balance yin and yang and to regulate the function of *qi*, blood and the *zang fu* organs as well as to loosen joints and relax muscles and tendons.

Dietary therapy

Chinese dietary therapy is an important part of life in the country as well as being included in many practitioners' prescriptions. Knowledgeable Chinese housewives often prepare special meals for common family ailments. Thus a patient suffering from insomnia due to a disharmony of heart and kidney might be advised to make a soup of lotus plumule (*lian zi xin*) to nourish the heart and include morus fruit (*sang shen zi*) to enhance kidney essence. These measures would be in addition to other TCM treatments, e.g. CHM and/or acupuncture.

Nutritional interventions may be of three types:[197]

- **Supplementation**: as well as various vitamins and minerals, the range may contain animal and plant products (e.g. algae or kelp).
- **Dietary modification**: this involves changes in dietary habits to exclude elements not considered nutritious or to establish better eating patterns.
- **Therapeutic systems**: the inclusion (or exclusion) of foods considered to have a contributory role to the patient's health.

Examples of diets with properties beneficial to health include:[199]

- **White rice porridge**: this regulates the bowels (constipation and diarrhoea), for nausea and loss of appetite.
- **Sweet and sour sauce**: considered to be an important constituent of diet because of its antiseptic properties.
- **Sweet and sour crispy noodles**: noodles are a good source of nutrients for athletes and growing children. The vinegar in the sauce has antiseptic properties.

Examples of dietary remedies for common illnesses include:

- **Acne**: infusion of the flowers of peach (*Prunus persica*) or almond (*P. amygdalus*) in water daily
- **Arthritis**: cinnamon tea (*Cinnamonum cassia*); for cold arthritis, sage steeped in rice wine sipped daily and for warm arthritis infusion of purslane (*Portalaca oleracea*) in water
- **Constipation**: fig wine, stewed pears and bananas eaten cold with honey
- **Flatulence**: seeds of mandarin orange chewed
- **Haemorrhoids**: simmer a mixture of almonds, peach kernels, pine nuts and sesame seeds in water and drink as a soup
- **Halitosis**: a few leaves of peppermint or the peel of a mandarin orange chewed.

Martial art therapy

This approach uses movements and exercises adapted from martial arts, such as *tai ji quan* and *kung fu*.[200] A case study report has indicated that a patient suffering from severe cervical stenosis improved after martial art therapy.[201]

Qigong

This is a meditative therapy with a history similar to that of Chinese massage. It is often combined with body movement and breathing exercises to achieve a balance of energy in the TCM meridian system. Xin et al. performed a systematic literature review of *qigong* intervention studies published in English or Chinese since 1980 and found that 11 studies were identified that met their criteria for an association between *qigong* and the management of type 2 diabetes.[202] They concluded that the exercise appeared to have beneficial effects on some of the metabolic risk factors but that methodological limitations made it difficult to draw firm conclusions about the benefits recorded.

Tai ji quan (tai c'hi)

Tai c'hi was created in the fourteenth century as a martial art and is practised widely in China. The term 'tai ji' refers to the balance of yin and yang. It consists of a series of slow flowing exercises inspired by the movement of animals, as reflected in the names given to the movements, e.g. 'white stork spreading wings'.

Though exercise reduces the risk of falls, the challenge is finding a programme that interests participants. Research shows that tai c'hi, with its oriental overtones, may be such a candidate.

Wolf et al., working in Atlanta, found that older people taking part in a 15-week tai c'hi programme reduced their risk of falling by 47.5%.[203] Wolf's group compared several factors before and after the interventions, and found improvements in certain key areas. The most notable change involved the reduction in the rate of falling for the tai c'hi group. The groups receiving computerised balance platform training did not have significantly lower rates of falling. The tai c'hi participants also took more deliberate steps and decreased their walking speed slightly compared with the other groups. Fear of falling was also reduced for the tai c'hi group. After the intervention, only 8% of the tai c'hi group said that they feared falling, compared with 23% before they had the training. In other work led by Wolf it was concluded that there was no statistically significant reduction in falls compared with wellness education.[204] The trial involved 287 people and lasted 48 weeks. It was suggested that tai c'hi does not begin to show a significant reduction in the risk of falling until after a number of months of regular participation. Fewer falls were observed in a subset of patients doing tai c'hi who had no history of fall fracture. Wolfson and colleagues found that several interventions to improve balance and strength among older people were effective.[205] These improvements, particularly in strength, were preserved over a 6-month period while participants did tai c'hi exercises.

The possible reduction in falls following participation in a tai c'hi programme was evaluated in a group of active individuals between the ages of 70 and 92 years.[206] Participants received three sessions of the exercise per week over 6 months when they were compared with a control group. They proved to have a lower incidence of falls and improved measures of balance.

There are other areas in which tai c'hi may be of interest to older patients. There is some evidence that tai c'hi improves the range of motion of the ankle, hip and knee in people with rheumatoid arthritis. A study showed that tai c'hi did not improve people's ability to carry out household chores, joint tenderness, grip strength or their number of swollen joints nor did it increase their symptoms of rheumatoid arthritis, but people felt that they improved when doing the exercises and enjoyed it.[207] It is still not known if it improves pain in rheumatoid arthritis or that person's quality of life. It is also not clear how much, how intense and for how long tai c'hi should be done to see benefits.

Wayne et al. evaluated the evidence for tai c'hi as an intervention to reduce rate of bone loss in postmenopausal women.[208] RCTs, prospective cohort studies and cross-sectional studies that included tai c'hi as an intervention, and had at least one outcome related to measurement of bone mineral density (BMD), were included. Conclusions on the impact of tai c'hi on BMD are limited by the quantity and quality of research to date. This limited evidence suggests that tai c'hi may be an effective, safe and practical intervention for maintaining BMD in postmenopausal women. In combination with research that indicates that tai c'hi can positively impact other risk factors associated with low BMD (e.g. reduced fall frequency, increased musculoskeletal strength), further methodologically sound research is warranted to better evaluate the impact of tai c'hi practice on BMD and fracture risk in postmenopausal women. However, less encouraging results emerged from an RCT carried out in Hong Kong.[209] The effects of tai c'hi (TC) and resistance exercise (RTE) were investigated on BMD, muscle strength, balance and flexibility in community living older people; 180 individuals (90 men, 90 women) aged 65–74 were involved. No effect was observed in men. No difference in balance, flexibility or the number of falls was observed between intervention and controls after 12 months.

Other traditional medicine related to TCM

Traditional Tibetan medicine

Tibetan medicine is reputed to be the most comprehensive form of Eurasian healthcare and the world's first integrative medicine.[210] Incorporating rigorous systems of meditative self-healing and ascetic self-care from India, it includes a world-class paradigm of mind/body and preventive medicine. Adapting the therapeutic philosophy and contemplative science of Indian Buddhism to the quality of secular life and death, traditional Tibetan medicine (TTM) features the world's most effective systems of positive and palliative healthcare. Based on qualitative theories and intersubjective methods, it involves predictions and therapies shown to be more accurate and effective than those of modern medicine in fields from physiology and pharmacology to neuroscience, mind/body medicine and positive health.

Tibetan medicine originated with the local folk tradition (known as *Bon*) that dates back to about 300 BC and was formally recorded by Xiepu Chixi, the physician to the Tibetan King Niechi Zanpu, in 126 BC.[211] Aspects of both the traditional Chinese and Indian (ayurvedic) medical systems were added later; ayurveda (see Chapter 7) has had the most profound influence on Tibetan medicine. The medicine of India was introduced to Tibet as early as AD 254, with the visit of two Indian physicians. During the following century several physicians from India reinforced the teachings. Other influences came from Persian (Unani), Greek and Chinese medical systems, and it continues to be practised in Tibet, India, Nepal, Bhutan, Ladakh, Siberia, China and Mongolia, as well as more recently in parts of Europe and North America. It embraces the traditional Buddhist belief that all illness ultimately results from the 'three poisons' of the mind: ignorance, attachment and aversion. Tibetan medical theory states that it is necessary to maintain balance in the body's three principles of function.

- *rLüng* (wind) the source of the body's ability to circulate physical substances (e.g. blood), energy (e.g. nervous system impulses) and the non-physical (e.g. thoughts).
- *mKhris-pa* (bile) is characterised by the quantitative and qualitative characteristics of heat, and is the source of many functions such as thermoregulation, metabolism, liver function and discriminating intellect.
- *Bad-kan* (phlegm) is characterised by the quantitative and qualitative characteristics of cold, and is the source of many functions such as aspects of digestion, the maintenance of our physical structure, joint health and mental stability.

The imbalances in an individual are revealed by a combination of reported symptoms, pulse diagnosis, tongue diagnosis, and urine analysis. The overall physical appearance of the person and information about their daily habits, and consideration of seasonal influences also contribute to the analysis. The Tibetan pulse diagnosis appears to be derived from the Chinese system, and is taken at the same artery of each wrist, but the method of feeling the pulse and the interpretations differ. Tongue diagnosis is simplified compared with the Chinese system (long disorders are characterised by red and dry tongue, chiba disorders by a yellowish tongue coating, and peigen disorders by a greyish and sticky coating with a smooth and moist texture). Urine analysis is unique to the Tibetan system and may have been introduced from Persia. Physicians inspect the colour, amount of vapour, sediment, smell and characteristics of the foam generated upon stirring, relying on the first urine excreted in the morning.

The modern materia medica of Tibet is derived from the book *Jingzhu Bencao (The Pearl Herbs)*, published in 1835 by Dumar Danzhen-pengcuo.[212] Its format includes two sections, one being in the style of the Buddhist sutra with praise of the medicines, and the other being a detailed classification of each substance, giving the material's origin, environmental conditions where it is found, quality, parts used and properties. The text included 2294 materials, of which 1006 are of plant origin, 448 of animal origin and 840 minerals. The heavier reliance on minerals and animals than on plants, compared with other traditional medical traditions, can readily be understood for a country at such high altitude which is very rocky and supports only small areas of plant growth over much of the terrain. About one-third of the medicinal materials used in Tibetan formulae are unique to the Tibetan region (including the Himalayan area in bordering countries), whereas the other two-thirds of the materials are obtained from India and China.

Although Tibetan herbal medicine includes the use of decoctions and powders, for the most part Tibetan doctors utilise pills that are usually made from a large number of herbs (typically 8–25 ingredients). Pills have the advantage of being easy to use and they can be prepared in advance at a medical facility where all the ingredients are gathered together. Due to the vast distances, rough terrain and limited development of Tibet, it was not possible to have the broad range of ingredients available to individual

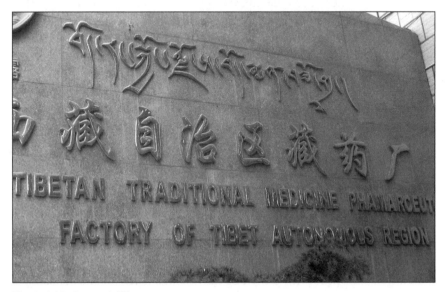

Figure 6.14 Factory in Tibet.

doctors who might compound formulae for decoction, as was often done in China. Instead, a relatively small variety of pills, prepared at central facilities, would be carried by the doctors to their patients. For many doctors, a collection of about two dozen principal formulae would have to suffice. In Lhasa, where there is a large manufacturing facility rivalling pharmaceutical manufacturing facilities in the west (Figure 6.14) doctors have access to about 200 types of pills.

In general, Tibetan remedies emphasise the use of spicy (acrid), aromatic and warming herbs. The climate has a substantial influence on these choices: the high altitude of Tibet means that cold and windy conditions prevail. The herbs help to compensate for this condition. Ayurvedic medicine relies heavily on spicy herbs for stimulating the digestive system functions, which is understood to be the key to health. Thus, among the commonly used Tibetan herbs are those derived mainly from the ayurvedic system, such as the peppers, cumins, cardamom, clove, ginger and other hot spices, complemented by local aromatics such as saussurea and musk. Also, the Tibetan system emphasises astringent herbs, possibly representing an attempt to conserve body fluids and alleviate any inflammation of the mucous membranes.

The 'king' herb of Tibetan medicine is the *chebulic myrobalan* (*Terminalia chebula*), an astringent herb that is said to possess all the tastes (different parts of the fruit have different tastes), properties and effects. Despite this emphasis on herbs with properties that are generally needed for the Tibetan climate, cooling and bitter herbs are often required to treat the disease manifestation, as inflammatory processes finally result if the pathogenic influences are not conquered or expelled.

Popular herbs used alone and in combination with other herbs are Tibetan rhodiola (*Rhodiola rosea*), known as stonecrop in the west, indicated for the treatment of dysentery, back pain, lung inflammation, painful and irregular menstruation, leukorrhoea and traumatic injuries, and *Hippophae rhamnoides* (sea buckthorn), claimed to be effective in treating ischaemic heart disease, eliminating phlegm, improving digestion and stopping coughs.

Traditional Mongolian medicine

Traditional Mongolian medicine (TMM) has developed over many years with some Mongolian doctors (*emchis*) becoming so adept in its practice that they became well known in Tibet and China. Mongolia is one of the few countries that officially supports its traditional system of medicine. However, Inner Mongolia, ruled by China, does not support TMM, and has even imprisoned people for practising it. Although herbs are the mainstay of Mongolian medicine minerals, usually in the form of powdered metals or stones, are also used. Mongolian medicine uses water as a medicine. Water is collected from any source, including the sea, and stored for many years until ready for use. Acidity and other stomach upsets were said to be amenable to water treatments.

Traditional Bhutanese medicine

The Himalayan kingdom of Bhutan is an independent state situated between China and India. It emerged as a unified polity in the early seventeenth century under the rule of an exiled Tibetan religious leader and much of its elite culture, including its medical traditions, were brought from Tibet during this period.[213] The Bhutanese traditional medical system subsequently evolved distinct characteristics that enable it to be viewed as a separate part of the Himalayan tradition of *Sowa Rigpa* ('the science of healing'), which includes what is now known as Tibetan medicine. Bhutan has evolved a state medical system in which their traditional medicine is an integral part and patients have the choice of treatment under traditional or biomedical practitioners.

As with Chinese and Tibetan medicine, the main methods of diagnosis in Bhutanese traditional medicine are feeling the pulse, checking urine, and examining the eyes and tongue, as well as interviewing the patient.[214] The Bhutanese rely on herbal combinations, limited acupuncture (including use of the golden needle), applications of heat (usually with metal rods) and minor surgical interventions, all done in the context of Buddhist ritual. A European Union project to support traditional medicine in Bhutan was initiated in the year 2000. According to data collected as part of this project, there are about 600 medicinal plants used in Bhutanese traditional medicines, out of Bhutan's 5600 identified species. About 300 of these herbs are used routinely and are at risk for ecological loss due to clearance of trees and over-collection of herbs. The EU has invested in having these herbs raised as cash crops to create jobs, provide a new medicine factory with raw materials and protect the environment.

Further reading

Bensky D, Clavey S, Stoger E, Gamble A, Bensky LL. *Chinese Herbal Medicine: Materia Medica*, 3rd edn. Vista, CA: Eastland Press, 2004.

Fan WJ-WA. *Manual of Chinese Herbal Medicine: Principles and practice for easy reference.* Boston, MA: Shambhala Publications Inc., 2003.

Maciocia G. *The Foundations of Chinese Medicine: A comprehensive text*, 2nd edn. London: Churchill Livingstone Elsevier, 2005.

MHRA. Using herbal medicines: Advice to consumers. UK MHRA website: http://tinyurl.com/6k7q9c (accessed May 2008).

More information

British Acupuncture Council: http://tinyurl.com/2hb9zo

British Medical Acupuncture Society: http://medical-acupuncture.co.uk
Chinese Medicine Advisory Service: http://tinyurl.com/yrmcg3
The Register of Chinese Herbal Medicine: www.rchm.co.uk
Karolinska Institutet Stockholm: www.mic.ki.se/China.html

References

1. Bliss B. *Chinese Medicinal Herbs*. San Francisco, CA: Georgetown Press, 1980: 3.
2. Curran J. The Yellow Emperor's Classic of Internal Medicine. *BMJ* 2008;**336**:777
3. Maoshing NI. *The Yellow Emperor's Classic of Medicine*. Boston, MA: Shambhala Publications, 1995: 318
4. Hoizey D, Hoizey M. *A History of Chinese Medicine*. Vancouver: University of British Columbia Press, 1993: 42.
5. Kaptchuk TJ. Acupuncture: theory, efficacy, and practice. *Ann Intern Med*. 2002;**136**: 374–83.
6. Williams T. *Chinese Medicine*. Shaftesbury, Dorset: Element Books, 1996.
7. Lyons A, Petrucelli RJ. *Medicine. An illustrated history*. New York: HN Abrams, 1987: 121–7.
8. Jobst KA, Shostak D, Whitehouse PJ. Editorial. *J Altern Complement Med* 1999;**6**: 495–502.
9. Selby A. *The Ancient and Healing Art of Chinese Herbalism*. London: Hamlyn, 1998.
10. Nicolai T. Important concepts and the approach to prescribing. In: Kayne SB (ed.), *Homoeopathic Practice*. London: Pharmaceutical Press, 2008: 50–1.
11. Williams T. *Chinese Medicine*. Shaftesbury, Dorset: Element Books, 1996: 31–3.
12. Kaptchuk TJ. *Chinese Medicine*. London: Rider, 2000: 105–41.
13. Fulder S. *The Handbook of Alternative and Complementary Medicine*. Oxford: Oxford University Press, 1996: 127–128.
14. Lao L. Traditional Chinese medicine. In: Jonas WB, Levin J (eds), *Essentials of Complementary and Alternative Medicine*. Baltimore, MA: Lippincott/Williams & Wilkins, 1999: 222–3.
15. Tang J-L, Zhan S-Y, Ernst E. Review of randomised controlled trials of traditional Chinese medicine. *BMJ* 1999;**319**:160–1.
16. Yu GP, Gao SW, Li Y, Gong W. A study of the quality of clinical trials in traditional Chinese medicine. *Chinese J Integrated Traditional Western Med* 1994;**14**:50–3.
17. Wu T, Li Y, Bian Z, Liu G, Moher D. Randomized trials published in some Chinese journals: how many are randomized? Trials 2009;**10**:46 Available online at http://tinyurl.com/msvcaa (Accessed 10 August 2009).
18. Houghton P. The role of plants in traditional medicine and current therapy. *J Altern Complement Med* 1995;**1**:131–43.
19. Wang G, Mao B, Xiong Z-Y et al. The quality of reporting of randomized controlled trials of traditional Chinese medicine: a survey of 13 randomly selected journals from mainland China. *Clin Therapeut* 2007;**28**:1456–67.
20. Tang J-L. Research priorities in traditional Chinese medicine. *BMJ* 2006;**333**:391–4.
21. Ulett GA, Han S, Han JS. Electroacupuncture: mechanisms and clinical application. *Biol Psychiatry* 1998;**44**:129–38.
22. Liang MX. *The Predicaments and Future of the Search for the Nature of Disease in Traditional Chinese Medicine*. Beijing: People's Medical Press, 1998: 1–48. (In Ulett et al.[20])
23. Devitt M. NCCAM Awards $9.5 million for acupuncture. *TCM Research Acupuncture Today* 2004;**5**. Available online at http://tinyurl.com/6f2fh6 (accessed 28 October 2008).
24. The State Administration of Traditional Chinese Medicine of the People's Republic of China. *Anthology of Policies, Laws and Regulations of the People's Republic of China on Traditional Chinese Medicine*. Shangdong: Shangdong University, 1997.
25. Anon. Acupunction. *Lancet* 1823;**i**:147–8.

26. Kaplan G. A brief history of acupuncture's journey to the West. *J Altern Complement Med* 1997;**3**:5–10.
27. Emslie M, Campbell M, Walker K. Complementary therapies in a local health care setting part 1: is there a real public demand? *Complement Ther Med* 1996; 4: 39–42.
28. MacDonald AJR. *Acupuncture: From ancient art to modern medicine.* Boston: George Allen & Unwin, 1982.
29. Janovsky B, White AR, Filshie J et al. Are acupuncture points tender? A blinded study of spleen 6. *J Altern Complement Med* 2000;**6**:149–55.
30. Fulder S. *The Handbook of Alternative and Complementary Medicine.* Oxford: Oxford University Press, 1996: 126.
31. Wang C, Xiong Z, Deng C, Yu W, Ma W. Miniscalpel-needle versus trigger-point injection for cervical myofascial pain syndrome: A randomised comparative trial (Letter). *J Altern Complement Med* 2007;**13**:13–18
32. White A. The safety of acupuncture techniques (Editorial). *J Altern Complement Med* 2007;**13**:9–10, 27.
33. Herbert R, Fransen M. Management of chronic knee pain (Editorial). *BMJ* 2007; **335**:786.
34. Marwick C. Acceptance of some acupuncture applications. *JAMA* 1997;**278**:1725–7.
35. Silvert M. Acupuncture wins BMA approval. *BMJ* 2000;**321**:11.
36. Moore RA, McQuay H, Oldman AD, Smith LE. BMA approves acupuncture. *BMJ* 2000;**321**:1220.
37. Vincent C, Furnham A. *Complementary Medicine. A research perspective.* Chichester: John Wiley, 1998: 160–1.
38. Godfrey CM, Morgan PA. A controlled trial of theory of acupuncture in musculoskeletal pain. *J Rheumatol* 1978;**5**:121–4.
39. Ceccherelli F, Gagliardi G, Rossato M, Giron G. Valuables of stimulation and placebo in acupuncture reflexotherapy. *J Altern Complement Med* 2000;**6**:275–9.
40. Kaptchuk TJ, Stason WB, Davis RB et al. Sham device v inert pill: randomised controlled trial of two placebo treatments. *BMJ* 2006;**332**:391–7
41. Ernst E. Clinical effectiveness of acupuncture: an overview of systematic reviews. In: Ernst E, White A (eds), *Acupuncture. A scientific appraisal.* Oxford: Butterworth-Heinemann, 1999: 107–27.
42. Hull SK, Page CP, Skinner BD, Linville JC, Coeyeaux RR. Exploring outcomes associated with acupuncture. *J Altern Complement Med* 2007;**12**:247–54.
43. Yamashia H, Tsukayama H, Hori N et al. Incidence of adverse reactions associated with acupuncture. *J Altern Complement Med* 2000;**6**:345–50.
44. Ernst E, White AR. Life threatening adverse reactions after acupuncture? A systemic review. *Pain* 1997;**71**:123–6.
45. Chen F, Hwang S, Lee H et al. Clinical study of syncope during acupuncture treatment. *Acupunct Electrother Res* 1990;**15**:107–19.
46. Brattberg G. Acupuncture treatments: a traffic hazard? *Am J Acupunct* 1986;**14**:265–7.
47. Ernst E. Adverse effects of acupuncture. In: Jonas WB, Ernst E (eds), *Essentials of CAM.* Baltimore, MA: Lippincott/Williams & Wilkins, 1999: 172–5.
48. MacPherson H. Fatal and adverse events from acupuncture: allegation, evidence and the implications. *J Altern Complement Med* 1999;**5**:47–56.
49. Rampes H, James R. Complications of acupuncture. *Acupunct Med* 1995;**11** 26–33.
50. Boxall EH. Acupuncture hepatitis in the West Midlands. *J Med Virol* 1978;**2**:377–9.
51. Hussain KK. Serum hepatitis associated with repeated acupuncture. *BMJ* 1974;**278**:41–2.
52. Vittecoq D, Metteral JF, Rouzioux C. Infection after acupuncture treatment. *N Engl J Med* 1989;**320**:250–1.
53. Castro KG, Lifson AR, White CR. Investigations of AIDS patients with no previous identification risk factors. *JAMA* 1988;**259**:1338–42.
54. Jeffreys DB, Smith S, Brennand-Roper DA, Curry PVL. Acupuncture needles as a cause of bacterial endocarditis. *BMJ* 1983;**287**:326–7.

55. Song JY, Sohn JW, Jeong HW et al. An outbreak of post-acupuncture cutaneous infection due to *Mycobacterium abscessus*. *BMC Infectious Dis* 2006;6:6.

56. Halvorsen TB, Anda SS, Naess AB, Levang OW. Fatal cardiac tamponade after acupuncture through congenital sternal foramen. *Lancet* 1995;345:1175.

57. Liou J-T, Liu F-T, Hsin S-T, Sum DCW, Lui P-W. Broken needle in the cervical spine: A previously unreported complication of *Xiaozendao* acupuncture therapy. *J Altern Complement Med* 2007;13:129–32.

58. White AR, Abbot NC, Ernst E. Self reports of adverse effects of acupuncture included cardiac arrhythmias. *Acupunct Med* 1996;14:121.

59. Ogata M, Kitamura O, Kubo S, Nakasono Q. An asthmatic death while under Chinese acupuncture and moxibustion treatment. *Am J Forensic Med Pathol* 1992;13:338–41.

60. Abbot NC, White AR, Ernst E. Complementary medicine. *Nature* 1996;381:361.

61. Fisher AA. Allergic dermatitis from acupuncture needles. *Cutis* 1976;38:226.

62. Castelain M, Castelain PY, Ricciardi R. Contact dermatitis to acupuncture needles. *Contact Dermatitis* 1987;16:44.

63. Norheim AJ, Fonnebo V. Acupuncture adverse effects are more than occasional case reports: results from questionnaires among 1135 randomly selected doctors and 297 acupuncturists. *Complement Ther Med* 1996;4:8–13.

64. Fujiwara H, Taniguchi J, Ikezono E. The influence of low frequency acupuncture on a demand pacemaker. *Chest* 1980;78:96–7.

65. Lyle CD, Thomas BM, Gordon EA, Krauthamer V. Electrostimulators for acupuncture: safety issues. *J Altern Complement Med* 2000;6:37–44.

66. Carron H, Epstein BS, Grand B. Complications of acupuncture. *JAMA* 1974;228: 1552–4.

67. Hung VC, Mines JS. Eschars and scarring from hot needle acupuncture treatment. *J Am Acad Dermatol* 1991;24:148–9.

68. Filshie J, White AR, eds. *Medical Acupuncture, A Western Scientific Approach*. Edinburgh: Churchill Livingstone, 1998.

69. Macdonald AJR. Acupuncture and analgesia and therapy. In: Wall PD, Melzack R (eds), *Textbook of Pain*, 2nd edn. Edinburgh: Churchill Livingstone, 1989.

70. White A. The principles behind acupuncture. *Health Matters Magazine* 1999;May:30–1.

71. Ernst E, White A. Acupuncture: safety first. *BMJ* 1997;314:1362.

72. Mann F. *Reinventing Acupuncture*. Oxford: Butterworth Press, 1993.

73. Cummings M. Acupuncture techniques should be treated logically and methodically. *BMJ* 2001;322:47b.

74. Ernst E, White AR. Acupuncture for back pain: a meta analysis of randomised controlled trials. *Arch Intern Med* 1998;158:2235–41.

75. van Tulder MW, Cherkin DC, Berman B et al. The effectiveness of acupuncture in the management of acute and chronic low back pain. *Spine* 1999;24:1113–23.

76. MacPherson H, Gould AJ, Fitter M. Acupuncture for low back pain: results of a pilot study for a randomised controlled trial. *Complement Ther Med* 1999;7:83–90.

77. Report on 10th Annual Symposium on Complementary Healthcare. *J Chinese Med* 2004;74:59.

78. Ratcliffe J, Thomas KJ, MacPherson H, Brazier J. A randomised controlled trial of acupuncture care for persistent low back pain: cost effectiveness analysis. *BMJ* 2006;333: 626.

79. Ernst E, Pittler MH. The effectiveness of acupuncture in treating acute dental pain: a systematic review. *Br Dental J* 1998;184:443–7.

80. Vickers AJ, Rees RW, Zollman CE et al Acupuncture for chronic headache in primary care: large, pragmatic, randomised trial. *BMJ* 2004;328:744.

81. Melchart D, Streng A, Hoppe A et al. Acupuncture in patients with tension-type headache: randomised controlled trial. *BMJ* 2005;331:376–82.

82. Vickers AJ, Rees RW, Zollman CE et al. Acupuncture for chronic headache in primary care: large, pragmatic, randomised trial. *BMJ* 2004;328:744.

83. White A, Foster NE, Cummings M, Barlas P. Acupuncture treatment for chronic knee pain: a systematic review. *Rheumatology (Oxford)* 2007;**46**:384–90.

84. Milgrom C, Finestone A, Eldad A, Shlamkovitch N. Patellofemoral pain caused by over-activity. A prospective study of risk factors in infantry recruits. *J Bone Joint Surg Am* 1991;**73**:1041–3.

85. Jensen R, Gothesen O, Liseth K, Baerheim A. Acupuncture treatment of patellofemoral pain syndrome. *J Altern Complement Med* 1999;**5**:521–7.

86. Ross J, White A, Ernst E. Western minimal acupuncture for neck pain: a cohort study. *Acupunct Med* 1999;**17**:5–8.

87. Irnich D, Behrens N, Molzen H et al. Randomised trial of acupuncture compared with conventional massage and 'sham' laser acupuncture for treatment of chronic neck pain. *BMJ* 2001;**322**:1574–9.

88. White AR, Ernst E. A systematic review of randomised controlled trials of acupuncture for neck pain. *Rheumatology* 1999;**38**:143–7.

89. Elden H, Ladfors L, Fagevik O et al. Effects of acupuncture and stabilising exercises as adjunct to standard treatment in pregnant women with pelvic girdle pain: randomised single blind controlled trial. *BMJ* 2005;**330**:761

90. Usichenko TI, Kuchling S, Witstruck T et al. Auricular acupuncture for pain relief after ambulatory knee surgery: a randomized trial. *Can Med Assoc J* 2007;**176**:179–83.

91. Avants SK, Margolin A, Holford TR, Kosten TR. A randomised controlled trial of auricular acupuncture for cocaine dependence. *Arch Intern Med* 2000;**160**:2305–6.

92. Margolin A, Avants SK. Should cocaine abusing, buprenorphine maintained patients receive auricular acupuncture? Findings from an acute effects study. *J Altern Complement Med* 1999;**5**:567–74.

93. Lu L, Fang Y, Wang X. Drug abuse in China: Past, present and future. *Cell Mol Neurobiol* 2007;**28**:479–90.

94. Diehl D. Acupuncture for gastrointestinal and hepatobiliary disorders. *J Altern Complement Med* 1999;**5**:27–45.

95. Beal MW, Nield-Anderson L. Acupuncture for symptom relief in HIV positive adults: lessons learned from a pilot study. *Altern Ther Health Med* 2000;**6**:33–42.

96. Chen HY, Shi Y, Ng CS, Chan SM, Yung KKL. Auricular acupuncture treatment for insomnia: A systematic review. *J Altern Complement Med* 2007;**13**:660–76.

97. Vickers AJ. Can acupuncture have specific effects on health? A systematic review of acupuncture antiemesis trials. *J R Soc Med* 1996;**89**:303–11.

98. Ernst E. Acupuncture as a symptomatic treatment for osteoarthritis – a systematic review. *Scand J Rheumatol* 1997;**26**:444–7.

99. Foster NE, Thomas E, Barlas P et al. Acupuncture as an adjunct to exercise based physio-therapy for osteoarthritis of the knee: randomised controlled trial. *BMJ* 2007;**335**:436.

100. Scharf HP, Mansmann U, Streitberger K et al. Acupuncture and knee osteoarthritis. *Ann Intern Med* 2006;**145**:12–20.

101. Vas J, Méndez C, Perea-Milla E et al. Acupuncture as a complementary therapy to the pharmacological treatment of osteoarthritis of the knee: randomised controlled trial. *BMJ* 2004;**329**:1216.

102. Minns Lowe CJ, Barker KL, Dewey M, Sackley CM. Effectiveness of physiotherapy exer-cise after knee arthroplasty for osteoarthritis: systematic review and meta-analysis of randomised controlled trials. *BMJ* 2007;**335**:812–15.

103. Lee H, Ernst E. Acupuncture for labor pain management: a systematic review. *Am J Obstet Gynecol* 2004;**191**:1573–9.

104. Smith CA, Collins CT, Cyna AM, Crowther CA. Complementary and alternative therapies for pain management in labour. *Cochrane Database Syst Rev* 2006;**4**:CD003521.

105. Elden H, Ladfors L, Olsen MF, Ostgaard HC, Hagberg H. Effects of acupuncture and stabilising exercises as adjunct to standard treatment in pregnant women with pelvic girdle pain: randomised single blind controlled trial. *BMJ* 2005;**330**:761.

106. Wedenberg K, Moen B, Norling A. A prospective randomized study comparing acupunc-

ture with physiotherapy for low-back and pelvic pain in pregnancy. *Acta Obstet Gynecol Scand* 2000;**79**:331–5.

107. Kvorning N, Holmberg C, Grennert L, Aberg A, Akeson J. Acupuncture relieves pelvic and low-back pain in late pregnancy. *Acta Obstet Gynecol Scand* 2004;**83**:246–50.

108. Gaudernack LC, Forbord S, Hole E. Acupuncture administered after spontaneous rupture of membranes at term significantly reduces the length of birth and use of oxytocin. A randomized controlled trial. *Acta Obstet Gynecol Scand* 2006;**85**:1348–53.

109. Anja Pinborg, Loft A, Andersen AN. Acupuncture with in vitro fertilisation (Editorial). *BMJ* 2008;**336**:517–18.

110. Manheimer E, Zhang G, Udoff L et al. Effects of acupuncture on rates of pregnancy and live birth among women undergoing in vitro fertilisation: systematic review and meta-analysis *BMJ* 2008;**336**:545–9.

111. Wang W, Check JH, Liss JR, Choe JK A matched controlled study to evaluate the efficacy of acupuncture for improving pregnancy rates following in vitro fertilization-embryo transfer. *Clin Exp Obstet Gynecol* 2007;**34**:137–8.

112. Kleinherz J, Streitberger K, Windeler J et al. Randomised clinical trial comparing the effects of acupuncture and a newly designed placebo needle in rotator cuff tendonitis. *Pain* 1999;**83**:235–41.

113. Dyson-Hudson T, Kadar P, LaFountaine M et al. Acupuncture for chronic shoulder pain in persons with spinal cord injury: a small-scale clinical trial. *Arch Phys Med Rehabil* 2008;**88**:1276–83.

114. White AR, Rampes H, Ernst E. Acupuncture for smoking cessation. *Cochrane Library* 1999;**4**:1–10.

115. Ernst E, White AR. Acupuncture as an adjuvant therapy in stroke rehabilitation? *Wien Med Wochenschr* 1996;**146**:556–8.

116. Gosman-Hedstroem G, Cleeson L, Klingenstierna U et al. Effects of acupuncture treatment on daily life activities and quality of life. *Stroke* 1998;**29**:2100–8.

117. Johansson K, Lindgren I, Widner H et al. Can sensory stimulation improve the functional outcome in stroke patients? *Neurology* 1993;**43**:2189–92.

118. Ernst E, White AR. Acupuncture as a treatment for temporomandibular joint dysfunction. *Arch Otolaryngol Head Neck Surg* 1999;**125**:269–72.

119. Yeh CH, Yeh SC. Effects of ear points' pressing on parameters related to obesity in non-obese healthy and obese volunteers. *J Altern Complement Med* 2008;**14**:309–14.

120. Law S, Li T. Acupuncture for glaucoma. *Cochrane Database Syst Rev* 2007;**4**: CD006030.

121. He L, Zhou M, Zhou D, Wu B, Li N. Acupuncture for Bell's palsy. *Cochrane Database Syst Rev* 2007;**4**:CD002914.

122. BMA Ethics Science and Information Division. *Acupuncture: Efficacy, safety and practice.* Amsterdam: Harwood Academic Publishers, 2000: 66–81.

123. Reilly DT. Young doctors' views on alternative medicine. *BMJ* 1983;**287**:337–9.

124. Anderson E, Anderson P. General practitioner and alternative medicine. *J R Coll Gen Practit* 1987;**37**:52–5.

125. Wharton R, Lewith G. Complementary medicine and the general practitioner. *BMJ* 1986;**292**:1498–500.

126. White AR, Resch K-L, Ernst E. Complementary medicine: use and attitudes among GPs. *Fam Pract* 1997;**14**:302–6.

127. Thomas K, Fall M, Parry G, Nicholl J. *National Survey of Access to Complementary Health Care via General Practice.* Department of Health report. Sheffield: Medical Care Unit, 1995.

128. Berman BM, Singh BK, Lao L et al. Physicians' attitudes toward complementary or alternative medicine: a regional survey. *J Am Board Fam Pract* 1995;**8**:361–6.

129. Hadley CM. Complementary medicine and the general practitioner: a survey of general practitioners in the Wellington area. *NZ Med J* 1988;**101**:765–8.

130. Marshall RJ, Gee R, Dumble J et al. The use of alternative therapies by Auckland general practitioners. *NZ Med J* 1990;**103**:213–15.

131. Easthope G, Beilby JJ, Gill GF, Tranter BK. Acupuncture in Australian general practice: practitioner characteristics. *Med J Aust* 1998;**169**:197–200.

132. Wonderling D, Vickers AJ, Grieve R, McCarney R. Cost effectiveness analysis of a randomised trial of acupuncture for chronic headache in primary care. *BMJ* 2004; **328**:747.

133. Canter PH, Thompson Coon J, Ernst E. Cost effectiveness of complementary treatments in the United Kingdom: systematic review. *BMJ* 2005;**331**:880–1.

134. Ratcliffe J, Thomas KJ, MacPherson H, Brazier J. A randomised controlled trial of acupuncture care for persistent low back pain: cost effectiveness analysis. *BMJ* 2006; **333**:626.

135. Maniadakis N, Gray A. The economic burden of back pain in the UK. *Pain* 2000;**84**: 95–103.

136. Thomas KJ, MacPherson H, Thorpe L et al. Randomised controlled trial of a short course of traditional acupuncture compared with usual care for persistent non-specific low back pain. *BMJ* 2006;**333**:623.

137. Reston J. Now about my operation in Peking. *The New York Times* 26 July 1971.

138. Kaptchuk TJ. Acupuncture: Theory, efficacy, and practice *Ann Intern Med* 2002;**136**: 374–83.

139. Cooper RA, Henderson T, Dietrich CL. Roles of non physician clinicians as autonomous providers of patient care. *JAMA* 1998;**280**:795–802.

140. Burke A, Upchurch D, Dye C, Chyu L. Acupuncture use in the United States: Findings from the National Health Interview Survey. *J Altern Complement Med* 2006;**12**:639–48.

141. Jarmey C, Tindall J. *Acupressure for Common Ailments*. London: Gala Books, 1991.

142. Marti JE. *Alternative Health Medicine Encyclopedia*. Detroit: Visible Ink Press, 1995: 3.

143. Bruce DG, Golding JF, Hockenhulkl N, Pethybridge RJ. Acupressure and motion sickness. *Aviat Space Environment Med* 1990;**61**:361–5.

144. Hu S, Stritzel R, Chandler A, Stern R M. P6 acupressure reduces symptoms of vection induced motion sickness. *Aviat Space Environment Med* 1995;**66**:631–4.

145. Murphy PA. Alternative therapies for nausea and vomiting of pregnancy. *Obstet Gynecol* 1998;**91**:149–55.

146. O'Brien B, Relyea MJ, Taerum T. Efficacy of P6 acupuncture in the treatment of nausea and vomiting during pregnancy. *Am J Obstet Gynecol* 1996;**174**:708–15.

147. Li-Chen L, Hsiah LL-C, Kuo C-H, Lee LH, Yen A M-F, Chien K-L, Chen TH-H. Treatment of low back pain by acupressure and physical therapy: randomised controlled trial. *BMJ* 2006;**332**:696–700.

148. Unschuld PU. *Medicine in China. A history of pharmaceuticals*. Berkeley, CA: University of California Press, 2000.

149. Harrison Nolting M, Cao Q. Introduction to the clinical use of Chinese prepared medicines. In: Pizzorno J Jr, Murray MT (eds), *Textbook of Natural Medicine*, 2nd edn. Edinburgh: Churchill Livingstone, 1999: 807–14.

150. Vickers A, Zellman C. ABC of complementary medicine – herbal medicine. *BMJ* 1999; **319**:1050–3.

151. Houghton P. Traditional Chinese medicine: does it work? Is it safe? *Chemist Druggist* 1999: vi–vii.

152. Mintel International Group. *Complementary Medicine. Mintel Report*. London: Mintel International Group, 2001.

153. Cassidy C. Chinese medicine users in the United States part 1: utilization, satisfaction, medical plurality. *J Altern Complement Med* 1998;**4**:17–27.

154. Lao L. Traditional Chinese medicine. In: Jonas WB, Levin J (eds). *Essentials of Complementary and Alternative Medicine*. Baltimore, MA: Lippincott/Williams & Wilkins, 1999: 215.

155. Ye Z. Future Issues with Complementary and Alternative Medicine Report of FIP Congress Beijing 2007. *Pharm J* 2007;**279**(suppl F8).

156. Dharmananda S. *Controlled Clinical Trials of Chinese Herbal Medicine: A review*. Oregon: Institute for Traditional Medicine, 1997.

157. Lampert N. Letter. *Lancet* 2001;**357**:882.

158. Sheehan MP, Rustin MHA, Atherton DJ et al. Efficacy of traditional Chinese herbal therapy in adult atopic dermatitis. *Lancet* 1992;**340**:13–17.

159. Bensoussan A, Menzies R. Treatment of irritable bowel syndrome with Chinese herbal medicine. *JAMA* 1998;**280**:1585–9.

160. Rasmussen P. Chinese herbs – more evidence. *NZ Pharm* 2008;**28**:16–17.

161. Sheehan MP, Atherton DJ. A controlled trial of traditional Chinese medicinal plants in widespread non-exudative eczema. *Br J Dermatol* 1992;**126**:179–84.

162. Hon KLF, Leung TF, Ng PC et al. Efficacy and tolerability of a Chinese herbal medicine concoction for treatment of atopic dermatitis: a randomized, double-blind, placebo-controlled study *Br J Dermatol* 2007;**157**:357–63.

163. Zhang M, Liu X, Li J, He L, Tripathy D. Chinese medicinal herbs to treat the side-effects of chemotherapy in breast cancer patients. *Cochrane Database Syst Rev* 2007;**2**: CD004921.

164. Wei X, Chen ZY, Yang XY, Wu TX. Medicinal herbs for esophageal cancer. *Cochrane Database Syst Rev* 2007;**2**.

165. Mok TSK, Yeo W, Johnson PJ et al. A double-blind placebo-controlled randomized study of Chinese herbal medicine as complementary therapy for reduction of chemotherapy-induced toxicity. *Ann Oncol* 2007;**18**:768–74.

166. Barnes J, Teng K. TCM: balancing choice and risk? *Pharm J* 2004;**273**:342.

167. Williams D. Greater expertise in TCM needed worldwide (Letter). *Pharm J* 2004;**273**: 221.

168. Bomme U, Bauer R, Fiedl F et al. Cultivating Chinese medicinal plants in Germany. *J Altern Complement Med* 2007;**13**:597–601.

169. Bateman J, Chapman RD, Simpson D. Possible toxicity of herbal remedies. *Scot Med J* 1998;**43**:7–15.

170. Chan TVK, Chan JCN, Tomlinson B, Critchley JAH. Chinese herbal medicine revisited: a Hong Kong perspective. *Lancet* 1993;**342**:1532–4.

171. Kao W-F, Hung D-Z, Tsai W-J et al. Podophyllotoxin intoxication: toxic effects of Bajiao-lian in herbal therapeutics. *Human Exp Toxicol* 1992;**11**:480–7.

172. Barnes J, Anderson LA, Phillipsson JD. *Herbal Medicines. A Guide for Health-care Professionals*, 3rd edn. London: Pharmaceutical Press, 2007.

173. Chan TKY. The prevalence, use and harmful potential of some Chinese herbal medicines in babies and children. *Vet Human Toxicol* 1994;**26**:238–40.

174. Thomson L. Chinese capsules face short shift. *NZ Pharm* 2001;**22**:8.

175. McGregoor FB, Abernethy VE, Dahabra S et al. Chinese herbs for eczema. *Lancet* 1989;**299**:1156–7.

176. Hughes JR, Higgins EM, Pembroke AC. Dexamethasone masquerading as a Chinese herbal. *Br J Dermatol* 1994;**130**:261.

177. Keane FM, Munn SF, du Vivier AWP et al. Analysis of Chinese herbal creams prescribed for dermatological conditions. *BMJ* 1999;**518**:563–4.

178. Vander Stricht BI, Parvais OE, Vanhaelen-Fastre RJ, Vanhaelen MH. Remedies may contain cocktail of active drugs. *BMJ* 1994;**308**:1162.

179. Press release: Serious health risk posed by Traditional Chinese Medicine 'Herbal Viagra' London: MHRA, 7 April 2009. Available online at http://tinyurl.com/dg7w4n (accessed 6 May 2009).

180. Kayne SB. Comment – *Aristolochia* – A case for exclusion. *Good Clin Pract J* 2001;**8**: 9–11.

181. Vanherweghem J-L, Depierreux M, Tielmans C et al. Rapidly progressing interstitial renal fibrosis in young women: association with slimming regimen including Chinese herbs. *Lancet* 1993;**341**:387–91.

182. Vanherweghem J-L. Misuse of herbal remedies: the case of an outbreak of terminal renal failure in Belgium (Chinese herb nephropathy). *J Altern Complement Med* 1998;**4**:9–13.

183. Depierreux M, Van Den Houte K, Vanherweghem J-L. Pathological aspects of newly

prescribed nephropathy related to prolonged use of Chinese herbs. *Am J Kidney Dis* 1994;**24**:172–80.

184. But PP. Need for correct identification of herbs in herbal poisoning. *Lancet* 1993;**341**: 637.

185. Van Haelen M, Van Haelen-Fastre R, But PPH, Vanherweghem ML. Identification of aristolochic acids in Chinese herbs. *Lancet* 1994;**343**:174.

186. *British National Formulary*, number 56. London: British Medical Association/Royal Pharmaceutical Society of Great Britain, September 2008.

187. McIntyre M. Chinese herbs: risk, side effects and poisoning: the case for objective reporting, and analysis reveals serious misrepresentation. *J Altern Complement Med* 1998;**4**:15–16.

188. Levi M, Guchelaar HJ, Woerdenbag HJ, Zhu YP. Acute hepatitis in a patient using a Chinese tea – a case report. *Pharm World Sci* 1998;**20**:43–4.

189. Working Party. *Report on Herbal Medicinal Products*. London: EMEA, 2000: 8.

190. Lord GM, Tagore R, Cook T et al. Nephropathy caused by Chinese herbs in the UK. *Lancet* 1999;**354**:481–2.

191. Chinese Herbal Medicines in Australia found to contain *Aristolochia. Report of Therapeutic Goods Administration*. Canberra: Department of Health and Aged Care, 1999.

192. Working Party. *Report on Herbal Medicinal Products*. London: EMEA, 2000: 4–5.

193. Ascher S. Mycotoxins in Herbal Medicinal Drugs. Report of Pharmacovigilance of herbal medicines – current state and future directions at the Royal College of Obstetrics and Gynaecology London from 26 to 28 April 2006. *Pharm J* 2006;**276**:543–5.

194. Kayne SB. Biodiversity and sustainability. In: *Complementary and Alternative Medicine. The traditional health care environment*. London: Pharmaceutical Press, 2009: 404–12.

195. World Wide Fund for Nature. *Prescription for Extinction: Endangered species and patented oriental medicines in trade*. Washington DC: Traffic, 1994.

196. Mills SY. Chinese herbs in the west. In: Evans WC (ed.), *Trease and Evans' Pharmacognosy*, 15th edn. Edinburgh: WB Saunders, 2002: 506–9.

197. Lao L. Traditional Chinese medicine. In: Jonas WB, Levin J (eds), *Essentials of Complementary and Alternative Medicine*. Baltimore, MA: Lippincott/Williams & Wilkins, 1999: 226–7.

198. Zollman VA. *ABC of Complementary Medicine*. London: BMJ Books, 2000: 36.

199. Windridge C. *Tong Sing, The Chinese Book of Wisdom*. London: Kyle Cathie, 1999: 211–19.

200. Massey PB. Medicine and the martial arts: a brief historical perspective. *Altern Complement Ther* 1998;**4**:128–33.

201. Massey PB, Kisling GM. A single case report of healing through specific martial art therapy: comparison of MRI to clinical resolution in severe cervical stenosis: a case report. *J Altern Complement Med* 1999;**5**:75–9.

202. Xin L, Miller YD, Brown W. A qualitative review of the role of qigong in the management of diabetes. *J Altern Complement Med* 2007;**13**:427–33.

203. Wolf SL, Barnhart HX, Kutner NG, McNeely E, Coogler C, Xu T. Reducing frailty and falls in older persons: an investigation of tai chi and computerized balance training. *J Am Geriatr Soc* 1996;**44**:489–97.

204. Wolf SL, Sattin RW, Kutner M, O'Grady M, Greenspan AI, Gregor RI. Intense tai chi exercise training and fall occurrences in older, transitionally frail adults: a randomized, controlled trial. *J Am Geriatr Soc* 2003;**51**:1693–701.

205. Wolfson L, Whipple R, Derby C et al. Balance and strength training in older adults: intervention gains and Tai Chi maintenance. *J Am Geriatr Soc* 1996;**44**:498–506.

206. Li F, Harmer P, Fisher KJ et al. Tai chi and fall reductions in older adults: a randomized controlled trial. *J Gerontol Med Sci* 2005;**60A**:187–94.

207. Han A, Judd MG, Robinson VA, Taixiang W, Tugwell P, Wells G. Tai chi for treating rheumatoid arthritis. *Cochrane Database Syst Rev* 2004;**3**:CD004849.

208. Wayne PM, Kielb DP, Krebs DE et al. The effects of Tai Chi on bone mineral density in postmenopausal women: a systematic review. *Arch Phys Med Rehabil* 2007;**88**:673–80.
209. Woo J, Hong A, Lau E, Lynn H. A randomised controlled trial of Tai Chi and resistance exercise on bone health, muscle strength and balance in community-living elderly people. *Age Ageing* 2007;**36**:262–8.
210. Loizzo JJ, Blackhall LJ, Rabgyay L. Tibetan medicine: a complementary science of optimal health. *Ann N Y Acad Sci* 2007;Sept 28 (PubMed).
211. Dharmananda S. *Tibetan Herbal Medicine.* Available at: http://tinyurl.com/2v5rnp (accessed 19 October 2008).
212. Wang Jinhui. The characteristics of the Jingzhu Bencao. *Chinese J Ethnomed Ethnopharm* 1995;**13**:4–5. (In Dharmananda.[210])
213. McKay A, Wangchuk D. Traditional medicine in Bhutan. *Asian Med* 2005;**1**:204–18.
214. Dharmananda S. *Traditional Medicine of Bhutan.* Available at: www.itmonline.org/arts/bhutan.htm (accessed 10 November 2008).

7

Indian ayurvedic medicine

Steven Kayne

The indigenous system of medicine in India is termed 'ayurveda' (*ayu* means life or longevity and *veda* means knowledge). Other related systems that are less well known in the west but may be just as popular in some areas of south and south-east Asia include unani, siddha and jamu. They are considered briefly at the end of this chapter.

Ayurveda and traditional Chinese medicine (TCM) have many commonalities. Both systems fundamentally aim to promote health and enhance the quality of life, with therapeutic strategies for treatment of specific diseases or symptoms in holistic fashion. Almost half of the botanical sources used as medicines have similarities; moreover, both systems have similar philosophies geared towards enabling classification of individuals, materials and diseases.[1]

The main focus of ayurvedic practice is found on the Indian subcontinent but there are other areas in the world where the system is evident too, as Figure 7.1 shows.[2]

Definition

Ayurveda is an ancient system of personalised medicine documented and practised in India since 1500 BC. According to this system an individual's basic constitution to a large extent determines predisposition and prognosis to diseases as well as therapy and life-style regime. Disease is considered to be an imbalance and its treatment involves diverse procedures to restore optimum function and balance. Practitioners use nutrition, yoga, exercise, complex herbal medicines and surgical techniques reactively as therapies and proactively for the preservation of health.

History

The origins of the 'science of life' have been placed by scholars of ancient Indian ayurvedic literature at somewhere around 6000 BC.[3] The teachings

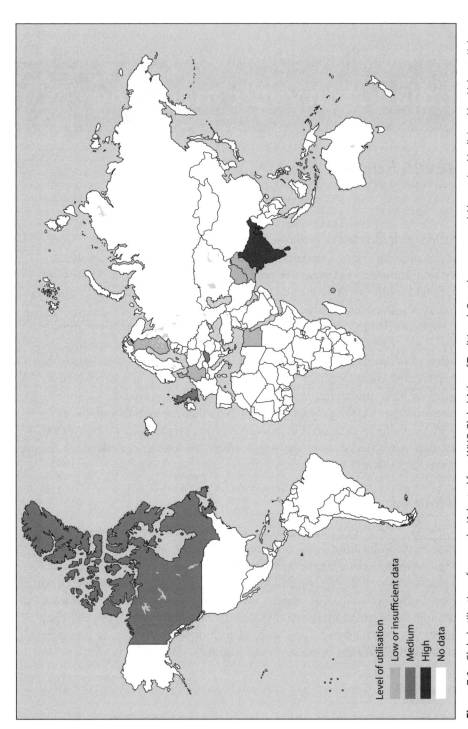

Figure 7.1 Global utilisation of ayurveda. (Adapted from WHO Global Atlas of Traditional, Complementary and Alternative Medicine, Map Volume. Kobe, Japan: WHO Centre for Health Development, 2005:47.)

were orally transmitted for thousands of years and then written down in melodic Sanskrit poetic verses known as *shlokas*. Ayurveda in its first recorded form (literature known as vedas) is specifically called atharveda.

Indian medicine spread across the eastern world to Tibet, central Asia, Indo-China, Indonesia and Japan, filling the same role in Asia as Greek medicine did in the west. The surgical and medical aspects of ayurveda developed separately around the eighth century BC, and were recorded in great detail in texts (*samhitas*). The surgical principles of ayurveda were explained by Sushruta, considered to be the father of surgery in his partic-ular samhita, a text known as the *Sushruta Samhita*. He described a number of techniques and instruments familiar to modern-day surgery: pre- and postoperative care, asepsis, suturing and sterilisation. He also described 141 types of surgical instruments and a number of surgical procedures, including the treatment of cataracts, haemorrhoids and bone problems, as well as techniques involved in cosmetic surgery such as rhinoplasty.[4]

The early medical aspects of ayurveda were collected and revised by Charak around the first century AD in his *samhita* and this work has provided the basis for future practice over the centuries. Charak's text described the significance of the *vata*, *pitta* and *kapha doshas*, elements that form the basis of *tridosha* physiology (see below), the seven tissues (*dhatus*) and the three excretions (*malas*), as well as giving information on the treatment of disease and the preparation of drugs. Other important compendia were written during the first and second centuries by Sushruta (also spelt Susruta) and Vagbhata, who together with Charak are considered to be the great three fathers of ayurveda.

Theory

Ayurvedic philosophy is based on the *samkhya* philosophy of creation. The word *samkhya* is derived from the Sanskrit *sat* (truth) and *khya* (to know). The main beliefs are as follows:

- There is a close relationship between humans and the universe.
- Cosmic energy is manifest in all things, both living and non-living.
- There are 24 elements of the universe.
- Cosmic consciousness is the source of all existence present as male (*shiva*, *purusha*) and female (*shakti*, *pakritt*) energy.

The general ayurvedic approach involves:

- determining the constitution of the patient and identifying the cause of the illness
- applying therapeutic measures to balance any disharmonies.

Determining the constitution and the cause of illness

Ayurveda embraces certain fundamental doctrines, known as the *darshnas*. The body is thought of as being composed of the following basic concepts:

- The five basic elements of life (*pancha mahabhutas*).
- The humours (*doshas*)
- The seven tissues (*dhatus*)
- The three waste products (*malas*)
- The gastric fire (*agni*).

Health is believed to comprise a balanced state of the *doshas* (made from five basic elements and senses), the *dhatus*, the *malas* and a gastric fire (*agni*), together with the clarity and balance of the mind, senses and spirit.

The basis of ayurvedic theory is summarised in Figure 7.2.

The five basic elements of life (*pancha mahabhutas*)

Ayurveda considers that the universe is made up of combinations of the five elements (*pancha mahabhutas*). These are *akasha* (ether), *vayu* (air), *teja* (fire), *aapa* (water) and *prithvi* (earth). The five elements can be seen to exist

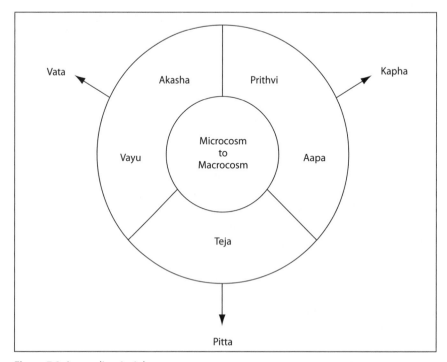

Figure 7.2 Ayurvedic principles.

in the material universe at all scales of life and in both organic and inorganic things. The five basic elements join together in different combinations to make up the three *doshas* (or humours):

- Ether (space), represented in the hollow spaces of the mouth, nose, gastrointestinal tract, thorax, capillaries and tissues – associated with the sense of hearing (ear and speech)
- Air, represented by movement of the various organs, i.e. expansion, contraction and pulsation – associated with touch (hand)
- Fire, the source of heat and represented by metabolism, digestion, body heat and intelligence – associated with sight (eyes)
- Water exists as secretions of the salivary glands and mucous membranes – associated with taste (tongue)
- Earth, represented by solid structures of the body, i.e. bones, cartilage and muscles – associated with smell (nose).

These five basic elements control all biological and psychological functions of the body, mind and consciousness. They are also responsible for emotions, including anger, compassion, fear, greed and love.

The humours (*doshas*)

Ayurveda believes that people may be of seven broad constitutional types (*prakritis*) each with a varying degree of predisposition to different diseases. It is believed that *prakriti* (*pra* means before and *akriti* means conception) is determined at conception and depends on the permutation and combination of the *doshas* (where *dosha* means a 'principle' that is protective in health or disease producing in ill-health). Among these, the three most contrasting *doshas*, *vata*, *pitta* and *kapha*, are known collectively as the *tridosha*. Ether and air are said to be the *vata dosha*, fire and water combine as the *pitta dosha* and earth and water combine as the *kapha dosha*. Various responsibilities are ascribed to the doshas:

- *Vata* is responsible for all body movement; it represents the nervous system and controls the emotions of fear and anxiety. *Vata* areas include the large intestine, pelvic cavity, skin and ears.
- *Pitta* governs digestion, absorption, nutrition, skin colour, intelligence and understanding. It arouses hate and jealousy. *Pitta* areas include the small intestine, stomach, blood, eyes and skin. It governs all heat, metabolism and transformation in the mind and body.
- *Kapha* is present in the throat, chest, head, sinuses, nose, mouth, etc. It governs body resistance and biological strength, promotes wound healing and supports memory. Psychologically *kapha* governs greed, envy and love.

A balance of the *doshas* is necessary for optimal health. In childhood *kapha* elements associated with growth predominate; in adulthood *pitta* is more important, while as the body deteriorates in old age *vata* becomes more important. When there is an imbalance or disharmony in health more than one *dosha* may be present.

Physical constitution

Bodily features may be characterised in terms of the doshas. For example, a person having a vata prakriti would be light-weight, tall and ill-nourished, a *pitta prakriti* would be characterised by moderate weight and a well-nourished appearance and a *kapha prakriti* would be typically associated with a heavily built person. Examples of *prakriti* are presented in Table 7.1.[5]

Mental constitution

Three *guras* or temperaments correspond to the humours that determine physical constitution, as described above, and are responsible for a person's behaviour patterns. They are, with brief examples of the main characteristics:

- *Satvas*: people with a *satva* temperament have healthy bodies and moderate behaviour. They are often very religious, compassionate and loving.
- *Rajas*: people who are interested in business, prosperity, power and prestige. They enjoy wealth and are extroverts.
- *Tamas*: people who are ignorant, lazy, selfish and show little respect for others.

In the realm of modern predictive medicine, efforts are being directed towards capturing disease phenotypes with greater precision for successful identification of markers for prospective disease conditions. Differences in biochemical profiles including liver function tests, lipid profiles and haematological parameters such as haemoglobin have been shown to exist between *prakriti* types.[6]

Disease

Allergies can result from an imbalance of any or all three of the *doshas* although typically one of them will characterise the reaction.[7] The *vata dosha* or bioenergetic principle of movement is always involved because an imbalanced *vata* lowers immunity, making one susceptible in the first instance. An incessantly runny nose, fatigue, continuous sneezing and throbbing headaches further indicate *vata*-type allergies. Heated, red eyes, sharp sinus headaches, fevers and itching skin indicate *pitta*-type allergies. A build-up of congested mucus indicates *kapha*-type allergies. The condition may be relieved by ayurvedic practices including nasal irrigation and breathing exercises.

Table 7.1 Examples of *pakriti* characteristics

Characteristic	Pitta	Vata	Kapha
Body size	Medium	Slim	Large
Body weight	Medium	Low	High
Eyes	Sharp, bright, grey–green	Small, sunken, black or brown	Big, blue
Nose	Long, pointed	Uneven shape	Short, round
Skin	Oily, smooth, warm	Thin, dry, cold	Thick, oily, cool
Teeth	Medium, tender gums	Protruding, thin gums	Healthy Strong gums
Appetite	Strong	Irregular, scant	Slow, steady
Digestion	Quick with burning	Irregular with wind	Prolonged with mucus
Taste preference	Sweet, bitter	Sweet, sour, salty	Bitter, pungent
Emotions	Anger, jealousy	Anxiety, fear	Greedy
Intellect	Accurate	Quick, careless	Slow, exact
Finance	Spends on luxuries	Poor, wastes money	Thrifty, astute

The seven tissues (*dhatus*)

The seven tissues are:

- plasma or cytoplasm (*ras*), which contains nutrients from digested food
- blood (*rakata*), which governs oxygenation
- muscles (*mamsa*), which maintain the physical strength of the body
- bone and cartilage (*asthi*), which give support to the body
- bone marrow and nerves (*majja*), which fill bony spaces and facilitate communication
- fat (*medas*) responsible for body bulk
- the sex hormones and immune system (*shukra*).

Each of the *dhatus* depends on its predecessor for good health, and for good health all must function correctly.

The three waste products (*malas*)

These are sweat (*svet*), faeces (*poorish*) and urine (*mutra*). They must be produced in appropriate amounts and eliminated through their respective channels.

The gastric fire (*agni*)

The final element important for healthy life is *agni*, the 'fire' that sustains vitality. *Agni* covers whole sequences of chemical interactions and changes in the body and mind. It has been compared to the digestive enzymes but is considered to be responsible for more than just the biochemical processes because it also maintains the health of the immune system, and is claimed to destroy microorganisms and toxins in the gut.

Applying therapeutic measures to balance any disharmonies – the practice of ayurveda

Specialties

Eight specialities have developed within ayurveda:

- General surgery (*shalya tantra*)
- Ear, nose and throat (*shalkya*)
- Medicine (*kaya chikitsa*)
- Psychiatry (*bhutvidya*)
- Obstetrics, gynaecology and paediatrics (*kumar-bhritya*)
- Toxicology (*agada tantra*)
- Geriatrics (*rasayans*)
- Fertility and sterility (*vajikaran*).

Choice of treatment

After a diagnosis has been made as to the particular dysfunction or disharmony present, there are many different types of treatment available to the ayurvedic practitioner, all of which may be used alone or to complement each other and include:

- dietary advice
- administration of medicines
- aromatherapy
- enemas
- massage
- mind–body interventions
- surgery.

Dietary advice

Just as with traditional Chinese medicine, Indian medicine places importance on diet. Diet is considered to be particularly important for both its direct effect on the individual's physiological state and its influence on the medicine. Inadequate digestion will result in the formulation of inter-mediary products. It is suggested that a build-up of these intermediate prod-ucts, collectively known as *ama*, might lead to disease. Ayurveda stresses the importance of avoiding this possibility through maintaining a diet appro-priate to one's constitution and recommends the application of measures to ensure correct digestion. Food should be clean and fresh, taken in small quantities and chewed well before swallowing.

Ayurveda identifies six tastes and says that each taste is associated with an organ in the body and, when found in excess, will adversely affect the organ. The six tastes and associated organs are:

- sweet – spleen, pancreas
- salty – kidney
- sour – liver
- pungent – lungs
- bitter – heart
- astringent – colon.

People are encouraged to take food appropriate to their constitution, e.g.:

- *Vata* is aggravated by astringent, bitter and pungent tastes, and balanced by salty, sour and sweet tastes. Generally most sweet fruit (including dates, figs and papaya) are found to be beneficial.
- *Pitta* is aggravated by pungent, salty and sour, and balanced by astringent, bitter and sweet tastes. Sweet fruit (e.g. apples, cherries and ripe mangoes) are beneficial here too.
- *Kapha* is aggravated by salty, sour and sweet, and balanced by astringent, bitter and pungent tastes. Cranberries and other astringent or sour fruit are beneficial.

Each person eats according to his or her own state of health in order to maintain harmony within the body. Thus an individual showing a *pitta prakriti* would benefit from 'cool' spices such as cardamom, mint and turmeric. Turmeric is especially beneficial to the liver because this is consid-ered to be a *pitta* organ. Similar to their Chinese counterparts, Indian house-wives choose – or perhaps 'prescribe' would be a better word – their dinner menus carefully with reference to prevailing environmental conditions and family activities, thus ensuring that their relations are kept in the best of health, both physically and mentally. Knowing this aim, one can appreciate the origin of the delicate balance of herbs and spices so characteristic of Indian cuisine. A number of dietary incompatibilities are recognised: milk is incompatible with bananas, fish with bread, while melons are claimed to be incompatible with most other foods.

For hypertension, the instructions might be to drink one cup of mango juice, followed an hour or so later by half a cup of warm milk, a pinch of cardamom and nutmeg, and a teaspoonful of *ghee*. *Ghee* is a butter curd product that increases the *agni* and improves assimilation. Cucumber *raita* may also help if taken with a meal. Cucumber is a diuretic and raita is a yoghurt-based spicy condiment that often features in Indian recipes. Ayurveda prescribes specific diets for several psychiatric disorders and for different drug therapies. For anxieties almond milk may be prescribed. It is made by soaking 10 raw almonds in water overnight, then peeling and blending them with a cup of warm milk. While in the blender a small pinch of nutmeg and saffron is added.

Administration of medicines

It should be noted that, as with Chinese herbal medicine, the term 'herbal medicine' includes animal and mineral products as well as products derived from vegetable sources. In common with other complementary and alternative therapies, the type and dose of medicine chosen are influenced by the individual's constitution as well as by the nature of the disease. Other factors governing the choice of medicine include the age and strength of the patient, digestive capacity, degree of tolerance and psychological state.

There are detailed descriptions of the methods by which medicines should be prepared. One technique, known as *samskara* (refinement), eliminates the toxicity of the source materials, rather like the aim of serial dilution in homoeopathy. Mixtures of medicines (*sumyoga*) may be administered to achieve a balanced preparation, one principle balancing another through synergism or antagonism, as with Chinese herbal medicine. Some ingredients enhance the action, while others reduce the toxicity. The ayurvedic formula *chyavanprash* combines more than 25 finely powdered herbs in a base of honey and ghee. It is taken with food as a tonic.

Plant-based medicines

These are used by ayurvedic practitioners in a number of ways, among which are the following examples:

- In the treatment of a gastric disturbance in a person exhibiting a *pitta prakriti* the usual remedies black pepper (*Piper rotundum*) and ginger (*Zingiber officinale*) would be administered judiciously or not at all, because they are both considered to increase *pitta* and may exacerbate the imbalance.
- Tonification, or supplementation therapy, uses herbs and foods that build and nourish tissues. This is prescribed for individuals who are

elderly, malnourished, chronically ill or emaciated. The timing of administration is also seen as being important. The particular formula given depends on the constitution of the patient.

- There is a range of herbal preparations available for treating problems specific to women. The Chinese herb *dong quai* (*Angelica sinensis*) is used in the treatment of many gynaecological ailments. It is said to regulate menstruation, 'tonify' the blood and relieve constipation. Again, there are various herbal mixtures tailored to the constitutional type. Table 7.2 illustrates remedies suitable for cramps in women.[8] One of the most popular herbal mixtures is known as *triphala* ('the three fruits'). This product is rejuvenating and strengthening for all three *doshas* and all seven *dhatus*. It is also a mild laxative. *Triphala* comprises three of the most popular ayurvedic herbs: *amalaki*, *bibbitakiu* and *haritaki*. It is normally taken alone, mixed with honey or as a tea an hour after the evening meal. However, being a mild diuretic, some people prefer to take it in the morning.

The medicines are supplied as mixtures of herbs in a dried form, or more usually with a suitable vehicle (*anupana*) to facilitate absorption. The most usual vehicles are water, milk, honey, aloe vera and ghee. People with high cholesterol levels should be wary about taking large amounts of ghee. Herbal oils are made by introducing active principles (cloves, garlic, etc.) into a suitable oily vehicle. Herbal oils, fine powders or ghee may be administered intranasally (*nasya*).

Until a few years ago most traditional Asian remedies used in the UK were imported from India. Only a few local *hakims* (traditional healers) produced their own remedies, using imported raw materials. However, there are now several companies producing ayurvedic medicines in the UK. Many of these remedies may be purchased over the counter, by mail order through Asian and English language newspapers and the internet, or brought back from visits to the subcontinent. Licensing of the herbal remedies will be

Table 7.2 Example of constitutional treatments for cramping in women

Vata	*Pitta*	*Kapha*
Blue cohosh	Chamomile	Black cohosh
Cramp bark	Cramp bark	Blue cohosh
Ginger	Peppermint	Chamomile
Pennyroyal	Skullcap	Cramp bark
Valerian	Squaw vine	Ginger
	Yarrow	

similar to Chinese herbal medicine (see Chapter 6). A range of ayurvedic toiletries, including soap and shampoo, is available on the UK market.

Animal products

There is some controversy about using animal products. However, finely ground deer horn as a paste may be applied to the thoracic region and is said to be of benefit in angina.

Metals

Despite its long history, ayurveda has not been averse to change. The Indian subcontinent has been subject to countless invasions during its history, with diseases being imported from other geographical locations and techniques absorbed from other cultures.[9] During the Middle Ages, for example, heavy metals, particularly mercury, entered the ayurvedic armamentarium and were used in the treatment of syphilis, which was brought by the Portuguese. The invention of new remedies is encouraged by modern practitioners.

For medicinal use metals are traditionally taken internally after undergoing rigorous purification to neutralise any toxic effects. The metals are boiled in water which is then reduced in volume by evaporation. Typically 5 ml of this water is taken orally two to three times daily. Some examples of the medical uses of metals are:

- Copper is a good tonic for the liver, spleen and lymphatics.
- Gold strengthens the nervous system.
- Silver has cooling properties and is beneficial in the treatment of excess *pitta*.
- Iron is beneficial for bone marrow and helps in anaemia.

There are safety issues associated with the use of heavy metals (see below).

Treatment with aromatherapy

Sweet warming aromas such as musk and camphor can balance *vata*, while *pitta* is soothed by calming aromas such as sandalwood, jasmine and rose. *Kapha* is pacified by warming stimulating oils together with pungent oils such as eucalyptus, sage and thyme.

Treatment with enema (basti)

Basti introduces medicinal remedies, including sesame oil or herbal decoctions, in a liquid medium into the rectum. Medicated enemas pacify *vata* and alleviate many *vata* disorders, such as constipation, backache, arthritis and various nervous disorders.

Treatment with massage

Oil massage (*Sanskrit: abhyanga*) is an important treatment. While a person may perform massage on his own as part of his daily routine, trained masseurs are required to perform this therapy when it is used for disease management. A massage that is part of the daily routine lasts for 5–15 minutes, but when it is performed for treating diseases it may take about 45 minutes.

Nauli is a method of massaging the internal organs, particularly the colon, intestines, liver and spleen. It also helps to maintain abdominal 'fire' and keep the colon clean. A warm ayurvedic oil massage is prescribed for anxiety. *Vatas* should use sesame oil, *pittas* sunflower or coconut oil and *kaphas* corn oil.

Indian head massage is another specialised form of massage, sometimes known as champissage from its Indian name *champi*, which is part of the wider ayurvedic medical approach. The head, neck and facial areas are massaged with the purpose of manipulating energy channels. The goal is to clear blocks in these energy channels that cause a build-up of negative energy which are purported to cause ailments. It claims to help stress, insomnia, ridding the body of toxins and promoting hair growth.

Interest in ayurvedic massage has been growing in the west with the general trend towards holistic medicines creating a big tourist attraction in the south Indian state of Kerala.[10] It has been claimed that ayurveda offered to tourists is often not genuine – and, as well as damaging ayurveda's reputation, could even harm the patients themselves. The devotees do not say that all commercialism is bad, but they do want ayurveda practised seriously, not turned into a side show for tourists. Boards advertising ayurvedic centres are dotted between the tourist cafés and souvenir shops on the beach at Kovalam. Most seem geared towards 1-hour massages, using oils, and most of the tourists here seem to see it as a chance to relax rather than a real medical treatment.

Mind–body interventions

Colour therapy

Ayurvedic treatments make use of colour in their healing procedures. As the colours of the rainbow are perceived as correlating with the body tissues (*dhasus*) and the *doshas*, the vibratory energy of the colours may be used to establish psychological harmony and peace of mind. As colour is so important, patients are told to illuminate themselves and their environment in the appropriate coloured lighting. An appreciation of the colours of nature is also considered to be important.

Colours have particular properties:

- Red is stimulating and warming (*kapha*).
- Orange is also warming; it gives energy and strength and is stimulating (*kapha*).
- Yellow relieves excess *vata* and *kapha*.
- Gold is a warming colour beneficial to *vata* and *kapha*.
- Silver is cooling and soothes *pitta*.

Treatment with precious and semiprecious stones

Gems are thought to have healing properties that can be harnessed by wearing them as jewellery or by placing them in a suitable liquid overnight and drinking the solution. It is believed that gems absorb the vitality of their owners, e.g.:

- Diamond strengthens immunity.
- Pearls have a cooling effect on wakening.
- Ruby strengthens concentration.
- Sapphire (blue) calms *vata* and *kapha* and stimulates *pitta*.

Treatment with meditation

Meditation, the art of bringing harmony to body, mind and consciousness, is used to soothe the body and reduce stress. Meditation is not concentration, quite the opposite. There should be no conscious effort – the mind should be allowed to relax completely ('float') as one listens to every sound.

Treatment with yoga

This is believed to calm the nervous system and balance the body, mind and spirit, as well as provide exercise. It is thought by its practitioners to prevent specific diseases and maladies by keeping the energy meridians open and maintaining life energy

Treatment with surgery

The father of Indian surgery is said to be Sushruta.[11] Controversy exists about the time when Sushruta lived, with estimates ranging from 1000 BC to the tenth century AD. Sushruta compiled his knowledge as the *Sushruta Samhita* (Sushruta's compendium). The book provides minute details of preoperative and postoperative care as well as other aspects of ayurvedic practice. Sushruta described surgery under eight headings:

- Incision (*bhedana*)
- Excision (*chedana*)
- Scarification (*lekhana*)
- Puncturing (*vedhya*)

- Probing (*esana*)
- Extraction (*ahrya*)
- Drainage or evacuation (*vsraya*)
- Suturing (*sivya*).

Treatment regimens

Rasayana and *Panchakarma* are examples of treatment regimens.

Rasayana

This is a specialised branch of clinical medicine in ayurveda meant for slowing the effect of ageing and to improve intelligence, memory, complexion, and sensory and motor functions. Numerous single and compound *rasayana* drugs possessing diversified actions, such as immuno-enhancement, free-radical scavenging, adaptogenic or anti-stress and nutritive effects, are described in ayurveda literature for their use in health promotion and management of diseases with improvement in the quality of life.

Panchakarma

This is a holistic rejuvenation therapy.[12] It comprises five different procedures described by the ayurveda texts for purification of the body:

- Therapeutic vomiting
- Purgation
- Enemas
- Nasal aspiration of herbs
- Therapeutic release of toxic blood.

Safety

Safety of administered medicines

Intrinsic toxicity[13]

The following examples illustrate the toxicity problems of certain traditional Indian medicines.

Khat (*Catha edulis*)

Khat, pronounced 'cot', and also known as *qat, gat, chat* and *miraa*, is a herbal product consisting of the leaves and shoots of the shrub *Catha edulis*.[14] It is cultivated primarily in East Africa and the Arabian peninsula, harvested and then chewed to obtain a stimulant effect. There are many different varieties of *Catha edulis* depending upon the area in which it is cultivated. The herb is chewed, smoked or drunk as an infusion. The active principles are the two alkaloids, norpseudoephedrine (cathinine) and cathinone. *Khat* produces a feeling of well-being and lessens fatigue. Although users say that the herb is not addictive, withdrawal has been known to cause lethargy and nightmares. In 1980 the World Health Organization classified *khat* as a drug of abuse that can produce mild-to-moderate psychological dependence, and the plant has been targeted by anti-drug organisations. It is a controlled/illegal substance in many countries. On the basis of the evidence presented to the UK Advisory Council on the Misuse of Drugs in 2005, it was recommended that *khat* should not be controlled under the Misuse of Drugs Act 1971. The Council report (http://tinyurl.com/mj4t85) stated that use of the substance was limited to specific communities within the UK, and had not, nor did it appear likely to, spread to the wider community. However, use of *khat* was not without detrimental effects and should be discouraged. Fresh leaves of *khat* contain the alkaloid stimulants cathinone (*S*-(−)-α-aminopropiophenone) and cathine (*S*,*S*-(+)-norpseudoephedrine) in addition to more than 40 alkaloids, glycosides, tannins and terpenoids. Although *khat* is not currently controlled under the UK Misuse of Drugs Act 1971, cathinone and cathine are classified as class C drugs under the Act. An offence is committed if they are extracted from the plant. Although this offence has been identified there have been no successful prosecutions to date.

The UK is a major destination for imports and exports of *khat* on to other countries in the world. In the first 6 months of 2005 there were imports each day of approximately 5–7 tonnes from Kenya, 500 kg from Ethiopia and 175 kg from Yemen (equates to roughly 25 000 bundles or doses), the bulk of which was held in transit for export to the USA where its use is illegal. *Khat* has a varied legal status across Europe. Most countries include cathinone and cathine under drug misuse legislation and they are listed in the UN Convention on Psychotropic Substances 1971.

Betel (*Piper betle*)

Use of betel is discouraged in western countries because of its alleged carcinogenic and perceived dysaesthetic properties; nevertheless, betel is widely available in the west.[15] The British Dental Health Foundation (www.dentalhealth.org.uk) has long advised betel users of the risks of mouth cancer. Warning signs include ulcers that do not heal within 3 weeks, red and white patches in the mouth, and unusual swellings or changes in the mouth and neck.

A betel quid comprises tobacco, *Areca catechu*, saffron and lime wrapped in a leaf from the plant *Piper betle*. The quid is placed in the buccal cavity, where it stimulates salivation. It is considered to have beneficial digestive properties. A number of the ingredients are reported to be carcinogenic. An associated practice involves chewing betel nuts, with a mixture of areca nut, lime (calcium hydroxide) and tobacco – known as paan in south-east Asia, where the practice is most common. The nut produces mild psychoactive and cholinergic effects, including a copious production of a blood-red saliva that users spit out. After years of chewing, the teeth may become red-brown to almost black.[3]

In 2009 Papua New Guinea's cultural obsession with chewing betel came under threat when the Governor of Port Moresby moved to ban betel nut chewing in public places, on health grounds.[16]

Heavy metals

Mercury,[17] lead[18] and arsenic have been detected in a substantial proportion of Indian-manufactured traditional ayurvedic medicines and cosmetics.[19] Twenty per cent of both US-manufactured and Indian-manufactured Ayurvedic medicines purchased via the internet have been shown to contain detectable lead, mercury or arsenic.[20] Metals may be present due to the practice of *rasa shastra* (combining herbs with metals, minerals and gems).

Lead is regarded as an aphrodisiac, and has been used to counteract impotence in men with diabetes. The following are other examples:

- The product *al kohl* is applied as an eye cosmetic; its main ingredient is lead sulphide.
- *Suma* powders contain over 80% lead and are applied as a cosmetic to the conjunctival surface of infants and children, from where they may be transferred to the mouth by the hands.
- *Sikor* is rich in lead and arsenic; it is used as a remedy for indigestion.

Kales et al. compared the relative haematopoietic toxicity of ayurvedic lead poisoning with a common form of occupational lead poisoning.[21] They found that ayurvedic poisoning produces greater haematopoietic toxicity than paint-removal poisoning. Ayurvedic ingestion should be considered in patients with anaemia. The authors recommend that these patients should be screened for lead exposure and strongly encouraged to discontinue metal-containing remedies.

Following a systematic strategy to identify all stores 20 miles or less from Boston City Hall that sold ayurvedic products, Dr Robert Saper and colleagues at Harvard Medical School estimated that one of five ayurvedic products produced in south Asia and available in the area under study contained potentially harmful levels of lead, mercury and/or arsenic.[22] It is suggested that users of ayurvedic medicine may be at risk from heavy metal toxicity, and testing of ayurvedic products for toxic heavy metals should be mandatory.

Drugs

Some years ago a report appeared of a patient presenting at a hospital in Birmingham with powders from the Punjab that he was using to self-treat psoriasis and were individually wrapped in newspaper.[23] High-performance liquid chromatography analysis of the powders revealed the presence of prednisolone, a prescription medicine that is potentially dangerous.

Identification of medicines

A number of problems that pharmacists and other healthcare providers may experience in identifying ingredients and assessing their potential toxicity in Asian remedies have been identified:[24]

- Typographical errors on the label
- Inaccurate phonetic transliteration
- Changes in nomenclature
- Absence of generic names on the label
- Undeclared ingredients and adulterants
- Assessing the literature and finding information.

Trease and Evans' Pharmacognosy,[13] to which frequent references are made in this chapter, provides an excellent and readily available source of information for traditional medicine practices.

Potential interactions

There is a substantial risk that patients will receive simultaneous western and traditional treatments. Patients seldom volunteer information concerning any traditional medicines being taken. A case has been reported in which a woman receiving chemotherapy for Hodgkin's disease supplemented her treatment with at least nine different ayurvedic medicines.[25] She suffered a thrombosis thought to result from an interaction between the orthodox and traditional medicines. Pharmacists can provide an extremely valuable function in this respect by intervening with advice whenever they consider it to be appropriate.

An interaction between the fruit karela (*Momordica charantia*), an ingredient of curries, and chlorpropamide has been reported.[26] Although this particular drug has been superseded by other hypoglcaemics, it serves to flag up a possible difficulty with concurrent treatment. Karela improves glucose tolerance and is therefore hypoglycaemic. There are a number of other close relatives of this plant that are also used by *hakims* to treat diabetes, including crushed seed kernels of the marrow (*Curcubita pepo*) and the honeydew melon (*Cucumis melo*). There is a danger that some patients may be treating their diabetes with both allopathic and traditional remedies without realising the risk of interaction.

Betel nut (see above) is prescribed by *hakims* either alone or in mixtures. There may be a risk of interactions between this herbal medicine and orthodox drugs.

Safety of surgical and manipulative procedures

The inclusion of surgical techniques adds another potential danger from non-sterile instruments and consulting environments, and incompetent procedures. There is also a risk from undue pressure or incorrect manipulation by inexperienced practitioners.

Evidence

There are difficulties in applying western methods to proving the effectiveness of traditional therapies. Data from both animal and human trials suggesting efficacy of ayurvedic interventions in managing diabetes have been published.[27] However, the reported human trials generally fall short of contemporary methodological standards. There are some encouraging results for its effectiveness in treating various ailments, including chronic disorders associated with the ageing process. Pilot studies have also been conducted on depression, anxiety, sleep disorders, hypertension, Parkinson's disease and Alzheimer's disease.[28]

The Indian Council of Medical Research has set up a unique network throughout India for carrying out controlled clinical trials of herbal medicines.[29] The programme is monitored by a scientific advisory group consisting of people from the ayurveda, unani and modern allopathic systems of medicine. This group contains experts in pharmacognosy, toxicology, pharmacology and clinical pharmacology, as well as clinicians and experts in standardisation and quality control. Trials are planned and protocols prepared by the whole group. All trials are comparative, controlled, randomised and double blind unless there is a reason for carrying out a single-blind study. The trials are planned by the whole group but carried out at the centres of allopathic medicine with established investigators. There are over 20 clinical trial centres throughout the country for carrying out the multicentre studies. Using this network the council has shown the efficacy of several traditional medicines, including *Picrorhiza kurroa* in hepatitis and *Pterocarpus marsupium* in diabetes.[30] As a result of these trials these traditional medicines can be used in allopathic hospitals.

The Central Council of India's systems of medicine oversee research institutes, which evaluate treatments. The government is adding 10 traditional medicines into its family welfare programme, funded by the World Bank and the Indian government. These medicines are for anaemia, oedema during pregnancy, postpartum problems such as pain, uterine and abdominal complications, difficulties with lactation, nutritional deficiencies and childhood diarrhoea.[31]

New regulations were introduced in July 2000 to improve Indian herbal medicines by establishing standard manufacturing practices and quality control. The regulations outline requirements for infrastructure, labour, quality control and authenticity of raw materials, and absence of contamination. Of the 9000 licensed manufacturers of traditional medicines, those who qualify can immediately seek certification for good manufacturing practice. The remainders have 2 years to comply with the regulations and to obtain certification.

The government has also established 10 new drug-testing laboratories for Indian systems of medicine and is upgrading existing laboratories to provide high-quality evidence to the licensing authorities of the safety and quality of herbal medicines. This replaces an ad hoc system of testing that was considered unreliable. Randomised controlled clinical trials of selected prescriptions for Indian systems of medicine have been initiated. These will document the safety and efficacy of the prescriptions and provide the basis for their international licensing as medicines rather than simply as food supplements.[32]

A randomised, double-blind, placebo-controlled, parallel-group monocentre trial with 182 patients investigated the efficacy and toxicity of an orally administered ayurvedic formulation for rheumatoid arthritis.[33] It was concluded that the preparation was not significantly superior to a strong placebo response except for joint swelling, although improvement in the group taking active medicine was numerically superior at all evaluation time points. Other trials have shown some promise in the treatment of bronchial asthma[34,35] and angina.[36] It is claimed that ayurveda can be used effectively in combination with modern medicine to provide better treatment of cancer.[37]

Practitioners

There are about 25–30 qualified ayurvedic physicians in the UK who are registered with the Ayurvedic Medical Association UK, and hold malpractice insurance and maintain a code of ethics. Most of the physicians are based in London but some of them are in areas that have a large Asian community such as Leicester, Birmingham and Bradford. In the USA legal licensure for any healthcare profession, including ayurveda, is under the jurisdiction of each individual state. Currently, none of the US states licenses ayurvedic physicians as primary care physicians. However, many ayurvedic physicians use their education and knowledge in combination with their other healthcare-related licensed credentials.

Integration with western medicine

The Indian Medicine Central Council was established by a 1970 act to oversee the development of Indian systems of medicine and to ensure good standards of training and practice. Training for Indian medicine is given in separate colleges, which offer a basic biosciences curriculum followed by training in a traditional system. Recently the Department of Indian Systems of Medicine has expressed concern over the substandard quality of education in many colleges, which in the name of integration have produced hybrid curricula and graduates, unacceptable to either modern or traditional standards. The department has made it a priority to upgrade training in Indian systems of medicine.[38]

Purists in ayurveda and unani oppose this trend to modernise their systems, particularly when such integration is carried out by experts in allopathy.[39] They have no objection to the use of modern concepts of the methodology of clinical trials in evaluating the efficacy and side effects of herbal preparations used in the traditional systems. Such clinical evaluation is essential because the remedies used in these systems will not be used in allopathic hospitals in a country such as India unless they have shown efficacy in well-controlled trials. However, carrying out randomised, double-blind, multicentre trials with standardised extracts is a slow and laborious process. Furthermore, not all herbal medicines need to undergo this rigorous trial because these preparations are already in use. The situation is still further complicated because the randomised trial may not be totally appropriate for the evaluation of medicines from the traditional systems, where the *prakriti* (ayurveda system) or *mijaj* (unani system) of the individual determines the specific therapy to be used.

Ayurvedic medicines

Herbal drugs constitute a major share of all the officially recognised systems of health in India: ayurveda, yoga, unani, siddha, homoeopathy and naturopathy. More than 70% of India's 1.1 billion population still use these non-allopathic systems of medicine.[39]

Forms of medicines

Ayurvedic medicines are made from herbs or mixtures of herbs, either alone or in combination with minerals, metals and ingredients of animal origin. The metals, animals and minerals are purified by individual processes before being used for medicinal purposes. Impurified materials are not allowed to be used as medicine. Many forms of ayurvedic medicaments may be identified including the following:

- *Quath*: crushed herbs, used as decoction or tea for internal and external uses
- *Churna*: fine powdered herbs, used as medicine with water or in food for internal and external uses

- *Tail*: herbs cooked in edible oil according to rules laid down for internal and external uses
- *Ghrat/Ghrit*: herbs cooked in special butter
- *Asav/Arista/Sura*: a kind of light wine obtained after fermentation of herbs
- *Arka*: a distillation of herbs
- *Rasausadhi/Kharliya rasayan*: herbs mixed with metals, minerals and animal ingredients
- *Bhasma*: ashes
- *Parpaty*: combinations of metals, minerals, animal ingredients and herbs
- *Kshar/Lavan/Salt/Drava*: these are specially prepared medicaments
- Medicaments based on *guggula* (the Indian bdellium tree *Commiphora mukul Engl.*)
- *Lauha bhasam*: *mandoor bhasam* (iron)-based medicaments
- *Avaleha/Modak/Paak/Prash*: herbs cooked in jaggery (traditional unrefined sugar) or sugar
- *Bati/Gutika/Goli*: mixtures of medicines shaped in pills, pillules or tablets for ease of administration
- *Pralep/Anjan/Varti/Dhoop*: liniments, drops, paint, paste, etc. for external uses.

Examples of common ayurvedic medicines

Some examples of herbal ingredients used in the preparation of common ayurvedic medicines in the UK are provided in Table 7.3.[13]

Examples of common applications of ayurvedic medicines[40]

By the very nature of the philosophy surrounding the practice of ayurveda it should not really be possible to treat conditions purely symptomatically. However, Table 7.4 gives a brief list of treatments to illustrate the general approach to treatment.

Figures 7.3 and 7.4 show examples of popular ayurvedic herbal products:

- *Trikatu* is a Sanskrit word meaning 'three spices'. It is the main stimulant compound used by ayurvedic doctors. Containing fruits of black pepper (*Piper nigrum*), Indian long pepper (*Piper longum*) and the rhizomes of ginger (*Zingiber officinalis*), it is a common combination used to stimulate and maintain the digestive and respiratory systems. This it does by reducing *kapha* and increasing *pitta* through the rejuvenation of low *agni* and the burning away of *ama* (toxins).

- *Triphala* is a *rasayana* formula comprising equal parts of three fruits: amalaki (*Emblica officinalis*), bibhitaki (*Terminalia bellirica*) and haritaki (*Terminalia chebula*). *Triphala* is used to promote appetite and digestion. When dissolved in the mouth, *Triphala* can be used to clear congestion and headaches.

Other related therapies

Unani

The word unani derives from the Arabic word for Greece: *al-Yunaan* and is used to refer to medicine of Graeco-Arabic origin. It is based on the teachings of Hippocrates, Galen and Avicenna. The system was introduced in India around tenth century AD with the spread of Islamic civilisation.

Unani medicine believes that diseases can be kept at bay by the use of clean and fresh water, breathing clean air and consuming fresh food. Likewise, a balance should be maintained between the mind and the body so that the metabolic process can take place easily and the body waste evacuated. Unani medicine also believes that all life forms have originated from the sea.

According to unani the human body is composed of seven natural and basic components, called *Umoor-e-Tabaiya*, that are responsible for maintenance of health. These are similar to those identified in ayurveda:

- Elements (*arkan*)
- Temperament (*mizaj*)
- Four humours (*akhlaat*) – blood, phlegm, yellow bile and black bile
- Organs (*aaza*)
- Vital forces or *neuro* (*arwah*)
- Facultie (*quwa*)
- Functions (*afaal*).

The loss of any one of these basic components or alteration in their physical state could lead to disease, or even death. It is highly essential to consider all these factors so as to reach the correct diagnosis and consequently the correct line of treatment.

The unani practitioner is called a *hakim*. There are ten specialised branches of unani medicine:

- Internal medicine
- Gynaecology including obstetrics and paediatrics
- Diseases of the head and neck
- Toxicology

Table 7.3 Examples of herbs used in the UK for ayurverdic medicines[13]

Source material	Indian name	Parts used	Main constituent	Example of use
Azadirachta indica	Neem	Seeds, oil	Alkaloids glycosides	Anthelmintic, antiseptic, astringent
Abrus precatorius	Ghungchi rati	Root, seeds	Alkaloids	Abortifacient Eye inflammation, oral contraceptive
Allium cepa	Tukhm piyaz	Seeds	Volatile oils (allyl sulphate)	Diuretic, expectorant Poultice
Artemesia absinthium Artemesia indica	Afsentin roomi Nagdoona	Leaves	Sesquiterpenes, lactones, bitters	Anthelmintic, tonic
Bombax celba	Mush simbhal	Gum, root	Glycosides, tannins	Hepatic dysfunction Menorrhagia
Cassia absus	Chaksu	Seeds	Alkaloids	Astringent Eye inflammation Ringworm
Crocus sativus	Zafran (saffron)	Flower styles	Volatile oil	Catarrh Enlarged liver
Cyperus rotundus	Nutgrass	Root, seeds	Sesquiterpenes	Antiemetic Anti-inflammatory Anti-pyretic
Ferula galbaniflua	Jawashir	Oleo-gum resin	Sesquiterpenes	Asthma, bronchitis Dysentery Menstrual irregularities
Ficus benghalensis	Anjir jangli	Root Bark	Glycosides Triterpenes	*Bark*: tonic, diuretic *Root*: diarrhoea and hypoglycaemic
Hedera nepalense	Bikh tablab	Fruit	Triterpenoid saponins	Rheumatism
Mallotus philippensis	Kamala	Fruit	Resin	Anthelmintic Oral contraceptive Red dye
Mentha piperita	Paparaminta	Leaves	Volatile oil	Cough and fever Diarrhoea, flatulence Nausea and vomiting
Quercus infectoria	N/A	Galls	Tannins	Haemorrhoids – ointments and suppositories
Rosmarinus officinalis	Rusmari	Leaves	Volatile oil	Pulmonary infections Oil: toothache, rheumatism

Table 7.3 *Continued*

Source material	Indian name	Parts used	Main constituent	Example of use
Salvia officinalis	*Bahaman surkh*	Leaves	Volatile oil	Gargle, gingivitis Treatment of thrush
Solanum indicum	*Bari-khatai, barhanta*	Fruiting plant	Steroidal alkaloids	Chest and urinary infections Skin conditions (paste)
Tephrosia purpurea	*Sarphunkha*	Whole plant	Flavonoids	Cystitis Dysentery Facial oedema
Vitex agnus-castus	*Remuka*	Fruit	Flavonols	Diuretic Stimulant
Zingiber officinalis	*Zanjibil*	Rhizome	Oleo-resin	Antiemetic, bronchitis Rheumatism

Table 7.4 Examples of ayurvedic treatments for some common conditions

Condition	Typical ayurvedic treatment	Other treatments
Acne	Herbs – *Andrographis* (known as *Chuan xin lian* in TCM), guduchi, shatavari Aloe vera juice Tea – cumin, coriander and fennel	Apply melon to the skin Yoga postures Breathing exercises
Anxiety	Calming tea – valerian, musta	Relaxing bath Almond milk Acupressure
Athlete's foot	Tea tree oil Aloe vera gel and turmeric	Wash with *neem* soap Neem oil applied
Boils	*Neem* powder paste *Triphala* wash For people with diabetes: *neem*, turmeric, *kutki* taken orally	Cooling, healing paste of sandalwood and turmeric Poultice of cooked onions to draw Liver cleanser (aloe vera gel)
Diarrhoea	Ghee, nutmeg, ginger, sugar Ginger powder with sugar. Mix and chew	
Eye problems	*Triphala* wash Rosewater	Cool water wash Gaze into the flame of a traditional ghee lamp
Jet lag	One hour before flight – ginger On flight – drink water After flight – rub warm sesame oil on scalp	
Sore throat	*Garge* – turmeric and hot water Ginger–cinnamon–liquorice tea	Avoid dairy produce Yoga postures Breathing exercises

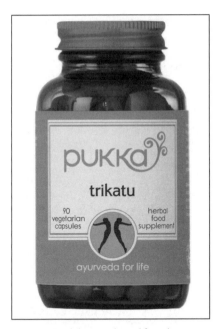

Figure 7.3 *Trikatu* packaged for sale. (Courtesy of Pukka Herbs.)

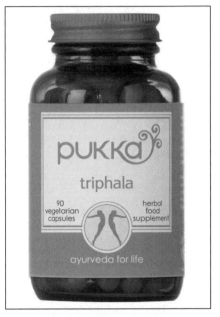

Figure 7.4 *Triphala* packaged for sale (Courtesy of Pukka Herbs.)

- Psychiatry
- Rejuvenation therapy including geriatrics
- Sexology
- Regimental therapy
- Dietotherapy
- Hydrotherapy.

The following treatments are used in unani:

- Regimental therapy: includes venesection, cupping, diaphoresis, diuresis, Turkish bath, massage, cauterisation, purging, emesis, exercise and leeching
- Dietotherapy: treating ailments by administration of specific diets or by regulating the quantity and quality of food
- Pharmacotherapy: using naturally occurring drugs, mostly material of animal and mineral origin. Single drugs or their combination in raw form are preferred over compound formulations.

In India, there are about 100 Unani medical colleges where the unani system of medicine is taught. It is a five-and-a-half-year course and the graduates are awarded a BUMS (Bachelor of Unani Medicine and Surgery) degree. There are about 10 unani medical colleges where a postgraduate degree is being given for BUMS doctors. All these colleges are affiliated to reputed universities and recognised by the government.

Siddha

Siddha medicine is a form of medical treatment of diseases developed by the ancient Tamils and is practised mainly in the south of the Indian subcontinent. It was described by the *siddhars* who wrote their recipes on palm-leaves for the use of future generations.

The siddha practitioner is expected to have knowledge of four basic concepts:[2]

- Alchemy (*vadham*)
- Medicine (*aithiyam*)
- Yoga (*yogam*)
- Philosophy (*thathuvam*).

The use of metals such as gold, silver, iron, lead and mercury, and extracts of corals and pearls, is a special feature of siddha medicine, which claims to detoxify metals to enable them to be used for stubborn diseases.

Jamu

Traditional Indonesian medicine (*jamu*) is thought to have originated from the Javanese royal palaces of Yogyakarta and Surakarta.[41] It is a holistic therapy with influences from Arabian, Chinese and Indian medicine. Jamu involves massage and the use of traditional herbal preparations made from the leaves, fruits, roots, flowers and bark of medicinal plants. Traditionally medicines were made freshly each day by boiling the prepared herbal ingredients (*jamu godok*) using a *lumpang* (small iron mortar), *pipisan*, *parut* (grater) and *kuali* (clay pot). Few households still maintain this tradition preferring to buy medicines from others or use products that have been packaged as teas. Important ingredients include species of ginger (e.g. *Zingiber officinale*, *Zingiber oronaticum* and *Zingiberb bevifalium)*, turmeric (*Curcuma domestica*) and cinnamon *(Gijeyzahyza glabra).*

There are two main applications of *jamu:*

- To maintain physical fitness, health and sexual performance
- To cure various kinds of illness.

Jamu is also used as a cosmetic. Some of the products are consumed, e.g. kepel fruit (a brown fruit the size of a chicken egg) is considered to be a natural deodorant. *Jambu mawar* (a kind of rose apple) gives a fresh breath. Other cosmetics are for topical application such as *bedak dingin* (cool powder) and *lulur* (scrubbing powder).

An examination on the microbiological quality of seven kinds of *jamu* and their raw materials was conducted according to the requirements of microbial contamination in traditional medicine, issued by the Department of Health of Indonesia.[42] Contamination was not significant. It was suggested that certain plants be scanned for antibacterial and antifungal activity.

More information

National Ayurvedic Medical Association: www.ayurveda-nama.org
National Institute of Ayurvedic Medicine: http://tinyurl.com/2qd89j
The Ayurvedic Institute: www.ayurveda.com
Unani Herbal Healing: www.unani.com
Ayurvedic Medical Association UK: 59 Dulverton Road, Selsdon, South Croydon, Surrey
    CR2 8PJ
Tel: 0208 657 6147
Fax: 0208 333 7904
Email: Dr. N.S.Moorthy@ayurvedic.demon.co.uk

Further reading

Godagama S. *Ayurveda*. London: Kyle Cathie, 2001.
Kapoor LD. *CRC Handbook of Ayurvedic Medicinal Plants*. Boca Raton, FL: CRC Press, 2000.
Williamson E. Ayurveda: introduction for pharmacists. *Pharm J* 2006;**276**:108–10.

References

1. Patwardhan B, Warude D, Pushpangadan P, Bhatt N. Ayurveda and traditional Chinese medicine: A comparative overview. *eCAM* 2005;**2**:465–73. Available at: http://tinyurl.com/yo8b32 (accessed 5 May 2009).
2. WHO. *Global Atlas of Traditional, Complementary and Alternative Medicine*. Kobe, Japan: WHO Centre for Health Development, 2005: 47.
3. Sodhi V. Ayurveda: the science of life and mother of the healing arts. In: Pizzorno J Jr, Murray MT (eds), *Textbook of Natural Medicine*, 2nd edn. Edinburgh: Churchill Livingstone, 1999: 257–8.
4. Rana RE. Arora history of plastic surgery in India. *J Postgrad Med* 2002;**48**:76–8.
5. Lad V. *The Complete Book of Ayurverdic Home Remedies*. London: Patkus, 1999: 18–19.
6. Prasher B, Negi S, Aggarwal S et al. Whole genome expression and biochemical correlates of extreme constitutional types defined in Ayurveda. *J Transl Med* 2008;**6**:48.
7. Healthmad. Ayurveda for Allergies. Available at: http://tinyurl.com/78ogva (accessed 20 April 2009).
8. Jonas WB, Ernst E. *Essentials of CAM. Introduction: Evaluating the safety of complementary and alternative products and practices*. Baltimore, MA: Lippincott/Williams & Wilkins, 1999: 89–107.
9. Glazier A. A landmark in the history of ayurveda. *Lancet* 2000;**356**:1118–22.

10. McGivering J. Traditional medicine being exploited. *BBC News* Tuesday 19 March 2002. Available at: http://tinyurl.com/5zx2ec (accessed 17 December 2008).

11. Tewari M, Shukla HS. Sushruta: 'The Father of Indian Surgery'. *Indian J Surg* 2005; **67**:229–30.

12. Packard CC. *Pocket Guide to Ayurvedic Healing*. Freedom, CA: Crossing Press, 1996: 111.

13. Aslam M. *Asian Medicine and its Practice in Britain*. In: Evans WC (ed.), *Trease and Evans' Pharmacognosy*, 15th edn. Edinburgh: WB Saunders, 2002: 489–41.

14. Report of the Advisory Council on The Misuse of Drugs. London: The Home Office, 2005. Available online at: http://tinyurl.com/6h7zck (accessed 1 May 2009).

15. Noeron SA. Betel: Consumption and consequences. *J Am Acad Dermatol* 1998;**38**:81–8.

16. Malkin B. Papua New Guinea bans betel nut. *Telegraph* online 7 January 2009. Available at: http://tinyurl.com/8dpp36 (accessed 8 January 2009).

17. Kew J, Morris C, Athie A et al. Arsenic and mercury intoxication due to Indian ethnic remedies. *BMJ* 1993;**306**:306–7.

18. Keen RW, Deacon AC, Delves HT et al. Indian herbal remedies for diabetes as a cause of lead poisoning. *Postgrad Med* 1994;**70**:113–14.

19. Aslam M, Davis SS, Healy MA. Heavy metals in some Asian medicines and cosmetics. *Public Health* 1979;**93**:274–84.

20. Saper RB, Phillips RS, Sehgal A et al. Lead, mercury, and arsenic in US- and Indian-manufactured Ayurvedic medicines sold via the Internet. *JAMA* 2008;**30**:915–23.

21. Kales SN, Christophi CA, Saper RB. Hematopoietic toxicity from lead-containing Ayurvedic medications. *Med Sci Monit* 2007;**13**:295–8.

22. Saper RB, Kales SN, Paquin J et al. Heavy metal content of ayurvedic herbal medicine products. *JAMA* 2004;**292**:2868–73.

23. Barnes AR, Paul CJ, Secrett PC. Adulteration of Asian alternative medicines. *Pharm J* 1991;**247**:650.

24. Aslam M. Problems of identity with traditional Asian remedies. *Pharm J* 1992;**248**:20–1, 23.

25. Fletcher J, Aslam M. Possible dangers of Ayurvedic herbal remedies. *Pharm J* 1991; **247**:456.

26. Aslam M, Stockley I H. Interaction between curry ingredient (Karela) and a drug (chlorpromamide). *Lancet* 1979;**i**:607.

27. Elder C. Ayurveda for diabetes mellitus: a review of the biomedical literature. *Altern Ther Health Med* 2004;**10**:44–50.

28. Sharma H, Chandola HM, Singh G, Basisht G. Utilization of Ayurveda in health care: an approach for prevention, health promotion, and treatment of disease. Part 2 – Ayurveda in primary health care. *J Altern Complement Med* 2007;**13**:1135–50.

29. Indian Council of Medical Research. *Annual Report of Council 1998–99*. New Delhi: Indian Council of Medical Research.

30. Atherton DJ. Towards the safer use of traditional remedies. *BMJ* 1994;**308**:673–4.

31. Kumar S. India's government promotes traditional healing practices. *Lancet* 2000;**335**: 1252.

32. Hoizey D, Hoizey M. *A History of Chinese Medicine*. Vancouver: University BC Press, 1993: 42.

33. Chopra A, Lavin P, Patwardhan B, Chitre D. Ayurvedic medicine reduces joint swelling in patient with rheumatoid arthritis. *J Rheumatol* 2000;**27**:1365–72.

34. Sekhar AV, Gandhi DN, Rao NM, Rawal UD. An experimental and clinical evaluation of anti-asthmatic potentialities of Devadaru compound (DC). *Indian J Physiol Pharmacol* 2003;**47**:101–7.

35. Gupta I, Gupta V, Parihar A, Gupta S, Ludtke R, Safayhi H. Effects of *Boswellia serrata* gum resin in patients with bronchial asthma: results of a double-blind, placebo-controlled, 6-week clinical study. *Eur J Med Res* 1998;**3**:511–14.

36. Kumar PU, Adhikari P, Pereira P, Bhat P. Safety and efficacy of Hartone in stable angina pectoris – an open comparative trial. *J Assoc Physicians India* 1999;**47**:685–9.

37. Garodia P, Ichikawa H, Malani N, Sethi G, Aggarwal BB. From ancient medicine to modern medicine: ayurvedic concepts of health and their role in inflammation and cancer. *J Soc Integr Oncol* 2007;**5**:25–37.
38. Vaidya AD, Devasagayam TP. Current status of herbal drugs in India: an overview. *J Clin Biochem Nutr* 2007;**41**:1–11.
39. Chaudhury RR. Commentary: challenges in using traditional systems of medicine. *BMJ* 2001;**322**:167.
40. Lampert N. Letter. *Lancet* 2001;**357**:802.
41. Williamson E. Systems of traditional medicine from south and south-east Asia. *Pharm J* 2006;**276**:539–40.
42. Limyati DA, Juniar BLL. Jamu Gendong, a kind of traditional medicine in Indonesia: the microbial contamination of its raw materials and end product. *J Ethnopharmacol* 1998;**63**:201–8.

8

Japanese kampo medicine

Haruki Yamada

Kampo medicine is a Japanese traditional herbal medicine that is based on Chinese herbal medicine (CHM). The name is derived from the Japanese symbols *kan*, which means China and *po*, which means medicine. Kampo remedies are very important in modern-day Japanese medicine.

History

Traditional CHM was introduced into Japan from China through cultural exchange between the fifth and sixth centuries and has been used for over 1000 years. Major classic textbooks of traditional Chinese medicine (TCM) include the following:

- *Koteidaikei* (*Huang di nei jing*: the *Yellow Emperor's Manual of Corporeal Medicine*)
- *Shinnohonzokyo* (*Shen non ben cao jing* – the *Materia Medica of the* Shen Nong)
- *Shokanron* (*Shang han lun*)
- *Kinkiyouryaku* (*Jin kui yao lue*) were completed in the Han period (202 BC to AD 220), and several medical textbooks originating from these works have been introduced from China.

Koteidaikei described the theory of yin–yang and the five elements, featured in the original philosophies of China. *Shinnohonzokyo* described the effects of medicinal herbs, and was composed of 365 medicinal herbs comprising animal, plant and mineral origins, and classified into three different (upper, middle and lower) grades depending on their safeties and efficacies. *Shokanron* and *Kinkiyouryaku* are both most important classic textbooks for the treatment by the decoction of traditional Chinese medicines. *Shokanron* has instructions on the diagnosis and treatment of typhoid-like acute febrile diseases, called *Shokan*. The symptoms of this disease are categorised in six stages according to the progress of the disease, and the pathological observation and corresponding suitable kampo formulae are described. In contrast to *Shokanron*, *Kinkiyoryaku* has been described various chronic diseases and the formulae for the treatment. Many popular kampo formulae appear in both classic textbooks as the major sources.

Chinese medicine underwent numerous modifications to make it better suited to the Japanese situation and kampo medicine was established in the Edo era during the eighteenth century. Except for limited trade with China and the Netherlands, Japan was a closed country during this time. Although Dutch medicine was introduced to Japan in the sixteenth century and administered alongside traditional medicine, its usage did not surpass that of the traditional medicine until end of the nineteenth century.

When Japan opened its door to western countries in 1867, the government would license only medical doctors for the practice of western medicine. As a result, the use of kampo medicine declined at this period.

Despite this unfavourable aspect of the period, kampo medicine continued to thrive through the efforts of a few medical leaders who recognised its benefits. With the progress of modern science and technology, modern medicine has greatly improved. Although incidences of numerous globally rampant infections had been reduced by the development of antibiotics, the latter half of the twentieth century saw a marked increase in chronic, endogenous, metabolic disorders. There has also been an increase in non-specific, constitutional or psychosomatic diseases. Some severe adverse effects associated with some natural and synthetic compounds have also resulted in occasional disillusionment with modern medicine. Against these social backgrounds, use of kampo medicines in Japan emerged as an alternative.

Consequently, kampo medicine now plays an important role in medical treatment in Japan. In 2001, The Ministry of Culture, Sports and Education of Japan confirmed the new core curriculum of the medical schools, and the education of kampo medicine was introduced into this new curriculum.

Principles of kampo medicine

Kampo medicine attempts to harness a state of harmony or equilibrium from the disturbed digestive, immune, endocrine and cardiovascular systems in the whole body to relieve or abolish symptoms related to the diseases.

It is based on a number of criteria that are used to assess each patient's overall condition of the whole body:[1]

- yin and yang for patient's constitution
- hypofunction and hyperfunction for the level of energy

- heat and cold for the character of the disease based on subjective feelings of heat (fever) and cold (chills)
- exterior or interior for the body area showing symptoms
- *ki* (vital energy), *ketsu* (blood) and *sui* (water) for the body's overall homoeostatic balance
- the theory of the pathogenesis of visceral disease
- the six stages in the progress of disease.

TCM is based on the theory of yin–yang and five elements (see Chapter 6). The yin–yang theory interprets all materials and phenomena as the contrasting results of two opposing abstractions: yin and yang. The theory of five elements aims to categorise these entities in terms of the five elements – wood, fire, earth, metal and water. Wood corresponds to hepatic function, fire to the heart or circulatory and autonomic nervous functions, earth to spleen and digestive function, metal to lung function, and water to kidney and urogenital function. Using a rationale based on these concepts, TCM explains the physiology and state of the viscera.

In kampo medicine, the disease state is observed to change over time. The *Shokanron* classifies the process of the disease into six stages, three each for yang and yin:

- Yang: *tai yang, shao yang* and *yang ming*
- Yin: *tai yin, shao yin* and *jue yin*.

Yang disease exhibits febrile and active reactions against pathological conditions whereas yin disease shows cold and passive reactions. Each stage has its primary sites where the disease appears:

- In *tai yang, shao yang,* and *yang ming* these appear in superficies (the outer surfaces of a body), mesoderm (the germ layer that forms many muscles, the circulatory and excretory systems, and the dermis, skeleton, and other supportive and connective tissue), and the interior of the body. The three stages of yang diseases are distinct in character because the primary sites all differ.
- Yin diseases are located mainly in the interior of the body.

Depending on the process of patient diseases, corresponding kampo herbal formulae are chosen for treatment.

Ki, ketsu and *sui* are concepts of three physiological factors that explain disturbance of the whole body. *Ki* (corresponding to the Chinese *qi)* is the vital energy and considered to correspond to the functions of digestion and absorption, and the neural system. Decreased *ki* becomes as weak in all of the activities as the human.

Ketsu corresponds to abnormality of blood such as abnormality of microcirculation and deficiency or stagnancy of the bloodstream. It is considered to be involved in the microadjustment of the body condition, circulation and endocrine functions.

Sui is considered to concern immunological and defence functions, and corresponds to the abnormality of water balance in the body. Compared with western medicines, *ki, ketsu* and *sui* are considered to be concerned partly with the neural, endocrine and immunological systems in the whole body system (Figure 8.1).

In kampo medicines, the theory of *ki, ketsu* and *sui* is the basis of assessing patients' clinical conditions. It is known that particular kampo formulae and their component herbs are able to normalise the abnormal state of *ki, ketsu* and *sui* as *ki* drugs, *kestu* drugs and *sui* drugs (Table 8.1).

Practice of kampo medicine

Kampo medicines are commonly used to treat many disorders including the following: hepatitis, menopausal disorders such as autonomic nervous and hormonal manifestations, defective coordination between the sympathetic and parasympathetic nervous systems, especially with respect to vasomotor activities (a condition known as 'autonomic imbalances'), bronchial asthma, cold syndrome, digestive disorders, atopic dermatitis, eczema, hypersensitivity to low temperatures, allergic rhinitis, general malaise, nephritis, constipation, chronic rheumatism, irritable bowel syndrome, hypertension, psychogenic pharyngeal symptoms, weak constitution, dermatitis, chronic bronchitis, diabetes, lumbago, neurosis, chronic paranasal sinusitis, neuralgia, sterility, degenerative joint disease and psychosomatic disorders.

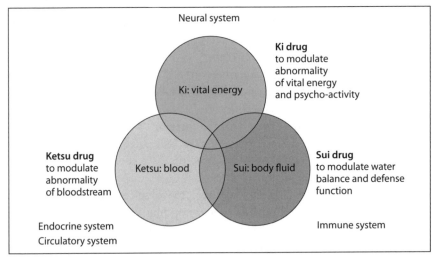

Figure 8.1 Harmony of *ki, ketsu* and *sui*.

Table 8.1 Kampo medicines for the disturbance of *ki, ketsu* and *sui*

Ki obstruction (abnormality of vital energy)	Symptoms	Kampo formulae
Deficiency of *ki*	Decline of vital activity: – listlessness – fatigue – loss of energy and appetite – decline of digestive function	*Shikunshito* *Hochuekkito* *Shokenchuto*
Obstruction of *ki*	Feeling of a small item of food obstructing the throat Fullness of abdomen	*Hangekobokuto* *Daikenchuto*
Rising of *ki*	Hot flush Palpitation attack starting from hypogastrium	*Keishikakeito*
***Ketsu* disturbance (abnormality of bloodstream)**		
Okestu syndrome (blood stagnation due to disability of microcirculation)	Menstrual disorders Turgescence of lower abdomen Tenderness of lower abdomen Congestion of skin mucosa and haemorrhoids	*Tokakujokito* *Keishibukuryogan* *Tokishakuyakusan*
Deficiency of *Ketsu*	Dry skin Pigmentation Anaemia Fatigue	*Shimotsuto* *Juzentaihoto* *Kyukikyogaito*
***Sui* disturbance (disorders of the body's fluid metabolism)**		
Accumulation of water	Edema Arthralgia Ascites	*Goreisan* *Boiogito*
Impaired water excretion	Urination disorder Abnormal pituitary secretions	*Seishinrenshiin* *Shoseiryuto*

Compared with the limited remedies offered by modern medicine, kampo medicine can relieve the suffering and discomforts inflicted by these diseases with relatively satisfactory effectiveness. Many of these diseases are multifactorial and still difficult to treat with only modern medicine; however, by correcting imbalance in the whole body, it is reported that kampo medicines are relatively effective in many cases, probably by affecting multiple target sites and recovering disturbance of whole biological systems (Figure 8.2).

This can be seen particularly in older people where diseases are caused by problems occurring simultaneously in several organs. Modern therapy

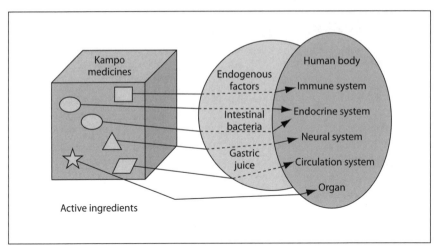

Figure 8.2 Active ingredients of kampo medicines.

treats these diseases with a variety of medicines. However, kampo medicine prescribes one individualised formula to treat the whole body, and eventually restore a normal physiological environment. In general, kampo medicines also have fewer adverse effects than modern medicines. Recently, some kampo medicines have been recognised as effective for the prevention of the progression of dementia such as Alzheimer's diseases and cerebrovascular disorders in Japan.[2,3] Kampo medicine does seem to be a very suitable treatment for older patients. The use of kampo medicines may also contribute to the reduction in medical costs.

Table 8.2 shows examples of component herbs of kampo formulae that are used or expected as medicines for the treatment of dementia.

More than 80% of practising physicians have experience of using the kampo system of medicine depending on the patient's clinical situation, either separately or to complement modern western medicines.[4]

Kampo medicines bring about benefit to the patients who:

- have diseases that affect physical functions
- have responded poorly to modern medical treatment or suffered side effects
- have improved on clinical examination, yet remained ill
- are normal on clinical examination, but remain affected
- are expected to show an improvement of the constitution or have a tendency towards psychosomatic disorders
- have decreased physical strength.

Table 8.2 Component herbs of kampo formulae associated with the treatment of dementia						
	KUT	**KKT**	**TSS**	**SMT**	**ORG**	**CTS**
Pinelliae tuber	O					O
Bambusae caulis	O					
Aurantii fructus immaturus	O					
Poria	O	O	O			O
Aurantii nobilis pericarpium	O					
Glycyrrhizae radix	O	O				
Scrophulariae radix	O					
Ginseng radix	O	O				O
Rehmanniae radix	O			O		
Zizyphi fructus	O	O				
Zizyphi semen	O	O				
Zingiberis rhizoma	O	O				O
Polygalae radix	O	O				
Atractylodis rhizoma		O				
Longan arillus		O				
Bupleuri radix		O				
Astragalis radix		O				
Angelicae radix		O	O	O		
Saussureae radix		O				
Paeoniae radix			O	O		
Cnidii rhizoma			O	O		
Atractylodis lanceae rhizoma			O			
Alismatis rhizoma			O			
Coptidis rhizoma					O	
Phellodendori cortex					O	
Scutellariae radix					O	
Gardeniae fructus		O			O	

Continued

Table 8.2 *Continued*						
	KUT	**KKT**	**TSS**	**SMT**	**ORG**	**CTS**
Uncariae uncis cum ramulus						○
Ophiopogonis tuber						○
Tachibana pericarpium						○
Chrysanthemi flos						○
Saphoshnikoviae radix						○
Gypsum fibrosum						○

CTS, *Chotosan*; KKT, *Kamikihito*; KUT, *Kamiuntanto*; ORG, *Ourengedokuto*; SMT, *Shimotsuto*; TSS, *Tokishakutyakusan*.

Diagnosis

Kampo diagnosis (*sho*) uses the holistic pattern of a patient's symptoms to determine the appropriate kampo formulae. The procedure investigates the following:

- The state of *ki*, *ketsu* and *sui*, yin–yang
- Any hypofunction and hyperfunction of body systems
- Any heat or cold in the superficies and interior of the body
- The five parenchymatous viscera (liver, heart, spleen, lung and kidney)
- The six stages of disease.

For example, *sho* of *Kakkonto (Ge-Gen-Tang)* is the symptom showing fever, neck and back pain, no sweat and aversion to wind. The pulse diagnosis is categorised as being 'floating and powerful'.

Four examination methods are used:

- Visual examination (overall, eyes, complexion, skin, nails, hair, lips and tongue)
- Examination by sense of hearing and smell
- Question and answer
- Sphygmopalpation (feeling the pulse) and abdominal palpation. Diagnosis of kampo medicine significantly differs from TCM in its use of abdominal diagnosis by palpation.

Traditional kampo medicines

Classification

Kampo medicines are classified by pharmacological activities into tonic, purgative, heat clearing, expelling superficial pathogenic factors, harmonising, regulating flow of *ki*, regulating flow of *ketsu* and dispelling dampness as a disease-inducing factor by the mode of actions for clinical use (Table 8.3).

Presentation

The medicines consist of a formulation of several different types of herbs. Examples of source materials for kampo medicines are shown in Figure 8.3. Minerals are included in the general term 'herbs'.

In the pharmacy these medicines are stored in wooden drawers and transferred with the use of special spoons (Figure 8.4). They are generally administered in the form of a decoction, prepared by extracting herbal material with warm water. When patients need such a decoction for treatment, they must prepare it by themselves. Each formulation has been named traditionally by putting *to* (meaning extract) as a suffix.

In order to adapt kampo medicines into modern-day therapy, several kampo extract pharmaceutical preparations with the same efficacy as the decoction have been developed. They are manufactured as granule forms by freeze drying the decoction prepared on a large scale. Consequently, these

Table 8.3 Classification of kampo medicines by mode of actions for clinical use	
Group of action	**Kampo formulae**
Tonic	*Shikunshito, Hochuekkito, Shimotsuto, Juzentaihoto, Rikkunshito, Hachimijiougan*
Purgative	*Daijokito, Daioukanzoto, Tokakujokito*
Heat clearing	*Orengedokuto, Byakkokaninjinto*
Expelling superficial pathogenic factors	*Maoto, Keishito, Kakkonto, Shoseiryuto*
Harmonising	*Shosaikoto, Hangeshashinto*
Regulating flow of *ki*	*Hangekobokuto, Kousosan*
Regulating flow of *kestu*	*Tokakujokito, Keishibukuryogan*
Dispelling dampness as a disease-inducing factor	*Goreisan, Boiogito*

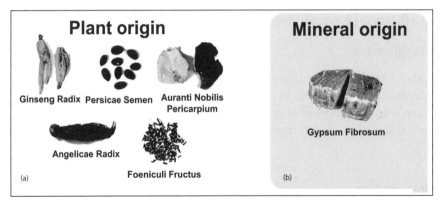

Figure 8.3 Examples of herbs prescribed for kampo medicines of (a) plant origin and (b) minerall origin.

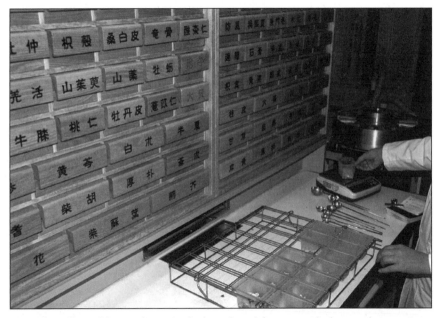

Figure 8.4 Chest of drawers for storing herbs and special spoons at the kampo pharmacy in the Oriental Medicine Research Center, Kitasato University.

drug forms are similar to western medicines. As these preparations are very convenient to use and highly portable, their current use is popular and extensive in Japan. However, the decoction of kampo medicines is still very useful as prescribed formulation because the ratio of component herbs in a decoction can be modified for a best fit to the patient's pathophysiological condition.

Kampo medicines have also been traditionally used as *gan* (pill form), *san* (powder form) and *kou* (ointment form), depending on the clinical applications.

In contrast to kampo medicines, Japanese folk medicines generally use a single Japanese herb, and its decoction has been taken orally for the treatment without any theoretical basis.

Quality control

Kampo extract pharmaceutical preparations, such as the granule form, have been quality controlled by good manufacturing practice (GMP) guidelines since 1988.

The Japanese pharmacopoeia

The pharmacopoeia of Japan lists 165 raw herbs used in kampo formulations and the *Japanese Herbal Medicine Codex* lists an additional 83 items.[4] For each herbal material listed in these two documents, the plant origin, physical properties and criteria for identification with respective testing methods are rigorously specified. Eleven kampo formulae have also been introduced into the Japanese pharmacopoeia. As natural plants, animal and mineral materials have been used as the raw material of ingredients in the pharmaceutical preparation, the quality control of these raw materials is required. This control includes the selection of high-quality herbs and their quality control including limits of contamination by pesticides and heavy metals, which are evaluated by morphological and physicochemical methods.

Quality

Quality control of herbs must be conducted by a qualified person who has special knowledge and experience with medicinal herbs. Preservation of herbs is very important for quality control. Process control and quality control for manufacturing of the final pharmaceutical preparation are also carried out in Japan.

As kampo formulae and their component herbs (crude drugs) contain multi-constituents, three-dimensional high-performance liquid chromatography (HPLC) analysis has recently been developed to compare the overall pattern of constituents through finger-printing analysis, in addition to the qualitative and quantitative analysis of the particular constituents that are specific in the herbs.

Evidence of effectiveness

Pharmacological studies

Although long-term clinical experiences suggest efficacy and safety, the mechanisms of action and active principles of kampo medicines have yet to be clarified scientifically.

Pharmacological studies of kampo medicines on a particular animal model of clinically related symptoms ought to be conducted.[5,6] The action of western medicine directs specifically to the nature and functions of a disease, whereas the action of kampo medicines attempts to harmonise the disturbed pathophysiological conditions of the patient (so-called *sho* clinically) as a whole to eventually balance a normal physiological environment in the system. Although it is difficult to clarify *sho* scientifically, pharmacological studies based on clinical effects are constructive for the evaluation of kampo medicines. Some kampo medicines are known to exhibit immunopotentiation activity when they are given to immunocompliant mice, but they also recover to normal level when they are administered to over-immunostimulated mice, such as those for adjuvant arthritis, even if they exhibit no effect on normal mice.

If western medicine and kampo medicines are compared using a globe, western medicine affects diseases divided by longitude, whereas kampo medicines affect several whole body systems, which are common in several diseases and divided by latitude. Thus the targets are different in both medicines.

Kampo medicines contain many constituents derived from component herbs. To control the quality of kampo medicines, the exact active principle(s) has to be identified. As kampo medicines are generally administered orally, some components may exist as precursors of active principles (see Figure 8.2). These 'inactive' compounds may be activated by endogenous factors such as gastric secretions, and intestinal enzymes and bacteria, e.g. although sennoside A or B in *Rhei rhizoma* (rhizome of *Rheum palmatum* Linne) is known to elicit a cathartic activity, such an effect is not produced when the sennoside is injected into mice. However, when either sennoside is administered orally, the cathartic activity is observed. In fact, rhein-anthrone, a metabolite formed by the action of intestinal bacteria, has been identified as the active component responsible for the catharsis.[7–9] In addition, rhein-anthrone is further metabolised to rhein which displays antibacterial activities against intestinal anaerobic bacteria.[10] As such, the action of intestinal bacteria affects the activities of *Rhei rhizoma*, and a certain feedback mechanism may be involved in mild catharsis (Figure 8.5). Therefore studies on the post-administration products or byproducts of orally administered kampo medicines are important in the elucidation of the mechanism(s) of action of a particular kampo formulation.

Orally administered glycyrrhizin of *Glycyrrhizae radix* produces a high concentration of its aglycone, glycyrrhetic acid, and a low level of glycyrrhizin in circulating blood of rat and human.[11] Therefore glycyrrhetic acid is an important active principle when kampo medicines containing *Glycyrrhizae radix* are administered orally. Efficacy of kampo medicines cannot be explained by the pharmacological activities of a particular active

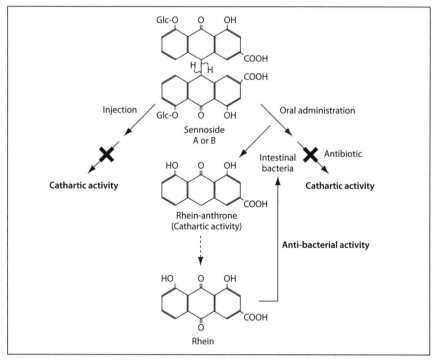

Figure 8.5 Cathartic activity and metabolite of sennosides from *Rhei rhizoma*.

principle. Several or all of the biologically active substances in a certain kampo medicine may influence the multiple target sites and the systems of the whole body via one or more combination effects (see Figure 8.2). As each kampo formulation contains many constituents derived from the component herbs, the action of the kampo medicine becomes very complicated when the preparation is administered orally. When the effects of sera taken from orally prednisolone-treated mice 1 hour after administration are compared with those of the control mice, the former inhibit lipopolysaccharide (LPS)-induced mitogenic responses dose dependently. These in vitro findings are similar to in vivo effects of prednisolone in rats. Although the approach is indirect, it is useful to employ sera obtained from animals administered orally with the test samples for in vitro investigations. When spleen cells are treated with *Shosaikoto* without LPS, mitogenic responses of spleen cells of mice treated orally with *Shosaikoto* were not observed and the addition of sera from similarly treated mice did not affect the responses.[12] However, only the direct addition of *Shosaikoto* to the culture medium reveals a mitogenic effect.[13] Therefore, an indirect in vitro effect may reflect the in vivo action of the formulation. As the serum samples contained active principles of orally administered kampo medicines, which are absorbed from the gastrointestinal tract, Tashiro advocates a similar approach for the in vitro evaluation of kampo medicines.[14] He further proposed this method to be categorised as serum pharmacology and serum pharmacochemistry.

As a kampo medicine contains many active ingredients, several combination effects are involved in their action. These combination effects can be classified as follows.

Pharmacological effects

These effects may include synergistic, additive and antagonistic actions, new pharmacological activity and reduction of adverse reaction.

Pharmaceutical effects

These effects affect modulations of taste and pH, absorption, enhancement of extraction and interaction among constituents.

Sometimes the decocted extract of the original prescription shows much higher effect than that of the mixture of extracts prepared individually from the respective component herbs at the designated similar ratio. Combinations of the component herbs in kampo medicines may also influence the content of active principles when decocted.

Combination effect of kampo medicines

If only one component herb is replaced in a formulation, the clinical application may be greatly changed. *Maoto*, *Makyokansekito* and *Makoyokkanto* are similar kampo formulations consisting of four component herbs. Three of the herbs (*Ephedrae herba*, *Ameniacae semen* and *Glycyrrhizae radix*) are common to both formulations but their indications for use are quite different (Table 8.4).

Maoto, *Makyokansekito* and *Makyoyokkanto* have all been used for the treatment of influenza, asthma and rheumatoid conditions, respectively. However *Maoto* is indicated where the patient has no sweating, high fever, muscle and joint pains, whereas *Makyokansekito* is indicated where there is natural sweating, cough and asthma. *Makyoyokkanto* is indicated where there are muscle and joint pains. Another Kampo formula, *Shosaikoto-gokeishikashakuyakusan* (TJ-960) has been studied for the effect of its component herbs on treating epilepsy induced by pentylenetetrazole injection in EI mice. TJ-960 shows very potent inhibitory activity of epilepsy. It consists of 10 component herbs, but when just one of component herbs was omitted from the original formulation, its activity became negligible.[15]

The foregoing examples show that a combination of several active principles in the component herbs of a kampo formulation is important for a kampo formulation to be effective.

Examples of studies on specific formulae

Three kampo formulae are introduced as examples of current pharmacological studies of kampo medicines.

Table 8.4 Combination effect of kampo medicines

Formulae	Typical indications	Major symptoms	Component herbs					
			Ephedra herba	Ameniacae semen	Glycyrrhizae radix	Cinnamomi cortex	Gypsum fibrosuim	Coicis semen
Maoto (Ma-Huang-Tang)	Influenza	No sweating High fever Muscle pain Joint pain	●	●	●	●		
Makyokansekiot (Ma-Xing-Gan-Shi-Tang)	Asthma	Natural sweating Asthma Difficulty in breathing	●	●	●		●	
Makyoyokkanto (Ma-Xing-Yi-Gan-Tang)	Articular rheumatism	Joint pain Muscle pain	●	●	●			●

Effects of *Juzentaihoto* on immunological and haematopoietic systems

Clinical effects of *Juzentaihoto* expect that it may improve constitution of the diseases related to immunological system. In vivo animal study suggests that *Juzentaihoto* has potent immunomodulating activity, such as stimulation of antibody production,[16] and the active ingredients were clarified to be 22 different pectic polysaccharides.[17] Helper T cells (Th) are known to separate into two subsets: Th1, which produces interferon-γ (IFN-γ) and interleukin (IL)-2, stimulates cellular immunity, and Th2, which produces IL-4 and IL-5, stimulates humoral immunity depending on the pattern of cytokine formation. Administration of *Juzentaihoto* pharmaceutical extract preparation (TJ-48) increased IFN-γ production remarkably, as well as IL-5 secretion from both mesenteric lymph node (MLN) and Peyer's patches (PPs), whereas IL-2 secretion was plainly reduced.[16] The ratio IFN-γ:IL-4 was shifted to Th1 domination in MLN and PPs relating to gastric mucosal immune system; however, little changed in the spleen relating to systemic immune system.[16] These observations indicate that *Jusentaihoto* regulates Th1:Th2 balance in gastric mucosal immune system. As kampo medicines have generally been taken orally, active ingredients may not only act by absorption from the intestine but also affect the mucosal immune system. Oral administration of TJ-48 activates T cells in PP cells, and stimulates the production of the haematopoietic factors such as IL-6 and GM-CSF (granulocyte–macrophage colony-stimulating factor) to proliferate bone marrow cells.[16] Oral administration of TJ-48 also regulates cytokine production from stimulated hepatic lymphocytes, and increases the population of NKT cells that are able to prevent cancer metastasis and autoimmune diseases.[16] NKT cells are a heterogeneous group of T cells that share properties of both T cells and natural killer (NK) cells. NKT cells seem to be essential for several aspects of immunity.

The effect of the active ingredients of *Juzentaihoto* on intestinal immune system-modulating activities was linked to a lignin–carbohydrate complex and a polysaccharide-containing arabinogalactan.[18,19] Although *Juzentaihoto* consists of two kampo formulae, *Shimotsuto* and *Shikunshito* with *Cinnamomi cortex* and *Astragari radix*, the activity appeared in the lignin–carbohydrate complex fraction of the decoction, which was prepared by combining *Shikunshito* (*Atractylodis lanceae rhizoma*, *Ginseng radix*, *Poria* and *Glycyrrhizae radix*) with *Cinnamomi cortex* and *Astragari radix*.[20] Therefore the intestinal immunity-modulating activity of *Juzentaihoto* is due to the combination effect of the component herbs.

Juzentaihoto also enhances peripheral blood counts in cancer patients who have been administered phase-specific drugs and/or have received radiation therapy. Oral administration of *Juzentaihoto* prolongs the survival of tumour-bearing mice injected with mitomycin C, and enhances proliferation of bone marrow stem cells, which may induce recovery from anaemia and reduce side effects of anti-cancer agents caused by bone marrow injury.[21]

Effects of *Hochuekkito* on upper respiratory mucosal immune system
In the mucosal immune system, if the intestinal immune system were activated by the oral administration of kampo medicines containing mucosal immune system-activating substance, the common mucosal immune system in nasopharyngeal-associated lymphoid tissue, bronchial-associated lymphoid tissue and urogenital-associated lymphoid tissue would be activated through activation of the intestinal immune system at the induction site. As the result, production of antigen-specific secretory IgA antibody is enhanced in local mucus if the antigen such as for influenza virus, is recognised. Therefore a mucosal immune system-enhancing activity may help respiratory infection and endogenous infection. When the influenza vaccine was immunised intranasally, antigen-specific secretory IgA antibody is produced in the nasal cavity.[22] Oral administration of *Hochuekkito* significantly enhances the influenza virus-specific IgA antibody titre in the nasal wash of aged mice, which were secondarily immunised by intranasal inoculation of the vaccine.[22] The upper respiratory mucosal immune system is known to maintain the function through targeting of the lymphocytes from the intestinal immune system in common mucosal immune system. Oral administration of *Hochuekkito* may partly contribute to enhancement of the IgA immune response against intestinal antigen through an increased population of L-selectin-positive B lymphocytes.[23] Therefore *Hochuekkito* may strengthen the defence system against various pathogens and food antigens in the local mucosal sites in intestine, lung and nasal cavity.

Improving effect of *Kamiuntanto* on brain cognitive function
The population of older people has been increased by improving health conditions. As a 'compensation' for longevity, chronic diseases, senile dementia, osteoporosis, general malaise and complex diseases (diabetes, hypertension, hyperlipidaemia, etc.) have increased in older people. For the diagnosis and treatment of these diseases imbalance of the whole body must be seen. Therefore kampo medicines would be suitable drugs for the treatment of older patients. There are now at least one million patients with senile dementia in Japan. Alzheimer's disease and cerebrovascular disorders are popular forms of dementia among older people, with the former characterised by memory loss and a progressive global impairment of intellect. Despite the great scientific advances in recent years, effective treatments for Alzheimer's disease are still limited. Some kampo medicines and herbal extracts were reported to improve the lesion of cognitive function in animal models for dementia, and memory-related behaviour and intellectual function of Alzheimer's disease patients.[24]

Alzheimer's disease patients are known to have decreased levels of acetylcholine and the acetylcholine-synthesizing enzyme, choline acetyltransferase (ChAT), and these levels correlate well with severity of dementia. When rat embryo septal cells were cultured with *Kamiuntanto*, a significant increase of ChAT activity was observed as seen with nerve growth factor (NGF).[24] When the 2-year-old rats, with decreased memory and learning activity on passive avoidance test, were given *Kamiuntanto* orally, mean latency was significantly increased similar to mature rats.[25] Oral administration of *Kamiuntanto* enhanced ChAT activity and the NGF mRNA expression in the frontoparietal cortex of the rats.[24] A clinical study showed that *Kamiuntanto* was well tolerated by Alzheimer's disease patients, and that it transiently restored cognitive function over baseline for an average of 9 months.[2] This study suggests that *Kamiuntanto* may be a safe and efficacious herbal medicine for the symptomatic treatment in mild-to-moderate Alzheimer's disease. When *Kamiuntanto* and donepezil, which is an anti-Alzheimer's disease drug, were taken together, after 12 weeks' treatment, a significant improvement in cognition was noted only in the combination therapy group, not in the monotherapy group. A significant increase in cerebral blood flow was also seen in the frontal region and lenticular nucleus only in patients who received the combination therapy. Therefore the combination of donepezil plus *Kamiuntanto* is safe and more effective in maintaining cognitive function than monotherapy.

The pharmacological activities of widely used kampo medicines are listed in Table 8.5.

Clinical studies

The Japanese Ministry of Health and Welfare requested clinical re-evaluation of eight kampo formulations by double-blind, placebo-controlled study in 1991. For the double-blind, placebo-controlled study, it is necessary to prepare placebo granules with similar taste and colour as the active preparation. In the case of a decoction, preparation of a control extract is very difficult.

Three formulae have been re-evaluated:

- *Shosaikoto (Xiao-Chai-Hu-Tang)* was evaluated for efficacy in chronic active hepatitis.
- *Daiokanzoto (Da-Huang-Gan-Cao-Tang)* was proofed for constipation.
- *Shoseiryuto (Xiao-Quing-Long-Tang)* was for bronchitis and perennial nasal allergy by double-blind, placebo-controlled study.

Rikkunshito (Liu-Jun-Zi-Tang) and *Shakuyakukanzoto (Shao-Yao-Gan-Cao-Tang)* were also reported as being effective for the treatment of dysmotility-like dyspepsia and the muscle cramps accompanying cirrhosis, respectively.

Table 8.5 Pharmacological activities of kampo medicines

Kakkonto
Suppression of fever
Anti-allergic action
Suppression of pneumonia due to influenza virus infection
Reduction of increased IL-1α level due to influenza virus infection

Hachimijiogan
Suppression of experimental diabetes
Suppression of the circulatory disorder
Inhibition of aldose reductase activity
Improvement of bone metabolism
Increment of testosterone level in testicle tissue
Diuretic action
Suppression of hypertension
Improvement of renal failure

Shosaikoto
Suppression of experimental hepatic injury
Suppression of decrease of bloodstream in liver
Enhancement of liver regeneration
Suppression of liver fibrosis
Immunomodulating activity
Clearance activity of immune complex
Antiallergic action
Anti-inflammatory action
Suppression of production of active oxygen molecules

Orengedokuto
Increment of blood circulation level in hippocampus of brain
Suppression of increased hypertension in SHR-SP
Decrease of total cholesterol, triglyceride and phospholipids level in heart
Suppression of platelet aggregation
Suppression of gastric mucous membrane injury
Anti-inflammatory activity
Suppression of lipid peroxidation
Improvement of experimental colitis

Shoseiryuto
Antiallergic activity
Anti-inflammatory activity
Suppression of chemical mediators (histamine, leukotriene, PAF) production on release
Increment of arachidonic acid metabolism (PGE$_2$ production)
Anti-influenza virus activity in allergic pulmonary inflammation model mice

Tokishakuyakusan
Action on hormones
Increment of progesterone production from ovarian cells by stimulation with hCG
Enhancement of LH and FSH secretions from rat ptosis cultured cells
Enhancement of estradiol secretion
Increments of uterus weight and number of oestrogen receptor in uterus
Induction of ovulation
Suppression of contraction of uterus
Action to blood coagulation

Continued

Table 8.5 *Continued*

Tokishakuyakusan *continued*
Decrease of urea protein in adenine induced renal failure in rat
Elimination of free radical
Inhibition of arachidonic acid cascade
Improvement of menopausal disorder
Enhancement of IL-6 secretion

Kamiuntanto
Neurotrophic-like activity (induction of ChAT activity of cerebral cortex)
Improvement of passive avoidance behaviour in basal brain-lesioned or aged rats
Increment of ChAT activity and NGF mRNA levels of the cerebral cortex
Increment of NGF secretion from astroglial cells

Keishibukuryogan
Modulation of hormone action (suppression of increases of wet uterus weight and uterus thymidine kinase activity by the action of estradiol)
Modulation of uterus action
Improvement of menopausal disorder

Bakumondoto
Anti-tussive action
Mucoregulatory action and airway clearance action
Suppression of contraction of bronchi by acetylcholine
Antiallergic action

Hochuekkieto
Immunomodulating activity
Effects on testis
Suppression of decrease of bone density under reduced physical strength
Anti-influenza activity on infectious model
Enhancement of serotonin receptor ($5HT_{2c}$) in brain

Rikkunshito
Anti-ulcer activity
Enhancement of locomotion of digestive tract
Suppression of experimental mucous injuries
Suppression of decrease of phosphoplipid in gastric mucous membrane
Increase of gastric mucus level
Elimination of active oxygen molecules
Suppression of decrease of bloodstream in gastric mucous membrane
Suppression of secretions of gastric acid and pepsin

Chotosan
Suppression of increased hypertension

Juzentaihoto
Immunopotentiating activity
Modulation of systemic immune system (increase of T-cell-dependent antibody response and phagocytosis, mitogenic activity against spleen B cells; anti-complementary activity)
Modulation of Th1:Th2 balance in gastric mucosal immune system
Modulation of hepatic immune system and induction of liver NKT cells
Anti-metastatic activity
Potentiation of haematopoietic system

Table 8.5 *Continued*

Shakuyakukanzoto
Maintenance of contractility against muscle clamping model

Shimotsuto
Anti-stress effect
Reversal effect of scopolamine-induced impairment in the radical maze performance
Delay of the development of the infarction and rarefaction following chronic ischaemia of the brain
Anti-metastatic activity

Saibokuto
Suppression of experimental allergic reactions
Suppression and antagonistic actions on release and production of chemical mediators
Suppression of decrease of β-receptor
Suppression of decrease of glucocorticoid receptor
Suppression of induction of IgE Fcε receptor II in lymphocytes from asthma patient
Improvement of tracheal mucociliary tract

Ninjinyoeito
Immunomodulating activity (suppression of decrease of NK activity in spleen cells)
Improvement of passive avoidance behaviour in hyoscine administered mouse

Saireito
Diuretic activity
Anti-inflammatory activity (increase of blood ACTH level, increase of corticosterone secretion from adrenal gland)

5HT, 5-hydroxytryptamine (serotonin); ACTH, adrenocorticotrophic hormone; ChAT, choline acetyltransferase; FSH, follicle-stimulating hormone; hCG, human chorionic gonadotrophin; Ig, immunoglobulin; IL, interleukin; LH, luteinising hormone; NGF, nerve growth factor; NKT, natural killer/T cells; PAF, platelet-activating factor; PG, prostaglandin; SHR-SP, stroke-prone spontaneously hypertensive rats; Th, T-helper cell.

In the case of *Rikkunshito*, a low-dose preparation was used as a placebo control because of difficulty in developing control granules.

In a separate double-blind, controlled study for re-evaluation, *Chotosan (Siao-Tang-San)* was also shown to have a beneficial clinical effect in the treatment of vascular dementia.[26]

Although kampo medicines have a long clinical experience, they also need an objective clinical evaluation as evidence-based medicine (EBM). However, kampo medicines have traditionally been used according to the disturbed pathophysiological conditions of the patient (so-called *sho* clinically), so clinical study of kampo medicines needs to consider the concept of *sho*.[27] In clinical trials, objects should be chosen depending on the status of *sho*, e.g. the trial can be limited to patients showing a hypofunctioning condition. The design of the trial is very important for clinical study of kampo medicine.

Kampo medicines have to consider two judgements in EBM: one is the most reliable scientific proof and the other is the specific clinical situation and value for each patient. Most reliable scientific proofs are obtained by re-evaluation of kampo extract preparations, objective clinical study and the importance of universality. When looking at EBM for kampo medicines, balance and harmonisation between both judgements are important for practical medical care.

The Japanese Society for Oriental Medicine has selected 95 EBM reports of kampo treatment, which were based on *sho* diagnosis and evaluation items in modern medicine, from the peer-reviewed published papers of the clinical studies of kampo medicines.[28] These EBM reports have been gathered for a variety of formulae.

Safety

Side effects of kampo medicines

If the *sho* diagnosis was correct, and the correct formulation was given to the patient, kampo medicines show relatively lower adverse reactions compared with western medicines. However, kampo medicines are also drugs, so they must be considered to have certain side effects depending on how they are used.

Furthermore it is important to note that, after taking kampo medicines, unexpected adverse drug reactions (ADRs) may happen before the symptoms improve. Some component herbs are known to cause ADRs depending on inappropriate use as follows.

Ephedrae herba

Ephedrae herba contains the adrenergic ephedrine, which activates both the sympathetic and central nervous systems, and may produce unwanted symptoms such as insomnia, palpitations, rapid pulse, excitement, elevation of blood pressure, hyperhidrosis, and dysuria. Therefore *E. herba* must not be used in patients who have ischaemic heart disease or angina pectoris. Kampo formulae containing *E. herba* are also generally not suitable for older people.

Glycyrrhizae radix

Glycyrrhizae radix contains glycyrrhizin. *G. radix* is prescribed in 15% of the 210 kampo formulations. Glycyrrhizin metabolises to the aglycone, glycyrrhetic acid, after oral administration, and glycyrrhetic acid facilitates potassium excretion and lowers total serum potassium.

Excess administration of *G. radix* causes oedema, hypertension and pseudoaldosteronism, so care must be taken if the plural kampo formulations containing *G. radix* are given together.

Rhei rhizoma

Rhei rhizoma contains sennosides that are prodrugs of rhein-anthrone, having cathartic activity. Therefore *R. rhizoma* is not suitable to give to patients who have hypofunctional symptoms.

Drug–drug interactions

Some western medicines are known to have potent adverse reactions, e.g. antitumour agents generally cause anaemia, decrease of leukocytes, and cause systemic weakness and vomiting. The use of western medicine with kampo medicines classified as tonic, such as *Juzentaihoto*, *Hochuekkito*, *Ninjinyoeito* and *Rikkunshito*, can reduce the adverse reaction to western anticancer drugs in patients and increase their quality of life. As one mechanism of action, it has been reported that *Juzentaihoto* enhances the proliferation of haematopoietic stem cells, and recovery of the haematopoietic system. Steroids also have side effects such as moon face (swelling), thrombus, infection and menopausal disorders.

Kampo medicines, such as *Shosaikoto*, *Saireito* and *Saibokuto*, can reduce these adverse reactions. It is also possible to decrease the daily dose of steroid and even to stop its use. It has been reported that these kampo medicines increase endogenous corticosterone concentrations in the body by affecting steroid metabolism.

It is known that several glycosides in kampo medicines show various biological activities as prodrugs, and aglycones, which are produced by the action of glycosidases from intestinal bacteria, can be absorbed into the blood and be active. Therefore, it is possible that some antibiotics may kill bacteria and affect the actions of kampo medicines when both are given together. As kampo medicines are very popular in Japan, drug interactions between kampo medicines and western medicine should be considered in order to avoid an undesired change in the efficacy.

Availability of kampo medicines

The first six kampo extract pharmaceutical preparations were developed in granule form in 1957. Since 1976, 147 kampo granular or powder formulations and one ointment have been approved for reimbursement by the Japanese national health insurance system. Their acceptance was based on clinical experience of efficacy and safety without any clinical validation studies. Herbs that are components of such kampo formulations are also covered by insurance.

In 1965, the Ministry of Health and Welfare of Japan designated 210 kampo formulations as over-the-counter drugs, chosen on the basis of favourable experiences by expert practitioners. In 2006, the number of drugs was increased to 298 traditional formulae in order to reflect societal changes with more elderly people, changing disease profiles and dietary habits as well as environmental changes.

Examples of major kampo medicines

Kampo formulae for immunological disease

Juzentaihoto (Si-Quan-Da-Bu-Tang)

Juzentaihoto consists of 10 component herbs: *Glycyrrhizae radix*, *Ginseng radix*, *Atractylodis rhizoma* or *Atractylodis lanceae rhizoma*, *Paeoniae radix*, *Cinnamomi cortex*, *Angelicae radix*, *Poria*, *Rehmanniae radix*, *Cnidii rhizoma* and *Astragalis radix*.

The preparation is known to influence the immune system specifically. *Juzentaihoto* is a tonifying drug, used to treat anaemia, anorexia, fatigue and general debilitation (caused by surgery, chronic diseases or child birth), night sweats and coldness of the hands and feet. In some patients, *Juzentaihoto* may also help in chronic fatigue syndrome, ulcerous colitis and atopic dermatitis.

Juzentaihoto reduces adverse effects associated with anticancer agents or radiation injuries. Table 8.6 shows examples of component herbs of kampo formulae that are used as tonifying drugs.

Hochuekkito (Bu-Zhong-Yi-Qi-Tang)

Hochuekkito consists of 10 component herbs: *Astragali radix*, *Ginseng radix*, *Atractylodis rhizoma* or *Atractylodis lanceae rhizoma*, *Angelicae radix*, *Aurantii nobilis pericarpium*, *Zizyphi fructus*, *Bupluri radix*, *Glycyrrhizae radix*, *Cimicifugae rhizoma* and *Zingiberis rhizoma*.

Hochuekkito has been used for the treatment and recovery of people who are overly concerned about their health ('valetudinarians'), and who have chronic diseases, tuberculosis, mild fever, night sweats, palpitation, fear, restlessness, weak feeble voice, slurred speech and disturbance of vision. It has been identified as an effective drug to improve the function of the digestive system and to strengthen the body's defences against various infectious agents.

Ninjinyoeito (Ren-Shen-Yang-Rong-Tang)

Ninjinyoeito consists of 12 component herbs: the 9 component herbs of *Juzentaihoto* listed above together with *Aurantii nobilis pericarpium*, *Polygalae radix* and *Schisandrae fructus*.

Ninjinyoeito has been used for the treatment of a debilitated general condition (caused by surgery or after illness), fatigue, malaise, anorexia,

Table 8.6 Component herbs of kampo formulae that are used as tonifying drugs

	JTT	HET	NYT
Ginseng radix	O	O	O
Atractylodis rhizoma or Atractylodis lanceae rhizoma	O	O	O
Glycyrrhizae radix	O	O	O
Poria	O		O
Zingiberis rhizoma		O	
Zizyphi fructus		O	
Angelicae radix	O	O	O
Paeoniae radix	O		O
Rehmanniae radix	O		O
Cnidii rhizoma	O		
Cinnamomi cortex	O		O
Astragalis radix	O	O	O
Aurantii nobilis pericarpium		O	O
Bupleuri radix		O	
Schisandrae fructus			O
Cimicifugae rhizoma		O	
Polygalae radix			O

HET, *Hochuekkito*; JJT, *Juzentaihoto*; NYJ, *Ninhinyoeito*.

night sweats, and coldness of hands and feet, especially in patients who are experiencing problems with their respiratory and central nervous systems.

Kampo formulae for psychosomatic diseases

Kamikihito (Jia-Wei-Gui-Pi-Tang)

Kamikihito is an extract of 14 kinds of component herbs: *Ginseng radix, Atractylodis rhizoma, Poria, Zizyphi spinosi semen, Longanae arillus, Bupleuri radix, Astragali radix, Angelicae radix, Gardeniae fructus, Polygalae radix, Zizyphi fructus, Glycyrrhizae radix, Saussureae radix* and *Zingiberis rhizoma*.

Kamikihito has been used to treat insomnia, anaemia, amnesia, anxiety and neurosis; accompanying constitutional characteristics of weakness, psychosomatic lassitude and a pale complexion may be recognised.

Kamiuntanto (Jia-Wei-Wen-Dan-Tang)

Kamiuntanto is an extract of 13 component herbs: *Dinelliae tuber, Phyllostachsis caulis, Aurantii fructus immaturus, Poria, Aurantii nobilis pericarpium, Glycyrrhizae radix, Ginseng radix, Rehmanniae radix, Ziziphi fructus, Ziziphi spinosi serum* and *Zingiberis rhizoma.*

Kamiuntanto has been used traditionally for psychoneurogical diseases. Suzuki et al. reported that the clinical application of *Kamiuntanto* for certain elderly patients with Alzheimer's disease slowed the rate of cognitive decline.[2] This observation supports earlier pharmacological studies of *Kamiuntanto* on brain cognitive function[24] and suggests that *Kamiuntanto* is useful as a potential therapeutic agent in diseases caused by cholinergic deficit.

Kampo formulae for cardiovascular diseases

Ourengedokuto (Huang-Lian-Jie-Tang)

Ourengedokuto is an extract of four component herbs: *Coptidis rhizoma, Phellodendri cortex, Scutellariae radix* and *Gardeniae fructus.*

The kampo formula has frequently been used for the treatment of hypertension. It also has efficacy in cases of facial flushing, sleeplessness, agitation, skin itching and gastritis.

Some clinical and basic research demonstrated that *Ourengedokuto* also improves decreased cerebral blood flow,[29] ischaemia-induced neuronal death[30] and damaged cognitive function.[31] These observations suggest that *Ourengedokuto* may be available as a potential therapeutic formula for treating cerebrovascular disorders.

Chotosan (Diao-Teng-San)

Chotosan comprises ten components, of which nine are herbs: *Pinelliae tuber, Poria, Ginseng radix, Zingiberis rhizoma, Uncariae ramulus et uncus, Ophiopogonis tuber, Aurantii nobilis pericarpium, Chrysanthem flos, Saphoshnikoviae divaricata* and the mineral gypsum fibrosum (considered to be a herb in kampo medicine).

Chotosan is administered to older patients with physical weakness and such subjective symptoms as headache, heavy feeling of the head, vertigo, hot flush, tinnitus, insomnia and painful tension of the shoulder.[26] It is suggested that these symptoms originate from disorders of the cerebrovascular system. Terasawa and co-workers demonstrated a double-blind, placebo-controlled clinical study of *Chotosan* in the treatment of vascular dementia.[26] Such items as spontaneity of conversation, lack of facial expression, decline in simple mathematical ability, global intellectual ability, nocturnal delirium, sleep disturbance, hallucination or delusion, and dressing and undressing were significantly improved at one or more evaluation points in those taking *Chotosan* compared with those taking placebo. The change in the revised version of Hasegawa's dementia scale from the start point in the *Chotosan* group tended to be higher than that in the placebo group with no statistical significance.

Kampo formulae for renal diseases

Saireito (Chai-Ling-Tang)

Saireito consists of 12 component herbs: *Bupleuri radix, Pinelliae tuber, Alismatis rhizoma, Scutellariae radix, Zizyphi fructus, Ginseng radix, Polyporus, Poria, Atractylodis rhizoma, Cinnamomi cortex, Glycyrrhizae radix* and *Zingiberis rhizoma*.

Saireito is a combined formulation of *Shosaikoto* and *Goreisan* that has been reported to be useful in improving nephritic syndrome. *Saireito* has also been used for the treatments of hydrodipsia (water thirst) and oliguria, renal diseases such as glomerular nephritis and nephrosis, hepatitis and oedema.

Kampo formulae for gynaecological disease

Tokishakuyakusan (Dang-Gui-Shao-Yao-San)

Tokishakuyakusan consists of six component herbs: *Angelicae radix, Paeoniae radix, Cnidii rhizoma, Atractylodis lanceae rhizoma, Alismatis rhizoma* and *Poria*.

Tokishakuyakusan has been used traditionally for gynaecological diseases such as ovarian dysfunction, endometriosis and menopausal syndrome in women. *Tokishakuyakusan* applies for the treatment of menoxenia, menstrual colic, sterility, abortion, vertigo, headache, oedema, anaemia, vasomotor imbalance, coldness of limbs and chilblains of the feet, nephritis and hypotonia.

Clinical studies have shown that treatment with the extract preparation of *Tokishakuyakusan* (TJ-23) improved the daily life of patients with Alzheimer's disease.[32–34] Sex differences in the ageing brain have been documented by clinically and epidemiologically suggesting that age-related changes in neural systems may result partly from hormonal changes. One of the major symptoms of menopausal women is dementia of Alzheimer's type. The symptoms are an impairment of intelligence and performance, impairment of memory and language disintegration. It was suggested that steroidal sex hormones seem to be one of the essential substances for maintenance of the limbic system and forebrain functions, which regulate memory, emotion, orientation of time and space, motivation and cognitive functions in menopausal women. Therefore *Tokishakuyakusan* may have therapeutic efficacy for the treatment of age-related deterioration and diseases such as dementia of Alzheimer's type.

Keishibukuryogan (Gui-Zhi-Fu-Ling-Wang)

Keishibukuryogan consists of five component herbs: *Cinnamomi cortex, Poria, Moutan cortex, Persicae semen* and *Paeoniae radix.*

Keishibukuryogan has been used for the treatment of coldness, hot flush, headache, stiff shoulder, vertigo, congestion in the small veins, telangiectasia, rough skin, discoloration of the tongue and gums, oppressive pain, resistance and fullness of the lower abdomen.

Shimotsuto (Si-Wu-Tang)

Shimotsuto is an extract of four component herbs: *Angelicae radix, Cnidii rhizoma, Paeonide radix* and *Rehmannia radix.*

Shimotsuto has been used traditionally for the treatments of fatigue after childbirth or abortion, abnormality of menstruation, climacteric disorder, coldness, chilblains and anaemia.

Kampo formulae for respiratory diseases

Bakumondoto (Mai-Men-Dong-Tang)

Bakumondoto consists of six component herbs: *Ophiopogonis tuber, Pinelliae tuber, Zizphi fructus, Glycyrrhizae radix, Ginseng radix* and *Oryzae fructus. Bakumondoto* has been used for the treatment of bronchitis and pharyngitis accompanying severe dry cough.

Kakkonto (Ge-Gen Tang)

Kakkonto consists of seven component herbs: *Radix puerariae, Zizyphi fructus, Glycyrrhizae radix, Zingiberis rhizoma, Ephedra herba, Paeoniae radix* and *Cinnamomi cortex.*

From ancient times *Kakkonto* has been applied for the improvement of symptoms in the acute phase of viral infection, such as common cold, influenza and varicella-zoster. *Kakkonto* is used in Japan to alleviate fever, headache, sore throat, chills and polyarthralgia in the acute phase of influenza, and shoulder pain.

Shoseiryuto (Xiao-Qing-Long-Tang)

Shoseiryuto consists of eight component herbs: *Pinelliae tuber, Glycyrrhizae radix, Ephedra herba, Paeoniae radix, Cinnamomi cortex, Schisandrae fructus, Asiasari radix* and *Zingiberis processum rhizoma.*

Shoseiryuto has been used clinically for the treatment of certain 'cold' syndromes: bronchitis, bronchial asthma, allergic rhinitis and rhinitis accompanying oedema, paroxysmal sneezing and watery nasal secretion relating to abnormal water balance. There is evidence from a double-blind clinical study that *Shoseiryuto* is effective in the treatment of allergic rhinitis

Saibokuto (Chai-Pu-Tang)

Saibokuto consists of 10 component herbs: *Bupleuri radix, Pinelliae tuber, Poria, Scutellariae radix, Ginseng radix, Zizyphi fructus, Magnoliae cortex, Perillae herba, Glycyrrhizae radix* and *Zingiberis rhizoma.*

Saibokuto has been used for the treatments of respiratory diseases such as paediatric asthma, bronchial asthma, bronchitis, cough, weakness of the constitution and anxiety neurosis accompanying unusual feelings in the throat and oesophagus, and depressed feeling, and occasionally palpitation, vertigo and nausea.

Kampo formulae for digestive disorders

Shosaikoto (Xiao-Chai-Hu-Tang)

Shosaikoto consists of seven component herbs: *Pinelliae tuber, Zyzyphi fructus, Glycyrrhizae radix, Ginseng radix, Bupeuri radix, Zingiberis rhizoma* and *Scutellariae radix.*

Shosaikoto is specifically used for treatments of patients with tenderness on pressure of the right subcostal region, and has been applied for cure and improvement of chronic dysfunction of the digestive system, dysfunction of liver diseases such as chronic hepatitis, infectious diseases with fever, common cold in a late stage and weak constitution of children, etc. *Shosaikoto* has been recognised as one of the biological response modifiers.

Rikkunshito (Liu-Jun-Zi-Tang)

Rikkunshito consists of eight component herbs: *Ginseng radix, Atractylodis rhizoma, Poria, Pinelliae tuber, Aurantii nobilis pericarpium, Zizyphi fructus, Glycyrrhizae radix* and *Zingiberis rhizoma.*

Rikkunshito has been used for the treatment of several complaints accompanied by digestive disorders such as gastric ulcer and chronic gastritis, and several digestive disorders after gastrectomy.

Kampo formulae for diseases involving metabolic and endocrine systems

Hachimijiougan (Ba-Wei-Di-Huang-Wang)

Hachimijiougan consists of eight component herbs: *Rehmanniae radix*, *Alismatis rhizoma*, *Poria*, *Discoreae rhizoma*, *Corni fructus*, *Moutan cortex*, *Cinnamomi cortex* and *Processi aconiti radix*.

Hachimijiougan has been used in older and elderly patients who exhibit weakness, cold and numbness in the lumbar region and lower extremities, together with nocturia. *Hachimijiougan* also has been used for the treatment of nephritis, diabetes, impotence, sciatica, lumbago, beri-beri, bleary eye, itch, oedema, bladder catarrh, prostatomegaly and hypertension.

Kampo formulae for pain

Shakuyakukanzoto (Shao-Yao-Gan-Cao-Tang)

Shakuyakukanzoto consists of *Paeoniae radix* and *Glycyrrhizae radix* (Figure 8.6).

Shakuyakukanzoto has frequently been used in patients with painful cramps. *Shakuyakukanzoto* has been shown to ameliorate cramp associated with cirrhosis in a double-blind clinical study. It has also been used for the treatment of sciatica, acute lumbago, gastrospasm, celiagra caused by gallstones or urinary calculus, myalgia, arthralgia and menstrual colic.

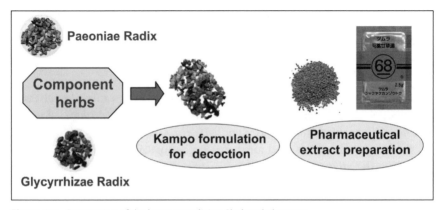

Figure 8.6 Preparation of the kampo medicine *Shakuyakukanzoto*.

References

1. Terasawa K, Itoh T, Nagasaka K et al. In: Sato Y, Hanawa T, Arai M et al. (eds), *Introduction to KAMPO–Japanese Traditional Medicine*. The Japan Society for Oriental Medicine: Elsevier Japan, 2005: 18–62.
2. Suzuki T, Arai H, Iwasaki K et al. A Japanese herbal medicine (Kami-Untan-to) in the treatment of Alzheimer's diseases: A pilot study. *Alzheimer's Report* 2001;4:177–82.
3. Terasawa K, Shimada Y, Kita T et al. Choto-san in the treatment of vascular dementia: a double-blind, Placebo controlled study. *Phytomedicine* 1997;4:15–22.
4. Yamada H. Japan. In: Bodeker G, Ong CK, Grundy C et al. (eds), *WHO Global Atlas of Traditional Complementary and Alternative Medicine*, Text Volume. Kobe: World Health Organization, Center for Health Development, 2005: 193–8.
5. Yamada H. Modern scientific approaches to Kampo medicine. *Asia Pacific J Pharmacol* 1994;9:209–17.
6. Yamada H. Introduction: What is Kampo medicine? In: Yamada H, Saiki I (eds), *Juzentaiho-to (Shi-Quan-Da-Bu-Tang) – Scientific evaluation and clinical application*. New York: CRC Press, 2005: 2 –6.
7. Hattori M, Kim G, Motoike S, Kobashi K, Namba T. Metabolism of sennosides by intestinal flora. *Chem Pharm Bull* 1982;30:1338–46.
8. Hattori M, Namba T, Akao T, Kobashi K. Metabolism of sennoside by human intestinal bacteria. *Pharmacology*, 1988;36(suppl 1):172–9.
9. Sasaki K, Yamauchi K, Kuwano S. Metabolic activation of sennoside A in mice. *Planta Medica* 1979;37:370–8.
10. Cyong JC, Matsumoto T, Arakawa K, Kiyohara H, Yamada, H, Otsuka Y. Anti-*Bacteroides fragilis* substance from rhubarb. *J Ethnopharmacol* 1987;279–83.
11. Hattori M, Sakamoto T, Kobashi, K, Namba T. Metabolism of glycyrrhizin by human intestinal flora. *Planta Medica* 1983;48:38–42.
12. Iwama H, Amagaya, S, Ogihara Y. Effect of shosaikoto, a Japanese and Chinese traditional herbal mixture, on the mitogenic activity of lipopolysaccharide: a new pharmacological testing method. *J Ethnopharmacol* 1987;21:45–53.
13. Iwama H, Amagai S, Ogihara Y. Effect of Kampo-hozai (traditional medicine) on immune responses, in vitro studies of Sho-saiko-to and Dai-saiko-to on antibody responses to sheep red blood cells and lipopolysaccharide. *J Med Pharm Soc WAKAN-YAKU* 1987;4:8–19.
14. Tashiro S. Growth inhibition of Sai-Rei-To on cultured fibroblast cells (in Japanese). *J Med Pharm Soc WAKAN-YAKU* 1985;2:108–9.
15. Hosoya E. Scientific reevaluation of Kampo prescriptions using modern technology. In: Hosoya E, Yamamura Y (eds), *Recent Advances of Kampo (Japanese Herbal) Medicines*. Amsterdam: Excerpta Medica, 1988: 17–29.
16. Matsumoto T, Yamada H. Immunological properties of Juzentaihoto. In: Yamada H, Saiki I (eds), *Juzen-taiho-to (Shi-Quan-Da-Bu-Tang) – Scientific evaluation and clinical application*. New York: CRC Press, 2005: 65–84.
17. Kiyohara H, Yamada H. The search for active ingredients of Juzen-taiho-to. In: Yamada H, Saiki I (eds), *Juzen-taiho-to (Shi-Quan-Da-Bu-Tang) – Scientific evaluation and clinical application*. New York: CRC Press, 2005: 115–39.
18. Kiyohara H, Matsumoto T, Yamada H. Lignin-carbohydrate complexes: Intestinal immune system modulating ingredients in Kampo (Japanese herbal) medicine, Juzen-taiho-to. *Planta Med* 2000;66: 20–4.
19. Kiyohara H, Matsumoto T, Yamada H. Intestinal immune system modulating poly-saccharides in a Japanese herbal (Kampo) medicine, Juzen-taiho-to. *Phytomedicine* 2002;9:614–24.
20. Kiyohara H, Matsumoto T, Yamada H. Combination effects of herbs in a multi-herbal formula: expression of Juzen-taiho-to's immuno-modulatory activity on the intestinal immune system. *eCAM* 2004;1:83–91.
21. Hisha H, Ikehara S. Hemopoiesis – stimulatory effect of Juzentaihoto. In: Yamada H,

Saiki I (eds), *Juzen-taiho-to (Shi-Quan-Da-Bu-Tang) – Scientific evaluation and clinical application*. New York: CRC Press, 2005: 85–103.

22. Kiyohara H, Nagai T, Munakata K, et al. Stimulating effect of Japanese herbal (Kampo) medicine, Hochuekkito on upper respiratory mucosal immune system. *eCAM* 2006; 3:459–67.

23. Matsumoto T, Noguchi M, Hayashi O, Makino K, Yamada H. Hochuekkito, a Kampo (traditional Japanese herbal) medicine, enhances mucosal IgA antibody response in mice immunized with antigen-entrapped biodegradable microparticles. *eCAM* 2007;doi: 10.1093/ecam/new/66.

24. Yamada H, Yabe T. Anti-dementia action of Kampo (Japanese herbal) medicines effects of Kampo medicines on central nervous system. In: Asakawa Y, Gottlieb OR, Hostettmann K et al. (eds), *Current Topics in Phytochemistry*, vol. 1. Trivandrum, India: *Research Trends*, 1997: 157–68.

25. Yabe T, Toriizuka K, Yamada H. Kami-untan-to (KUT) improves cholinergic deficits in aged rats. *Phytomedicine* 1996;2:253–8.

26. Terasawa K, Shimada Y, Kita T et al. Choto-san in the treatment of vascular dementia: a double-blind, Placebo controlled study. *Phytomedicine* 1997;4:15–22.

27. Kita T, Terasawa K. Kampo and EBM (in Japanese). *Shinryoukenkyu* 2000;359:1–8.

28. EBM Special Committee, The Japan Society for Oriental Medicine. Evidence reports of Kampo treatment. *Kampo Medicine* 2005;56(suppl):1–120.

29. Kogure H, Kawashima, K, Nagasawa H. Effect of Oren-gedoku-to on cerebral vascular accident. *Pharma Medica* 1988;6:33–6.

30. Yoshinaga S, Kimura M, Tanaka A, Tomonaga M. The effects of Kampo medicine 'Oren-gedoku-to' on clinical manifestations and cerebral blood flow in chronic stage of cerebro-vascular diseases. *Jpn J Med Pharm Soc Wakan-Yaku* 1992;9:22–7.

31. Iwasaki K, Ohgami Y, Ueki, A, Fujiwara M. Effect of Orengedokuto and Chotosan on disruption of spatial cognition (in Japanese). *Jpn J Med Pharm Soc Wakan-Yaku* 1991;8:476–7.

32. Mizushima N, Ikeshima T. Efficacy of Tokishakuyakusan on senile dementia (in Japanese). *Jpn J Med Pharm Soc Wakan-Yaku* 1989;6:456–7.

33. Yamamoto T, Kawano K. Kampo treatment of Alzheimer's type dementia (in Japanese). *Jpn J Med Pharm Soc Wakan-Yaku* 1989;6:454–5.

34. Yamamoto T. Kampo treatment for dementia (in Japanese). *Jpn J Med Pharm Soc Wakan-Yaku* 1991;8:478–9.

9

Korean medicine

Seon Ho Kim, Bong-Hyun Kim and Il-Moo Chang

The history of Korea dates back approximately 4000 years ago (Figure 9.1). Geographically, Korea is a neighbouring country of China. However, most Korean people are of Mongolian trait and are different ethnologically from the genuine Chinese race. In addition, the Korean language is Altaic and entirely different from the Chinese language. According to Chinese historical literature, the Korean people have been called the 'Eastern Bowmen' or the 'Eastern Barbarians' with the characteristics of the horse-riding people from the ancient Chinese dynasties of Xia and Yin (Shang) about 2000 BC.

History

Historical records show that there has long been interaction between Korea and China from ancient times: cultural exchanges, trade, immigration of peoples and even many wars. This was especially true during the three-kingdom period in Korean history, in which Kokuryo (37 BC–AD 668), Baekje (18 BC–AD 610) and Shilla (57 BC–AD 668), including the Unified Shilla (AD 668–935), occupied the north-eastern part of the current Chinese land (Manchuria) and the Korean peninsula. The time period of the three kingdoms of Korea corresponded with the periods from the Han dynasty (206 BC–AD 220) to the Tang dynasty (AD 618–907) in China. In this period, a variety of cultural exchanges occurred. Confucianism, Buddhism, Taoism and much classical literature written in the Chinese alphabet were introduced and widely accepted during the three-kingdom period in Korea. During this time period, it was most likely that the traditional Chinese medicine and its medical classics such as the *Huang Ti Nei Ching* (the *Yellow Emperor's Classic of Internal Medicine*), *Shang Han Lun*, and *Shen Nung Pen Chao Ching* were introduced and widely practised along with acupuncture and herbal therapies. Moreover, it is obvious

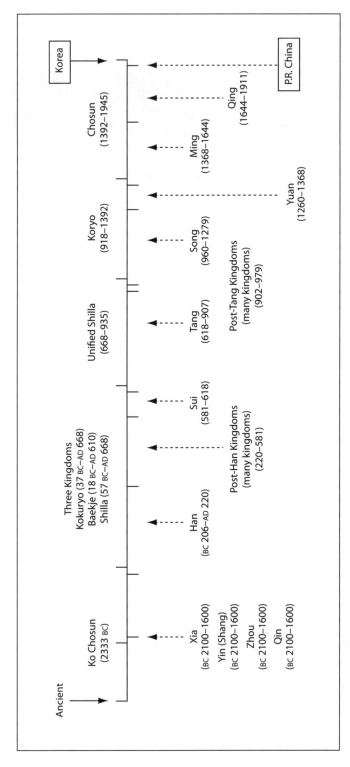

Figure 9.1 Korean and Chinese historical timeline.

that the Oriental view of cosmology, which is known as 'yin–yang and the five phases' (see Chapter 6), was also introduced and adopted not only for the theoretical basis of traditional Korean medicine (TKM), but also for the broad spectra of social and political systems of the three kingdoms, and even for the daily life of the Korean people as it was in China.

Due to its geographical location and developed maritime capabilities with a naval force during the three-kingdom period, Korea played the role of the cross-road culture between China and Japan. Several medical books of TKM written by Korean authors of the Baekje, Shilla and Unified Shilla kingdoms were sent to Japan, according to the Japanese historical literature, and valuable medicinal materials, the ox bezoars (ox gallstones or *Calculas bovis*), were supplied to China for preparing various herbal formulae (Figure 9.2).

After the fall of the three kingdoms in Korea, the Koyo dynasty (AD 918–1392) succeeded them, and occupied the whole Korean peninsula. The English pronunciation of Korea was actually derived initially from the Kokuryo kingdom, and then the Koryo dynasty. The Koryo dynasty period corresponded with the period of the Song, Jin and Yuan dynasties in China. For the Koryo dynasty of Korea, and especially the Jin and Yuan dynasties of China, very significant advances and mutual collaborations in traditional medicines were made in both countries. In China, new theories for traditional medicine evolved and were advocated by different groups of doctors who formed their own schools, and many new herbal formulae were developed and used for treatments of various ailments. In Korea, the metal printing blocks were invented and used for various publications, and thus the easy dissemination of TKM literature was possible. Also, the *Hyang Yak* (indigenous herbal plant sources in Korea) were searched out and substituted for the imported Chinese herbal materials being supplied to the public. There were also improvements in the cultivation method of ginseng (*Panax ginseng*), and further developments of the preparation methods of red ginseng for the purpose of longer preservation. By developing these methods of ginseng cultivation, a number of tonic formulae could be prepared in both Korea and China.

The Chosun dynasty (AD 1392–1910) succeeded the Koryo dynasty and occupied almost the same territory as the Koryo had on the Korean peninsula. Its time period corresponded with the period of the Ming (AD 1368–1644) and Qing (AD 1644–1911) dynasties in China. This time period also corresponded to the Renaissance in the Occidental world, a period when the use and development of modern medical technologies and chemical drugs, which differed from those of the dark Middle Ages, began to blossom. In the Oriental world in the period of the late seventeenth to the early eighteenth century, a new medical theory on infectious diseases evolved and was advocated by a group of medical doctors who were frustrated by the fact that the old, conventional ways of therapeutic doctrine, based on the *Shang Han Lun*, which had been

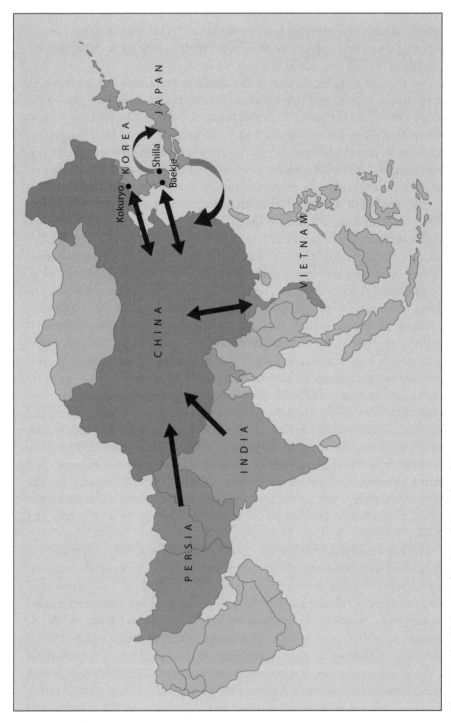

Figure 9.2 Establishment of traditional Oriental medicine.

used for more than 1000 years, were no longer effective. These doctors then began to seek a new view on the causative factors of infectious diseases.

Subsequently, they tried to define the newly infectious diseases, and proposed a hypothesis called 'warm-climate disease' by which all infectious diseases arise in or are due to a warm climate environment. None the less, it is very interesting that those medical doctors had not known of the existence of microorganisms, and some of these virulent microorganisms were responsible for a variety of infectious diseases that plagued many Oriental societies until the late nineteenth century. During the late Renaissance period, a number of Christian missionaries arrived in China, Japan and Korea; they brought various western diseases, but they also brought various western medicines, and some of the missionaries even performed surgical operations. There was an episode in which a Chinese emperor of the Qing dynasty had a malaria infection, and the royal family doctors tried to cure him, but failed with the traditional formulae. Interestingly, when a missionary father had the chance to give him a drug containing quinine, which was derived from the bark of the Cinchona tree, the emperor completely recovered from the malaria infection. This is an example by which the Oriental world became aware of the realities and efficacies of modern western medicine. However, looking more closely at the story, it becomes a bit more controversial because there had already been a traditional herbal medicine with superior effectiveness in malaria infection, artemisine, the active ingredient isolated from *Artemisia annua*, and now used for malaria resistant to quinine. However, it is not known why the royal family doctors did not use *Artemisia annua* for the Emperor at that time.

During the 500-year period of the Chosun dynasty in Korea, TKM flourished in both aspects of the development of its own identity and the great expansion of its use for the health benefits of the general public. These outcomes were largely a result of the Great King Sejong's policies on science and technology development in the early Chosun dynasty. In that period, various scientific and technological innovations and advances were made: the development and adoption of a standard calendar, the establishment of a standard metrology system for the units of weight and measurement and, most importantly, the invention of the *Han Geul* (Korean alphabet). *Han Geul* is based on phonetic letters, entirely different from the ideographic Chinese alphabet, and basically consists of 14 consonants and 10 vowels. The invention of the Korean alphabet made the dissemination of TKM information and practices rapid and easy. Consequently, several epoch-making contributions for the advancement of traditional Oriental medicines were also achieved. These are summarised in the next section.

Medical classics on the bibliographical view in the Chosun dynasty

According to medical historians on TKM, about 200 medical books were written and published in Korea during the period from the three kingdoms to the Chosun dynasty. Half of these books were lost, and the remaining half were collected and are preserved at the Kyu Jang Gak Library (formally the Chosun Dynasty Royal Library) at Seoul National University and the Han Dok Museum of Medicine and Pharmacy which was founded by a private collector.[1,2] These medical classics cover an extensive area of medical therapies: basic theory, paediatrics, obstetrics and gynaecology, smallpox, measles, ophthalmology, forensic medicine, acupuncture technology, herbal medicines, and even veterinary medicine for horses and cattle. Of these medical classics, there were several famous books that significantly influenced the progress of traditional medicines in Korea as well as in China and Japan.

Eui Bang Yoo Chui (the Classified Assemblage of Medical Prescriptions)

This book is a series of compilations of almost all herbal formulae and medical theories available in Korea and China. It consisted of 264 volumes and took more than 30 years to be printed (AD 1445–1477). Only 30 copies were printed, but 29 copies were lost during the Korea–Japan wars (AD 1592–1598), and the Japanese general Kato Kiyomasa took one copy. This last copy is now kept in the Japanese royal library located in the Japanese king's palace. There is no doubt that this book contributed to the progress of traditional Japanese medicine (kampo).

Hyang Yak Chae Chui Wol Ryong (the Harvest and Collection of Indigenous Herbal Plants during the Four Seasons)

This book is a kind of guidebook for identifying and collecting indigenous herbal material in each month of the year across the Korean peninsula. It consisted of one volume and was published by the Great King Sejong (AD 1431). The purpose of publishing this book was to supply domestic needs for commonly used herbal materials with indigenous herbal plant sources. Subsequently, this book was the basis for establishing various herbal formulae using Korean herbal materials.

Hyang Yak Jib Seong Bang (the Compendium of Traditional Korean Herbal Formulae with Indigenous Herbal Materials)

This book consists of 30 volumes and was published in AD 1431. It comprises 57 chapters in which 959 disease patterns are well classified, and their pathological characteristics and therapeutic treatments are also described, with a total of 10 706 herbal formulae and 1416 kinds of acupuncture applications. In addition, a special chapter is dedicated to Korean herbal formulae with indigenous herbal materials for the treatment of various diseases. In the annex, various methodologies for processing herbal materials in order to remove the toxic components out of the herbal constituents are described in detail. Such processing methodologies are unique and characteristic pre-treatments of crude herbal materials and for prolonging the preservation of herbal materials. This information is a research source for preparing the standard processing methodology in the herbal medicine industry at the present time.

Dong Eui Bo Gam (the Treatise on Eastern Asian Medicine)

This book was written by a royal family doctor, Heo Jun (AD 1610). It has 25 volumes in which he discussed and commented on various traditional Korean and Chinese medical theories based on actual clinical experiences, and listed more than 6800 herbal formulae and some acupuncture therapies. This book has been recognised to be a sort of medical bible in the area of traditional Oriental medicine, and many copies were published in China, Japan and Taiwan. This book shows very accurate citations with a total of 83 reference books that were previously published in Korea and China (Figure 9.3).

Sa Am ascetic's summary of acupuncture–moxibustion therapy

Sa Am is the pseudonym of a monk who led an ascetic life during the middle of the Chosun dynasty. His real name is unknown. He wrote the above book, but it was not accurately known when the book was printed. He established a new methodology of acupuncture therapy on the basis of the five-phase theory of the Oriental cosmology. His method, which had been outside the mainstream for a long period, has been re-discovered in recent years, and further developed. Now clinical applications have been widely performed by TKM doctors due to its high effectiveness on various diseases occurring at the five viscera and six bowels. More detailed information is given below.

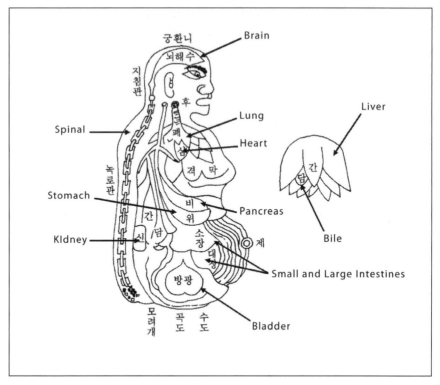

Figure 9.3 Sketch of human anatomy of Dong Eui Bo Gam (AD 1610).

Dong Eui Soo Se Bo Won (the Textbook of Oriental Medicine for Longevity and Life Preservation)

The above book consisted of four volumes, and was written by Lee, Je Ma. This book was printed by his students after his death (AD 1901). He proposed a new theory, the so-called four constitutional medicines, based on the physiological and functional differences of the human body according to the external shape, emotional activities, and size of the internal viscera and bowels. Such physiological and functional differences are categorised into four constitutions by which all humans can be classified: the Greater Yang person, the Greater Yin person, the Lesser Yang person and the Lesser Yin person. In his theory, patients with the same disease should be treated differently according to their constitutional characteristics. More detailed information is provided below.

Unique acupuncture therapy and a new theory of four constitutional medicines in TKM

Sa Am ascetic's acupuncture therapy

As described above, the Sa Am ascetic's acupuncture therapy was developed in Korea. It is characterised by the following two distinct requisites:

- First, the therapy follows the five-phase theory by engendering or restraining the functions of the viscera and bowels, which were rendered defective by certain diseases. As the acupuncture is applied to the proper acupoints, the patient's emotional conditions are also considered.
- Second, unlike classic acupuncture therapy, Sa Am ascetic's acupuncture is applied only at various acupoints located below the arm to the hand, and below the knee to the foot (Figure 9.4).

In addition, relatively small-sized needles are clinically applied to, at most, the eight acupoints located on the arm–hand and knee–foot areas. Therefore, patients feel the acupuncture therapy safe and comfortable and its therapeutic potency appears to be very effective in clinical practice. Recently this acupuncture therapy has been widely practised in clinics, and much clinical research has been conducted in TKM hospitals.

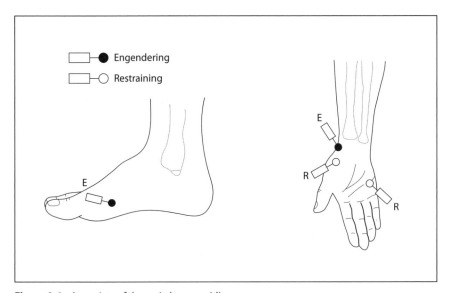

Figure 9.4 Acupoints of the main lung meridians.

The *Sa Sang* medicine: four constitutional medicines proposed by Lee, Je Ma

In Lee's four constitutional medicines (FCM), humans are classified into four types: the Greater Yang, the Greater Yin, the Lesser Yang and the Lesser Yin. The Greater Yang person has large lungs and a small liver; the Greater Yin person has small lungs and a large liver; the Lesser Yang person has a large spleen and small kidneys; and the Lesser Yin person has a small spleen and large kidneys. These different sizes of the viscera and subsequently related physiological functions lead to different clinical treatments. In addition, size difference and physiological function are also directly associated with the emotional behaviour. Therefore, a patient's state of mind is considered to have as important an impact as the FCM treatments, e.g. based on FCM, the practitioner would say that the Greater Yang person's behaviour is easily inclined to anger. When the Greater Yang person gets sick with a high fever, a unique herbal formula is given both to reduce the fever and to soothe the anger during the initial treatment.

In his book, there are just a little over 100 herbal formulae available for various illnesses of the four constitutional types. Actually, he did not fully complete his proposed theory in terms of clinical evidence during his life, so various scientific efforts have been continued to objectify its effectiveness, e.g. in order to make a standard diagnosis in terms of the FCM, just one questionnaire with a series of questions is given to patients to identify their constitutional type. Along with the questionnaire, routine check-ups including a pulse diagnosis are also given. Currently, most TKM doctors tend to perform classic treatments together with the FCM treatments in clinical practices in Korea. In addition, a number of research groups of the TKM schools have investigated the possibility of a relationships between the FCM theory and genetic disorders. Through the use of modern experimental tools, they aim to examine the feasibility of personalised treatments.

Current status and perspective of TKM

Education

From the late 1960s, two medical educational systems and practices have been conducted in tandem in Korea: 40 western-type medical schools and 12 TKM schools are operated and both schools provide a 6-year curriculum and, after graduation, the graduates have to take the national examination to obtain the doctoral licence; they then are allowed to practise as an Oriental medical doctor. Currently about 800 graduates take the national examination every year. In the 6-year curriculum, about half the courses are allocated to modern life-science courses such as biochemistry, microbiology, anatomy, physiology and pharmacology, and the remaining half are devoted to various TKM courses and clinical training. This curriculum is aimed at least in part to ensure that the graduates of the TKM schools become able to provide expertise as a TKM doctor along with a comprehensive knowledge of traditional and modern medical sciences. This educational system for TKM schools is apparently unique in Asian countries, and ultimately has some advantages in the ability to treat patients jointly and effectively with western doctors.

On the issue of the educational system, it is worth mentioning that Hong Kong's health authority benchmarked the TKM educational system when establishing a higher traditional medical school, and made the decision to adopt the Korean system a decade ago after surveying the Chinese, Japanese and Vietnamese systems. For postgraduates, most TKM schools offer the Masters (MS) and advanced degree (PhD) programmes.

Research organisations and recent achievements

Most research activities have been carried out at the university level. Kyung Hee University's College of Oriental Medicine and the East–West Medical Research Institute have been recognised as among the leading institutions in clinical and acupuncture research. The latter has been designated as one of the WHO collaborating centres for traditional medicine in Korea for 10 years. One example of the innovative work being done in acupuncture research is the result of the cooperation between Kyung Hee University and the University of California (Davis): they revealed physiological brain responses for the first time using brain functional magnetic resonance imaging (fMRI) as acupuncture therapy was being performed on human acupoints.[3] In the field of herbal medicine research, the Natural Products Research Institute, Seoul National University, which has been also designated as a WHO collaborating centre for traditional medicine, laid one of the cornerstones by constructing a comprehensive database of traditional herbal medicines that consists of several groups of information with more than 12 000 herbal formulae. The database includes the chemical information of ingredients along with three-dimensional images of chemical structures, taxonomy of component herbs, pharmacological and toxicological information, and processing methods for some toxic herbal material. This database provides services in Korean, Japanese and English under the name TradiMed[4] through the internet.

One of the significant achievements made by a research group of the Natural Products Research Institute, Seoul National University, was the development of an English coding system for herbal formula titles.[5] More than 100 herbal formulae have been developed in China, Japan, Korea and Vietnam over a period of 2000 years. These formulae range from single-herb to multiherb formulae with up to 40 or more different component herbs. All of the formula titles are expressed in the Chinese alphabet with ideographic meanings. If an attempt had been made to translate the meanings of the formula titles into English, it probably would have been impossible for western scientists to understand them. Another option would have been for western scientists to learn the Chinese alphabet, but this feat would take an inordinate amount of time. Therefore, we opted for a new approach. To start, the naming patterns of the formula titles were sorted into seven groups, and then we developed the English coding system which comprises:

(one or two Principal component herbs with major pharmacological action) + (Pharmacological indication) + (Dosage form) + (Numbers of component herbs)

By preparing this type of code, it was possible to construct the English version of the TradiMed database. This coding system is currently under further study to match the Anatomy Therapeutic Code (ATC) drug system of the WHO, with the interested groups including Tokyo University and Uppsala University's WHO collaborating centre. In addition to the afore-mentioned research organisation, a newly created organisation, the Korea Institute of Oriental Medicine (KIOM), was founded in 1994 to promote the research capabilities in TKM through a governmental research organisation. KIOM has mainly conducted basic research and has collaborated widely with many domestic TKM schools and foreign schools through government-funded support.[6]

Perspectives

There is no possibility that TKM can substitute for mainstream western medicine and fulfill all the requirements of the national health system. However, it can make a significant and important contribution in a complementary and alternative role. When a combination therapy of western medicine and TKM is practised for certain groups of diseases, there are frequently superior outcomes in terms of effectiveness, tolerability and cost. In order to develop the cooperative treatments between the two medicines, called 'integrative medicine', it has been agreed to develop methods to verify the effectiveness of TKM therapy based on scientific evidence. Thus many TKM hospitals have begun to try to implement the global standard for clinical trials, commonly referred to as good clinical practice (GCP of ICH), into TKM therapies. In addition, one of the 'modernising' steps has been to move away from the old-fashioned dosage forms, such as a large volume of water decoctions and large pills, to the modern dosage forms such as tablets, capsules and granules. These new dosage forms are produced under the good manufacturing practice (GMP) of the International Conference on Harmonisation of Technical Requirements for Registration of Pharmaceuticals for Human Use (known as the GMP-ICH regulations). To integrate these new dosage forms, bioequivalence tests are a prerequisite and, correspondingly, there is much research activity going on in both academic and industry spheres.

In the light of such current research trends, it can be hypothesised that more integrative medical practices will be found and implemented in the near future for the benefit of the general public.

References

1. Kyu Jang Gak Institute of Korean Studies. Available at: http://tinyurl.com/cpoeem (accessed 6 May 2009).
2. Han Dok Museum of Medicine and Pharmacy. Available at: http://tinyurl.com/cud2k2 (Korean) (accessed 5 May 2009).
3. Cho ZH, Chung SC, Jones JP et al. New findings of the correlation between acupoints and corresponding brain cortices using functional MRI. *Proc Natl Acad Sci USA* 1998; 95:2670–3.
4. TradiMed (Traditional Chinese Medicine). Available at: www.tradimed.com (accessed 5 May 2009).
5. Yi YD, Chang I-M. An overview of traditional Chinese herbal formulae and a proposal of a new code system for expressing the formula titles. *eCAM* 2004;1:125–32.
6. Korea Institute of Oriental Medicine. Available at: www.kiom.re.kr/index.jsp (accessed 5 May 2009).

10

Traditional medicines in the Pacific

Rosemary Beresford

This chapter considers the traditional approaches to sickness and health in four countries in the South Pacific region shown in Figure 10.1 – Australia, Fiji, Samoa and New Zealand – highlighting both similarities and differences where these exist. It identifies the impact of European colonisation on the health of these Pacific nations, the difficulties experienced in using traditional methods to treat new and unfamiliar sicknesses, and also the ways in which indigenous peoples adapted their old ways to deal with the new problems.

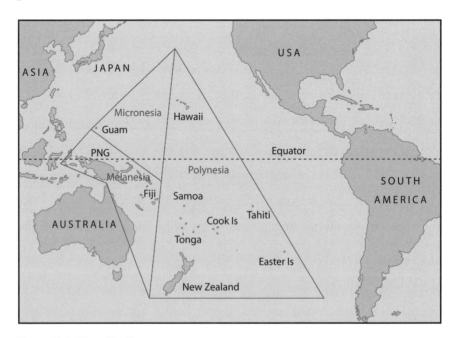

Figure 10.1 Map of Pacific ocean.

Finally it discusses some of the work that has been carried out more recently to separate the folk law elements of traditional medicine usage from the more evidence-based practice of contemporary western society and shows that, surprisingly, there may be considerable commonality between the two.

The setting

Australia

Australia (similar to New Zealand) is often considered as an enclave of European culture and traditions, thousands of miles away from the source of its traditions. This culture is, however, of fairly recent origin, a matter of only a few hundred years. Before the arrival of European adventurers and settlers, the two countries enjoyed the traditions of their own indigenous peoples. Australasia, although sometimes considered to consist of just Australia and New Zealand, does in fact encompass many other neighbouring islands in the South Pacific ocean, many of which share similar traditions, including those associated with the recognition and treatment of illness.

The Australian subcontinent is huge, encompassing a landmass of 7.5 million square kilometres, a physical geography that ranges from snow-capped mountains through arid deserts to tropical swamps. Its climate too is extreme, scorching hot and dry in the centre, hot and humid in its northern regions, and almost temperate in its coastal southern parts. Its native people, the Aborigines, have lived in its land for thousands of years, living in tribal units in a nomadic lifestyle, not cultivating land or crops as a rule but moving from one area to another as availability of food sources dictated. The tribes spoke in many different languages or dialects and had no formal written means of transmitting information from one group to another or from one generation to the next. Although some pictorial means were used, most information was passed on by word of mouth. When someone became sick, an elder in the tribe, a traditional healer (*ngangkari*), would be called in to identify the problem, specifically the evil spirit responsible for the sickness. This spirit would be driven away by ritualistic dancing and chanting by the revered elder who would dress in distinctive garb for the occasion. To aid the driving away of the evil spirit, the ill person could also be treated with a concoction of herbs and herbal extracts considered effective for the purpose.

Fiji and Samoa

These are two small (groups of) islands in the South Pacific. Both were settled by their indigenous Melanesian or Polynesian people about 3000–4000 years ago and each became the focus of western attention in the mid-nineteenth century when the British and others became aware of the richness of the vegetation of the islands and their potential for trade.

Fiji

Fiji became a British colony in 1874, after which time the population mix of the country was altered by the influx of Indians who were brought in by the British as contract labourers. Fiji's many islands are now home to about 900 000 people, about half of whom are Melanesian–Fijian and most of the remainder Indo-Fijian.

Samoa

Samoa was also settled by British as well as German and American entrepreneurs, although Britain ceded its territory to Germany in the early twentieth century in exchange for the right to retain control over Fiji. New Zealand took over from Germany after 1918 and controlled it until Samoan independence in 1962. At this time, the name Samoa was accepted by the United Nations as the official name of the two largest, western islands of the country. Tuitila and other smaller islands to the east are still known as American Samoa because they remain an unincorporated and unorganised territory of the USA. The customs and practices of the 180 000 or so mainly Polynesian people of the islands are very similar, however, as is their approach to medicine.

New Zealand

New Zealand is a little larger than the UK but is populated by just over 4 million people. It is made up of a number of islands, the major ones being known as North Island and South Island, respectively. Its native population, the Maoris, arrived about 1000 years ago and its European (British) settlers in the mid-nineteenth century (although it had been visited first by Dutch explorers in the mid-seventeenth century). It is currently also home to a number of other immigrant groups, notably Polynesian and Asians, mainly from south-east Asia. Europeans are the predominant ethnic group now, totalling about 78% at the last (2006) census, while Maoris make up 10%, Asians 9% and Polynesian Pacific Islanders 6%. (The greater than 100% total occurs because people of Maori descent can identify as both European and Maori.)

Perceptions of health

Indigenous people in each of the four countries discussed considered ill-health to be the result of an imbalance, often as a consequence of an offence against some spiritual teaching or being. Traditional treatment of ill-health thus generally took the form of a variety of approaches: physical manipulation, herbal medicine and oversight by a spiritual healer. Specific information about such treatments has been difficult to obtain, largely because of the lack of a written language in each country before the arrival of European colonists and other visitors.

Accounts of treatments before this time were largely penned by temporary visitors such as explorers, missionaries and whalers who were not necessarily aware of the complexities of the societies that they were observing nor of course the subtleties of languages with which they were not at all familiar.

This changed after these countries were settled by the colonists, who spent more time with the native populations, learning their languages and observing their customs, including their methods of treating illnesses. Although these early settlers brought with them the means – mainly herbal extracts – of treating illness then available in Europe, they also began to experiment with local flora to extend their armamentarium of possibly medicinally active plants. They also planted seeds of European plants, either deliberately or accidentally, and used them where applicable. At the same time, the local populations observed the customs of the settlers, including their methods of treating European sicknesses. When they in turn became infected with the diseases brought in by the settlers, they too began to adopt European methods of treating themselves using the herbal medicines of their own country and those introduced by the settlers. As a consequence, when information about traditional medicines was later recorded in written documents there was often some confusion between those that were originally used and those developed only after colonisation.

Australia

Before the influx of Europeans in the late eighteenth century, it seems probable that Aborigines enjoyed relatively good health, despite the rigours of the Australian climate and the scarcity of some food sources. The ill-health that they experienced was largely brought about by living in close proximity to each other, leading to many skin problems and respiratory disorders. Their diet was necessarily poor and they would frequently encounter sharp objects in their wanderings in the form of either plants stumbled over or objects wielded by other people. They did not, as far as we can ascertain, suffer from most of the infectious diseases of the west, diseases such as smallpox, cholera, tuberculosis, sexually transmitted infections, mumps and measles. Nor did they experience life-threatening cardiovascular disorders. They were therefore quite unprepared for the devastating impact of foreign microorganisms which killed them in their thousands, and they were also not prepared for the equally devastating impact of western society on their own, less structured way of life.

Traditional remedies

There are many uncertainties about the use of herbal medicines pre-European times. Not only were there no written records, but there was also little clarity about the botanical identification of plants used, the specific part to be used and how this part was to be applied. Those Europeans who tried to find out more about the plants used in earlier times were sometimes misinformed through Aboriginal willingness to please.

> Aboriginals are sometimes so very willing to give names of plants to the traveller that, rather than disappoint him, they will prepare a few for the occasion.[1]

On other occasions information was difficult to obtain because:

> Aborigines take a long time to get to know a person and they don't really trust a stranger, because, in the old days, a stranger was quite often an enemy . . . .[2]

Digestive problems are very common in people whose ability to preserve food is limited and whose understanding and practice of good hygiene measures are poor. The nineteenth century settlers noted that Aborigines were well acquainted with these conditions and employed a number of plants to remedy them. The gummy exudates (known collectively as *kino*) from various species of eucalyptus, notably *Eucalyptus siderophloia* and other trees or bushes, were regularly chewed to slow down or stop diarrhoea. Many of these *kino* exudates have since been shown to contain tannins or other astringent compounds that inhibit secretions of the gastrointestinal tract. Other eucalypt exudates had a laxative action, notably that of *E. viminalis*, which has since been shown to contain the sweet tasting substance, mannitol.

> . . . a pleasant purgative, so gentle in its operation that it can be given to the tenderest infant.[3]

Toothache was a problem for many and the remedy most often used was the exudate (the composition of which is still uncertain) from what was popularly known as the toothache tree (*Euoidia vitiflora*). The wood of this tree has what is described as a 'nauseating odour' but its resinous exudates, when placed in tooth cavities, did relieve the pain of toothache.

Many other plants, including several species of acacia, were used as painkillers for both internal and external sources of pain. A number of these also had sedative properties, especially those in the Solanaceae and Lobeliaceae families, the best known of which is the plant known as 'pituri' (*Duboisia hopwoodii*). This has been shown to contain a number of alkaloids, including nicotine. The leaves of pituri were chewed in much the same manner as is tobacco and produced a number of similar effects, initially stimulation of activity, followed by lethargy and fatigue. The plant grows in many parts of Australia and its use by Aborigines was so well known that it was considered to be like:

> . . . what opium is to the Chinaman, what whisky is to the Scotch man . . .[4]

Skin disorders were also common, although the vague descriptions of many of these make it difficult for us to identify their specific cause. Many were probably the result of living in close proximity to others. Under these conditions fungal and viral infections could spread rapidly, as did parasitic infestations such as scabies. Warts also appear to have been common and were removed by inserting sharp spines of an acacia under them and then pulling away the withered wart an hour or so later. The milky sap of the native fig was used to treat ringworm, as were resins of the eucalypt species, red blood wood and a *Myristica* species, the Queensland nutmeg. The Aborigines used many plants to treat general infections although these were not widespread before the arrival of the Europeans. Nevertheless, 43 remedies were listed in a 1903 bulletin entitled 'Superstition, magic and medicine'.[5] These remedies were generally extracted into water (which initially would have been cold or just warm because the Aborigines had no means of boiling water until the Europeans introduced them to metal utensils). Such extracts were then taken internally or used to bathe the skin, eyes or other affected parts. *Melaleuca* (tea tree) spp., for example, were used for general infections and, more specifically, for respiratory ones (Figure 10.2). Eucalypts were also widely used to ease disordered breathing by breaking up phlegm and reducing the swelling of mucous membranes.

The settlers investigated the medicinal value of a number of indigenous plants basing their choices on similarities that they observed between these and the European plants with which they were more familiar. One of the first to be identified as being medicinally useful was a species of eucalyptus (*E. piperita*), the Sydney peppermint tree, the crushed leaves of which emit an odour strongly reminiscent of the peppermint herb (*Mentha piperita*).

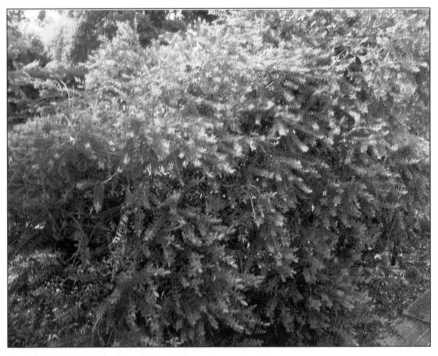

Figure 10.2 *Melaleuca* (tea tree).

The volatile oil of the eucalyptus plant (Figure 10.3) was then used for similar respiratory problems as that of the peppermint plant. The Australian oil has a much stronger smell than its European counterpart and so was used in smaller quantities – happily as it turns out because eucalyptus oil is chemically different from peppermint oil and a great deal more toxic.

Tonics were very fashionable in European circles in the nineteenth century. These often contained small quantities of quinine or other bitter-tasting substances and were used to stimulate saliva flow and thus promote general well-being. Aborigines appeared not to have used their plants for such purposes but the settlers identified – after some trial and error – that a number of Australian plants could substitute for remedies used in Europe. Some plants such as *Centaurium spicatum* were 'pleasantly bitter'; others such as bitter bark, *Alstonia constrica*, were much less pleasant leaving a long-lasting bitter after-taste in the mouth.[6]

When the Aborigines were confronted with European diseases they not only tried their own old remedies and those that the Europeans had brought with them but also investigated the value of other native plants. A number of them appear to have been chosen on the *similia similibus curantur* or 'like treats like' principle, one favoured by many cultures in different regions and at different times. This was especially evident in their choice of some plants

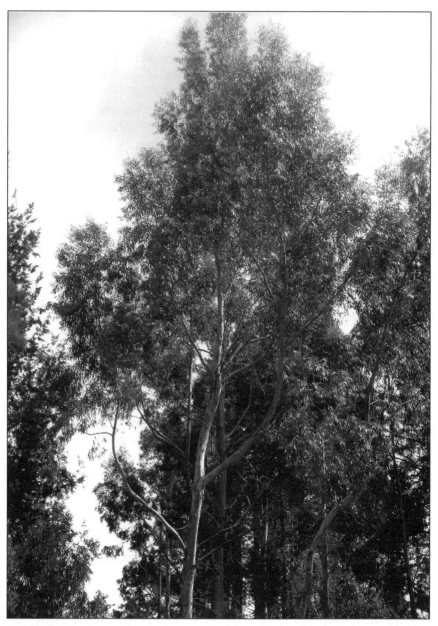

Figure 10.3 Eucalyptus tree.

to treat genitourinary diseases. Plants that grew close to water were thus used to treat those people who had pain or difficulty with urination. Plants such as *Euphorbia drummondii,* which produced a sticky exudate, were used to treat gonorrhoea, a disease with a pus discharge of similar appearance.

Present day

Pharmaceutical companies have utilised Aboriginal knowledge in the development of a number of commercially viable entities. Much of the world's supply of hyoscine now comes from species of *Dubosia*. The volatile oil, tea tree oil, which is extracted from *Melaleuca alternifolia*, is widely promoted as an antiseptic, antibacterial and antifungal agent, and is included in numerous cleaning and cosmetic products, as are the oils of many *Eucalyptus* species. The kangaroo apple bush, *Solanum aviculare*, is a source of alkaloids related to the steroids produced in the Mexican yam, and which could also become a viable source of the starting materials for oral contraceptive synthesis.

These commercial successes, together with the increasing trend in western society to utilise herbal medicines, has revived interest in Australia's flora and traditional herbal medicine history. A systematic search of information in Australia's Northern Territory about Aboriginal use of plants led in 1988 to the compilation of the first Aboriginal pharmacopoeia of the Northern Territories.[7] This provides botanical and chemical information about 70 plants used by Aborigines for medicinal purposes and includes both the conditions for which these plants were recommended and the various types of preparations most commonly used. More recent research has compared the efficacy of certain traditional remedies with western preparations used for the same conditions, and has found them to be at least as effective, especially when used to treat skin problems such as boils and other general surface infections. As traditional remedies are often more acceptable than western ones to some Aboriginal communities, such medicines may be used to improve the often very poor general health of people in these communities.

It is ironic that a people whose culture is so ancient and who live in a country with a flora that is at least potentially so medicinally active should have such poor health that their life expectancy is almost 20 years less than that of 'immigrant' Australians. One of several strategies being employed to help reduce this inequity has been the recent introduction of support for traditional healers and other Aboriginal health workers in Aboriginal communities. The hope is that their use of a combination of traditional and western medicine will help promote a greater sense of ownership, pride and thus self-worth in the people of these communities, and thus ultimately better general health.

Fiji

It is difficult to determine which of Fiji's flora are indigenous and which introduced by its human inhabitants. The forest plants seem, however, to be the oldest surviving species while later ones appear to include most of the food and medicinally active species. Many of these are not specific to Fiji but are found throughout tropical regions in south-east Asia and the Pacific. Those used by the Indo-Fijian population are generally the ones favoured by the ayurvedic tradition of medicine (discussed in Chapter 7). Those discussed here are used mainly by indigenous Fijians.

The health of pre-European Fijians appears to have been generally good, although diseases such as yaws, filariasis, malaria and other fever-producing conditions were recorded. Post-European settlement, however, the Fijians suffered from imported diseases such as gonorrhoea, diphtheria and measles, so much so in fact that it was feared that the population might even die out completely. Early Europeans could obtain little information about plants used as medicines by the local population. One such person writing in the 1860s complained that the women who seemed to have knowledge of medicinally useful plants could not be induced to part with this knowledge because it was a source of income for them.[8] Later authors, however, seem to have been more persuasive and a number of comprehensive accounts have since been published.[9]

Traditional remedies

Fijians generally have a strong respect for tradition and traditional remedies, relying on a combination of physical and supernatural means to treat sickness. Minor problems such as coughs and colds, headaches or earache, otherwise known as *mate vayano*, were just accidental occurrences that were thus responsive to physical treatments whereas *mate ni vanua*, 'diseases of the land' were due to spirit interference and as such could be treated only much more rigorously, usually with the assistance of sorcerers (*dauvakatevoro*) as well as those who had knowledge of the medicinal plants required. The ceremonies involved in treating such conditions, similar to many other ceremonial occasions in Fiji, usually included the use of infusions of *yaqona*, a drink prepared from the powdered root of the kava plant (*Piper methysticum*). This drink is a mild sedative which is said to be effective in the treatment of many different conditions, ranging from coughs and colds to filariasis[10] (Figure 10.4).

Most plants were (and still are) used to treat a number of different complaints. Leaves and bark were frequently used, generally by soaking in hot or boiling water. Sometimes, as above, the root and stem would be used as the medicine and might be crushed before extraction to provide a stronger preparation. Leaves could be chewed and their 'juices' swallowed or the saliva-softened product used as a poultice. Pastes and ointments were also prepared, by mixing powdered plant material with a little water or coconut oil, respectively.

Vesi (*Intsia bijuga*) is a coastal tree that grows to a height of about 12 metres which has spreading branches that were used to make the traditional

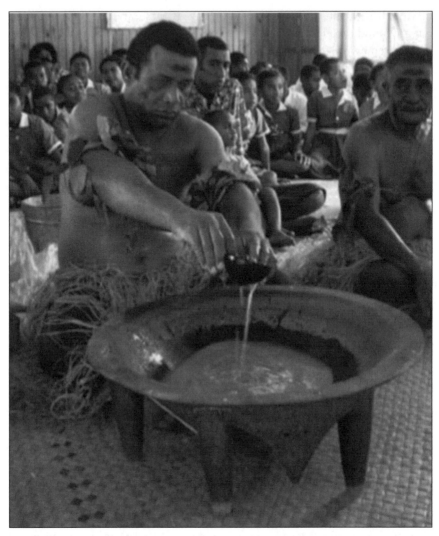

Figure 10.4 Kava ceremony.

four-legged kava bowls, as well as canoes, clubs and other objects. It was considered to be a sacred tree so medicines prepared from it were thought to be very efficacious (against *mate ni vanua* as well as *mate vayano* illnesses). Decoctions of powdered bark or the juice expressed from the inner bark is used to treat the aches and pains of rheumatism whereas the steamed and thus softened bark is used to immobilise and heal bone fractures. Other parts of the plant are used to treat respiratory disorders such as asthma as well as milder colds (and a decoction of leaves was thought to drive out unwanted spirits).[9]

Gasau (*Miscanthus floridulus*) is a common, perennial reed that is used as a house-building material as well as a medicine for both internal and external problems. Its stems and leaves are used to treat diarrhoea and urinary problems (just as were water-related Aboriginal plants). Leaves and leaf buds are also used to treat eye problems, both injury and age related.[9]

Wa yalu (*Epipremnum pinnatum*) is an ornamental, large-leafed plant that is common throughout the Pacific. A decoction of its leaves is used to treat constipation and other gastrointestinal problems (and it is said that US troops stationed in the Pacific found this so effective that they sent sacks of the leaves to the folks back home). Other problems for which the plant has been claimed to be effective are a range of skin conditions, including infected wounds, boils and infestation with scabies. It has also been used for contraception, irregular or painful periods, and infertility.

Niu (*Cocos nucifera*) is familiar to us in imagination at least as the coconut palm that is the most common coastal tree of Fiji and other South Pacific islands. The shell is used as a container, fuel and source of wood for ornaments. The nut itself is crushed for its oil and the liquid inside used as a 'milk' drink or the starting material for an alcoholic drink known as 'palm toddy'. Coconut oil is used alone as a massage oil and is also incorporated into ointments with other ingredients. Used as massage oil, it is said to relieve the aches and pains of rheumatism, pregnancy and exercise-induced over-exertion of muscles. Its emollient properties, when used either alone or with other ingredients, are promoted in many different cosmetic preparations. Coconut milk is used to treat mothers whose breast milk is too yellow and is recommended to be drunk frequently and in large quantities by people with blackwater fever (other examples of *similia similibus* perhaps?).

Wabosucu (*Mikania micrantha*) is known colloquially as 'mile a minute' because of the speed at which this creeping plant can grow. The juice of the leaves is a popular remedy for cuts and bruises; crushed leaves relieve the pain of wasp and other insect stings, and a poultice of leaves is used to treat boils, especially those that are located in the armpits.

Yaqona, kava (*Piper methysticum*), is cultivated as both a garden and commercial plant in Fiji. Its use as a mild, sedative narcotic in ceremonial occasions, including the treatment of *mate ni vanua*, has already been mentioned but it is also used medicinally for a wide range of everyday conditions such as coughs and colds, headaches and sore throats, as well as for more unpleasant conditions such as filariasis.

Present day: kava – a case study

Kava has been used in Fiji and other Pacific islands for generations and had not excited any controversy until its sedative and mild anxiolytic properties were recognised by westerners who began using kava products provided by herbal medicine companies. A number of spontaneously reported cases of liver damage associated with kava use were reported in several European countries from the late 1990s,[11] the upshot being that the German Federal

Institute for Drugs and Medical Devices banned its use in that country.[11] Other countries followed Germany's lead, with the result that kava-containing products (which were commercially available as 'food supplements') were banned from sale in Australia, Canada, Switzerland and the UK. Regulatory authorities in other countries were less confident of a link between kava and liver disorders. New Zealand, for example, accepted the advice of its expert advisers and did not withdraw kava from general sale.[13]

More recently the Food and Drug Administration (FDA) in the USA has questioned the original concerns regarding the hepatotoxicity of the product after a number of investigative studies carried out in the USA and elsewhere. Although the debate has not yet ended, the picture that is emerging is of a twofold problem with kava's non-traditional compared with traditional use. Kava use in Pacific countries such as Fiji generally follows well-established procedures in which the root of the plant is powdered and extracted with water and the resulting beverage drunk.[14] No other potentially active substances would normally be consumed concurrently. The kava products used in non-traditional societies were often prepared from the leaves and stem peelings of the kava plant,[13] and the resulting extracts ingested by people who might also be using other medicines that were themselves potentially hepatotoxic. The potential for kava to interact with other medicines, especially those that inhibit the cytochrome CYP450 system, has consequently attracted a great deal of attention.[15]

The experimental studies cited by the FDA include analyses of the chemical constituents of extracts prepared from different parts of the plant and in vivo studies of the pharmacological effect of such extracts. The sedative activity of kava appears to be related to its kavalactones, most of which are concentrated in its roots. The hepatotoxicity that has been demonstrated is confined to extracts prepared from the leaves and stem peelings of the plants, which contain the alkaloid, pipermethystine.[16] This alkaloid is not found in root extract.

The whole episode is a cautionary tale of what can go wrong when traditional usage of a medicinally active plant is extrapolated (and exploited) beyond its boundaries by people who are unaware that, although some information may not be written down, the way in which certain products are used has not been arrived at by chance but by long-established observation and experience.

Samoa

The practice of medicine in Samoa, similar to that in the other countries discussed in this chapter, appears to have been little documented before the arrival of the European settlers in the nineteenth century. There were no written records from before that time and what was recorded by the very earliest settlers makes little reference to medicinal plants. What does seem clear, however, is the fact that, before the arrival of these Europeans, the health of the Samoan population was reasonably good, and similar to that of Fijian, Aboriginal and Maori populations. The health problems that they did experience were largely the result of the way in which they lived and the climate of Samoa, which is hot and humid – a breeding ground for fungal and other infections as well as numerous biting insects. Families lived in large units, in close proximity to each other, on a diet that, although quite varied, was deficient in many vitamins and other essential foodstuffs. Skin problems were thus very common as were various respiratory and gastrointestinal ailments. Those problems that had an obvious external cause were treated physically where possible or with herbal medicines. Those problems that were internal and/or had no obvious cause were thought to be the due to the displeasure of the gods (*atua*) or spirits of ancestors (*aitu*) and had to be treated by spiritual means, through the intercession of the spiritual healer (*taulaitu*).[17]

The arrival of the Europeans was followed by the arrival of European diseases and, just as had happened in other Australasian countries, the death of large numbers of the native population. Western (or *Palagi,* foreign) diseases, the Samoans noted, could sometimes be treated with *Palagi* herbal medicines so it was after this time that Samoan plants were investigated more intensively by the local population for their ability to treat both Samoan and *Palagi* diseases. After a flurry of such investigations in the late nineteenth and early twentieth centuries, the situation settled into what it remains effectively today, with both Samoan and western medicine coexisting in relative harmony and Samoan people choosing to use local medicine for Samoan sicknesses and western ones for *Palagi* problems.

Samoans believe that good health is dependent on a balance of three worlds: natural, social and spiritual. When these are out of balance, sickness ensues, the treatment depending on which of the three worlds is most out of line. If the condition is one that will respond to Samoan treatment, the patient or their family may use one of their own folk medicines or seek out a traditional healer (*fofo*). (A family may often 'own' a particular folk medicine but a *fofo* will generally be knowledgeable about a much wider range of possibilities, as well as having massage and other skills.) All traditional remedies are prepared simply and usually from fresh materials gathered by the healer or their assistants. Leaves may be pounded or squeezed, and roots, barks and stems scraped into powders and applied as is or dissolved/suspended in water.

Traditional remedies

The plant that is most frequently used in Samoan herbal medicine is the Indian mulberry (*Morinda citrifolia*), which is known in Samoa as *nonu*. This small tree, which is widely distributed throughout Polynesia, is used to treat skin infections such as boils, styes and infected wounds. It has also been used to treat some respiratory and urinary tract infections (and the unpleasant odour of the fruit is thought to repel the spirits responsible for causing certain ailments).[11] *Nonu* (or '*noni*', as it is also known) is becoming increasingly popular in the west as an all-purpose preventive medicine and is reported by its proponents to have a broad range of therapeutic effects, including antibacterial, antiviral, antifungal, antitumour, anthelmintic, analgesic, hypotensive, anti-inflammatory and immune-enhancing effects. Many of these effects are supported by in vitro and in vivo studies and, more recently, by a number of clinical trials.[18] Many more clinical studies need to be carried out, however, before the claims made for its wide range of therapeutic efficacies can be substantiated.

Another plant that has been used traditionally – although only occasionally – as an infusion of crushed leaves or bark to treat urinary and gastrointestinal infections is *mamala, Homalanthus nutans (*formerly known as *Omalanthus nutans)*. This small tree may prove to have a more important role in the future because it is currently being investigated for its possible efficacy against viral diseases, notably HIV, the virus that causes AIDS.[19,20] Although the plant is rarely used in Samoa to treat viral infections, it was apparently identified by local healers to a visiting American botanist as one that might be used to treat hepatitis. The active ingredient in the plant was identified as a protein kinase C compound, prostratin.[21] Subsequently, a profit-sharing collaboration has been set up between a university and research institute in USA and the Samoan government, the village and the families of the two healers who helped in the discovery.[21]

Not everyone is happy with the arrangement, however, and the legal wrangles that are continuing at present serve as a warning that development and exploitation may be two sides of the same coin.

Other plants that are found mainly in Samoa and used medicinally are *fue manogi (Piper graeffei)*, a sweet-smelling tree climber that is used to treat mouth ulcers, sore throats and infected wounds (especially if the latter have been caused by spirits), and *matalafi (Psychotria insularum)*, which is used to treat many different conditions, whether these are believed to be caused by *aitu* or natural means. Infusions of *matalafi* bark are rubbed onto the skin to treat inflammation and infected wounds and, as indicated by its botanical name, to alleviate 'possession' by driving away the causative spirits.

Many plants that are used in Samoa are also found in other Pacific island countries and are generally used for the same purpose in each. Thus Samoan people, similar to those in Fiji, are also familiar with the actions of *Piper methysticum* and *Mikania micrantha*, although these are known in Samoa as *ava* and *fue saina* respectively.[17]

Present day

Samoa is a very conservative country, one that places great importance on family and other traditional values. Samoan medicine, including herbal medicines, still has an important place in Samoan society, coexisting harmoniously alongside western medicine even though some of the treatments used appear to owe as much to the placebo effect of the healer as to the medicines themselves. The value to the community of these medicines has been recognised by government and other agencies because they work to slow down the loss of native forests and thus the plants of medicinal as well as other economic importance. Indeed, should *mamala* be shown to have anti-HIV activity that can be commercially exploited, then it and possibly other plants will be valued even more for their medicinal and economic importance.

New Zealand

As was the case in the other countries described in this chapter, the health of the Maoris of New Zealand was not improved by the arrival of the British settlers. Indeed, there were fears in the late nineteenth century that the Maori population might disappear altogether, so severely had they suffered from the many epidemics produced by strains of unfamiliar microorganisms. Fortunately this did not eventuate and New Zealand's Maori numbers continue to increase each year. However, the health of Maoris is not as good as that of those of European descent. The reasons for this disparity in health status are hotly debated but do appear to be the result of a combination of socio-economic and cultural factors. From the arrival of the settlers in the mid-nineteenth century until about the middle of the twentieth century, most Maoris lived on the ancestral lands, close to families. Maori urbanisation occurred rapidly after this, however, and with it the gradual loss of community support, which is held to be at least partially responsible for some of the current situation. More recently, Maoris in these urban areas have been re-evaluating their past and reinstituting traditional customs and practices, including those of Maori health (*Hauora Maori*).

Traditional remedies

Maoris, similar to Samoan people, also believe that good health results when there is a balance between the various worlds that they inhabit. Maoris, however, recognise four factors – spiritual, physical, emotional and psychological – as being crucial for good health. *Hauora Maori* encompasses all of these and Maori medical practice includes a combination of treatments such as massage, counselling and medicines, many of which are derived from native plants. The use of plants for healing is known as *Rongoa Maori*.

New Zealand is home to about 1970 plant species, of which around 1600 are considered indigenous.[22] At least some of these plants may have been used for generations by Maoris, although the identification and specific usage of these have been hampered by the lack of a written Maori language before European settlement in the nineteenth century.[23,24]

Earlier European visitors, such as whalers and missionaries, had noted that a number of plants were used to treat wounds and other skin problems while some were used to treat digestive problems. They did not record plant usage for other conditions. Joseph Crocome, for example, who was the first medically qualified person to practise in Otago (among the whalers and missionaries in Waikouaiti in 1838), is reported:

> . . . when his own scanty stock of drugs failed him [to have] turned to the Maori for some of their medical lore and remedies. *Koromiko* [Figure 10.5] for internal troubles, infusion of *Phormium tenax* [flax] and the slippery gum from around the roots and leaves as a bath for severe wounds, an infusion of ngaio for severe purpose: these simples sopped into flax fibre, and teased out ribbonwood 'jacket' packed over swellings and lumps, made useful substitutes for dressings of abscesses and tumours.[25]

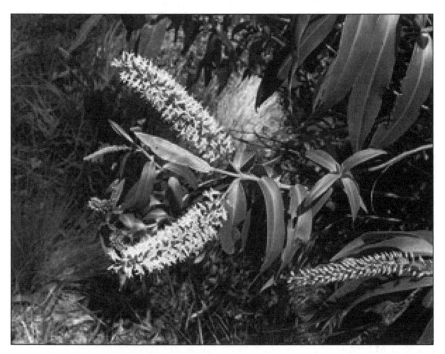

Figure 10.5 Koromiko (*Hebe salicifolia*).

Later visitors observed that plants were used during the treatment of many internal medical problems. Some of these writers considered that plants were used mainly as adjuncts during the largely ritualistic treatment of these conditions, possibly because Maoris at that time did not recognise disease as a cause of death. Disorders of the body were thought instead to be caused by the influence of evil spirits and as such could be removed only by the power of the 'priest'/healer (*tohunga*):[23]

> . . . there was no science of medicine in Maoriland. The native belief that all bodily ailments were caused by evil spirits, or came as a punishment from the gods, effectually prevented research in even simple lines such as herbal remedies. When they at last received the knowledge of internal medicine from Europeans the natives were captivated by the new mode of exorcising evil spirits. They took to medicine as a duck to water, and swallowed any nostrum they could procure, be it ever so vile. Ere long, they began to concoct strange herbal remedies for themselves.[24]

Other writers have, however, suggested that Maoris did indeed have extensive knowledge of many plants that could be and were used as medicines, knowledge that might, however, have been kept deliberately from the incoming 'foreigners':[24, 27]

> . . . that we can estimate . . . their dexterity or versatility in compounding drugs is impossible owing to the great secrecy with which such manipulations were carried out. The tohunga pretended to be instructed by his god as to the herbs he should select and the manner of combining them . . . .[28]

Although Joseph Banks, the botanist who accompanied Cook on his 1779 voyage to New Zealand, is reported to have remarked that 'the health of the natives was so sound that probably their need of physic was small',[27] the average Maori in pre-European times 'had a short, harsh life [to about 30 years of age] but a short inventory of serious diseases to be treated'.[29]

The accounts written by explorers, missionaries and other early settlers do appear to confirm that a number of different plants were used to treat various skin disorders such as wounds, 'itch' and 'growths'. Others were used internally to treat what might be described in general terms as gastrointestinal or breathing problems. Many could have been related to the living conditions of most Maoris at the time, when food was scarce, especially in winter months, and living conditions were often crowded and close.

Skin and some internal problems were treated by means of steam or vapour baths. Heated stones were placed in a form of an earth oven, sprinkled with water and then covered with the plant(s) supposed to be efficacious in the treatment of the specific condition.[30,31]

Other treatments included direct application of plant tissue to wounds, followed by bandaging or application of hot poultices of plant extracts:

> We once observed a man who, accidentally, inflicted a severe cut upon his leg with an axe; he immediately squeezed the juice of a potato into the wound and tied it up, and in a few days it was quite well.[32]

The well-travelled missionary, William Colenso, wrote that he doubted whether 'the New Zealanders ever used any vegetable as an internal medicine before their intercourse with Europeans; for severe burns, however, they applied outwardly the ashes and charcoal dust of burnt fern fronds' as well as many other plants such as *harakeke, rengarenga* and *rangiora* for the treatment of what he described as sores, unbroken tumours and abscesses, while flax leaves and sheets of dry totara bark were used as splints for 'broken bones, the New Zealanders being far better surgeons than physicians'.[33]

Despite Colenso's assertion that plants were not used as internal remedies before the arrival of Europeans, a sufficient number of other accounts refer to the treatment of constipation (with flax root) and diarrhoea (with *koromiko*) to indicate that treatments did exist for these conditions at least before European settlement.[22] What is not in doubt, however, is that after this they 'began to find curative properties in different plants',[28] activities that led to the production of a number of articles, pharmacopoeias and other books in which the medicinal uses of indigenous plants were described at length (although not always uncritically).[35,36]

Leaves of *koromiko* (veronica, *Hebe salicifolia*), which were used widely to treat diarrhoea: 'Astringent, for dysentery, etc. The decoction is good for ulcers, and for venereal disease.'[36]

So well known was this remedy, that a tincture of the plant was included in Volume I of the *Extra Pharmacopoeia* of 1915 as a 'remedy for chronic dysentery and diarrhoea'.[37] Its curative properties were valued in more recent days when young leaf tips were sent to the Maori Battalion in the Middle East during World War II, to treat the dysentery and diarrhoea that afflicted so many of the troops.

The bark of *kowhai* (*Sophora microphylla, macrophylla*), when 'taken only from the sunny side of the tree', could be: 'infused, mixed with wood ash . . . rubbed onto skin for various rashes; steeped in boiling water for several hours, for bruises, newly set fractures; or, with manuka bark, rubbed onto patients with backache.' The leaves could be boiled and then drunk for colds and sore throats.

Its almost miraculous effect on George Nepia, an All Black rugby player whose leg had been so seriously damaged that it seemed that amputation might be the only treatment, is vividly described in his biography:[38]

> What a contrast, I thought. A *pakeha* [European] doctor had told me that I would not play again during the season. The injury was too serious, he said. A Maori woman, using Maori treatment had cured me. Play soon, she said.

And he did, 10 days later.

Captain Cook used the dried leaves of manuka (*Leptospermum scoparium*) to make a tea, 'which has a very agreeable bitter taste and flavour when they are recent'.[29] Not surprisingly, therefore, this plant is known popularly as tea tree although it is quite different botanically and chemically from its Australian namesake. The leaves and bark of manuka were used as a decoction to treat urinary problems, and to reduce fever. Infusions of the inner bark were used to promote sleep and ease pain, and its seed capsules chewed to relieve colic pains and diarrhoea. (Today, in Europe as well as New Zealand, manuka honey is prized – and priced above all other honeys – for its antibacterial properties, which are utilised in wound treatments and for peptic ulcers.)

Another plant used to treat pain was *horopito* or pepper tree (*Pseudowintera colorata*), known to the early European settlers as the 'Maori painkiller/bushman's painkiller'.[28] Leaf extracts were used to treat the skin rash known as 'paipai', stomachache and sexually transmitted infections, while whole leaves were chewed for toothache. Bark extracts were used as a quinine substitute (tonic) and also to treat burns.

Harakeke (*Phormium tenax*), the New Zealand flax, was used for shelter, clothing, baskets, mats and general healing. So important was this plant to nineteenth-century Maoris that they were reported to have been astonished when they discovered that it did not grow in England and to have asked how the English managed to live without it. (Now of course they do not because the New Zealand flax has become a striking, exotic addition to many a British garden.) Leaves were used by Maoris as splints and bandages and, after boiling, as a poultice for skin problems and general aches and pains. The boiled liquid of both leaf bases and roots were used internally as a purgative.

Present day

In New Zealand, as in the other three countries discussed in this chapter, more recognition is being given to the therapeutic value of traditional medicines, including the use of medicines derived from local flora. Although some knowledge has inevitably been lost over time, the increasing interest in *Rongoa*

Maori by both Maori and non-Maori New Zealanders is ensuring that current knowledge is both stored and expanded. Traditional uses of plants have been taken as indicators of chemical content and pharmacological activity and hence possible commercial value. There is disquiet among some older Maoris that this research involving use of local knowledge might be exploited by overseas interests to the detriment of New Zealand people and certainly this is a factor that must be recognised as a potential problem in all countries not yet protected by international agreements. Overall, however, the future for traditional medicine is looking bright as more and more people are recognising the value of such treatments, to be used not instead of 'western' medicines but as complementary to them.

Further reading

Brooker SG, Cambie RC, Cooper RC. *New Zealand Medicinal Plants*. Auckland: Reed Books, 1998.

Cox PA, Banack SA. Eds. *Islands, Plants and Polynesians*. Portland, OR; Dioscorides Press, 1991.

Cribb AB, Cribb JQ. *Wild Medicine in Australia*. Sydney: Fontana/Collins, 1983.

Macpherson C, Macpherson L. *Samoan Medical Belief and Practice*. Auckland: Auckland University Press, 1990.

Southwell I, Lowe R, eds. *Tea Tree. The Genus Melaleuca*. Melbourne: Harwood Academic Publishers, 1999.

Weiner MA. *Secrets of Fijian Medicine*. Berkeley, CA: University of California Press, 1984.

Whistler WA. *Polynesian Herbal Medicine*. Hawaii: The National Tropical Botanical Garden, 1992

More information

Te Rongoa – Maori Herbal Medicine: http://pharmacy.otago.ac.nz/rongoa/index.html (accessed November 2007)

Fallon F, Enig MG. *Australian Aborigines – Living off the Fat of the* Land: www.weston-aprice.org/traditional_diets/australian_aborigines.html (accessed November 2007)

Dittmar A. *Samoan Herbal Medicine*: www.dittmar.dusnet.de/english/esamoa.html (accessed November 2007)

Moulds RFW, Jalani J. Kava: herbal panacea or liver poison? (Electronic) *Med J Aust* 2003;**178**:451–3. Available at: www.mja.com.au/public/issues/178_09_050503/mou 10043_fm.html (accessed November 2007)

References

1. Maiden JH. *The Useful Native Plants of Australia*. Sydney: Turner & Henderson, 1889. Cited in Lassak and McCarthy,[2] p 13.
2. Lassak VA, McCarthy T. *Australian Medicinal Plants*. Sydney: Reed New Holland, 2001: 13
3. Maiden JH. *The Forest Flora of New South Wales*, vol 4. Sydney: 1911. Cited Lassak and McCarthy,[2] p 106.
4. Maiden JH. *The Forest Flora of New South Wales*, vol 7. Sydney: 1922. Cited in Lassak and McCarthy,[2] p 22.

5. Roth WE. Superstition, magic and medicine. *North Queensland Ethnography Bulletin No. 5*. Brisbane: Government Printer, 1903. Cited in Lassak and McCarthy,[2] p 194.
6. Lassak VA, McCarthy T. *Australian Medicinal Plants*. Sydney: Reed New Holland, 2001: 75.
7. Barr A, Chapman J, Smith N, Beveridge M. Aboriginal Communities of the Northern Territory of Australia. *Traditional Bush Medicines. An Aboriginal Pharmacopoeia*. Santa Clarita, CA: Greenhouse Publications, 1988.
8. Seeman B. *Flora vitiensis: a description of plants of the Viti or Fiji Islands with an account of their history, uses and properties*. London: L Reeve & Co., 1865–73. Cited in Cambie and Ash,[9] p 2.
9. Cambie RC, Ash J. *Fijian Medicinal Plants*. Clayton South, Victoria: The Commonwealth Scientific and Industrial Research Organisation, 1994.
10. Parham JW. *Plants of the Fiji Islands*, revised edn. Suva: Government Printer, 1972.
11. Strahl S, Ehret V, Dahm, HH, Maier, KP. Necrotizing hepatitis after taking herbal remedies. *Dtsch Med Wochenschr* 1998;**123**:1410–14.
12. Stickel F et al, Hepatitis induced by Kava (*Piper methysticum rhizoma*). *J Hepatol* 2003;**39**:62–7.
13. New Zealand Association of Medical Herbalists. *Submission on Proposed Reclassification of Kava as a Prescription Medicine*. Auckland: New Zealand Association of Medical Herbalists, 2005.
14. Whistler WA. *Polynesian Herbal Medicine*. Auckland: National Botanical Tropical Garden, 1992.
15. Anke J, Ramzam I. Pharmacokinetic and pharmacodynamic drug interactions with Kava (*Piper methysticum* Forst.f.). *J Ethnopharmacol* 2004;**93**:153–60.
16. Lim STL, Dragull K, Tang CS et al. Effects of kava alkaloid, pipermethystine, and kavalactones on oxidative stress and cytochrome P450 in F-344 Rats. *Toxicol Sci* 2007;**97**:210–21.
17. Whistler WA. *Samoan Herbal Medicine*. Honolulu: Isle Botanica, 1996.
18. Wang MY, West BJ, Jarakae CJ et al. *Morinda citrifolia* (Noni): A literature review and recent advances in Noni research. *Acta Pharmacol Sin* 2002;**23**:1127–101.
19. Cox PA, Balick MJ. The ethnobotanical approach to drug discovery. *Sci Am* 1994; June:82–7.
20. Biancotto A, Grivel J-G, Gondois-Rey F et al. Dual role of prostratin in inhibition of infection and reactivation of human immunodeficiency virus from latency in primary blood lymphocytes and lymphoid tissue. *J Virol* 2004;**78**:10507–15.
21. Prostratin Press Release. AIDS Research Alliance, 13 December 2001.
22. Brooker SG, Cambie RA, Cooper RC. *New Zealand Medicinal Plants*, 2nd edn. Auckland: Heinemann, 1987.
23. Best E. Maori religion and mythology. *Dominion Museum Bulletin* 1924:**10**.
24. MacDonald C. *Medicines of the Maori*. Auckland: Collins, 1973.
25. Fulton R. Medical practice in Otago and Southland in the early days. *Otago Daily Times*, Dunedin, 1922.
26. Best E. *The Maori*. Wellington: Government Printer, 1924. (Polynesian Soc. Mem. 5)
27. Riley M. *Maori Healing and Herbal*. Paraparaumu, New Zealand: Viking Sevenseas NZ Ltd, 1994.
28. Goldie, WH. Maori medical lore. *Trans Proc NZ Inst* 1905;**37**:1–120.
29. Hooker JD. *Journal of the Right Hon. Sir Joseph Banks, Bart. KB, PRS, during Captain Cook's first voyage in HMS Endeavour in 1768–71 to Terra Del Fuego, Otahite, New Zealand, Australia and the Dutch East Indies, etc*. Macmillan: London, 1896.
30. Cook J. *A voyage towards the South Pole and around the world*. London: Strahan & Cadell, 1777.
31. Polack JS. *Manners and Customs of the New Zealanders*. London: Madden, 1840.
32. Cruise RA. *Journal of a Ten Months' Residence in New Zealand (1820)*, 2nd edn. London: Longman, Hurst, 1824.

33. Colenso, W. On the botany of the North Island of New Zealand. *Trans Proc NZ Inst* 1869;1(pt 3 – essays):1–58. 1875;233–83.

34. Buck P. (*Te Rangi Hiroa.*) *The Coming of the Maori.* Christchurch: Whitcombe & Tombs Ltd, 1949.

35. Kerry-Nicholas, JH. *The King Country*, 3rd edn. London: Sampson Low, Marston, 1884.

36. Neil JF. *The New Zealand Family Herb Doctor.* Dunedin: Mills, Dick, 1889. (2nd edn 1891)

37. *The Extra Pharmacopoeia*, Vol I, 16th edn. London: Martindale & Westcott, 1915.

38. Nepia G, Mclean T. *I, George Nepia.* Wellington: AH & AJ Reed Ltd, 1961.

11

Traditional Jewish medicine

Kenneth Collins

The Jewish people have always seen medicine and faith as inextricably linked.[1] There has been continuing Jewish fascination with medicine from earliest times, usually associated with reverence for the healer with an understanding that treatment and cure carry with them something of the divine. Traditional medicine, sometimes also referred to as popular or folk medicine, occupies the ground between the use of natural medicinal substances and the traditional religious quest for the victory of the forces of good in an uncertain world. Although the pharmacology of Biblical and Talmudic medicine, as well as that of mediaeval Jewish practitioners, may seem strange to the modern health consumer, Jewish folk practices have remained remarkably persistent, surviving to the present day.

Jewish popular medicine has often been seen as the superstitious legacy of the encounter between Jews and their neighbours, especially in the mediaeval Christian and Arab worlds, over millennia of dispersion. Thus, at times this tradition has been seen as primitive, the product of an era best forgotten, whereas others, less disparagingly, see elements of a rich historical tradition in these practices. In recent years, especially following the movement of the previously marginalised Jews from eastern communities into the political mainstream in Israel, there have been serious attempts to understand this folk medicine culture in its proper context.[2]

Jewish popular medicine is firmly based within the Jewish religious tradition. It utilises the canon of Hebrew scriptures in the *Tanach* as understood in the voluminous commentaries and discourses of the rabbis recorded in the *Mishna* and *Gemara*. Together, these works, known collectively as the Talmud, have formed the basis for further rabbinic elaboration over the millennium and a half since the final redaction of the *Gemara*. Jewish traditional medicine also uses the rich symbolism inherent in Jewish ritual and the Hebrew language. Thus, the fragrant herbs used at the *havdalah* ceremony at the end of the Sabbath could be used as an inhalation for colds, and a treatment for diarrhoea, high blood pressure, hair loss and pestilence during the following week.[3]

The land of Israel was strategically placed on the trade routes of antiquity and was especially open to the medical practices and traditions of its many neighbours. These included Egypt, where the Israelites lived for some centuries, to Mesopotamia, home of the Jewish patriarchs. In differing periods Egyptian and Mesopotamian medicine were highly esteemed even though many of the medications came with their own associated religious and cultural practices, often inimical to that of Israel. Further, Israel enjoys a special climate located between sea and desert, with such remarkable land features as the Dead Sea and the River Jordan, and is located at the conjunction of three continents with their varied plant and animal populations.

Medicine in the Bible

The Hebrew Bible records that the *kohenim* (priests) supervised cases of contagious diseases but, unlike in other contemporary cultures, did not perform the functions of a physician. The prophets, however, occasionally practised the art of healing. Elijah and his disciple Elisha both restored life to a child who appeared to have died (I *Kings* xvii:17–22 and II *Kings* iv:18–20, 34–35). Isaiah cured King Hezekiah, at the direction of God, of an inflammation by applying a plaster made of figs (II *Kings* xx:7). Ben Sira wrote in the Apocrypha:

> Honour a physician with the honour due unto him for the uses which ye may have of him, for the Lord hath created him . . . . The Lord has created medicines out of the earth; and he that is wise will not abhor them. . . . And He has given men skill that He might be honoured in His marvellous works. . . . My son, in thy sickness be not negligent; . . . give place to the physician; . . . let him not go from thee, for thou hast need of him. (*Ecclesiasticus* 38:1–12)

Although the Bible is clearly not in any way a medical text, its voluminous account of the early history of the Jewish people and their constant religious struggles contains a number of references of a medical nature. However, it is difficult to find any reference to any medication taken for internal use, although many of the products that are mentioned throughout its text do have a medicinal component. There are indications of the understanding of quarantine and health protection, and sanitary regulations concerned the eating of meat, the quick carrying out of burials and social hygiene. There were practising midwives as well as physicians. Treatments included bathing, anointing with oils, wine, balm and medicinal compresses, and splinting for fractures. The health benefits of music were already known in Biblical times. The minstrel's music enabled the prophet to be more receptive to the Divine Message while David played on his harp to drive away the melancholy from King Saul.[4] *Proverbs* describes trust in God as 'potions, *sku'I*, for the bones'. *Ezekiel* 47:9 talks of waters flowing from Jerusalem as 'wherever the waters come they shall be healed and everything lives wherever the river comes'.

The Bible also records the traditional plants of the area. The *Book of Genesis* relates that when Joseph was sold into slavery in Egypt the Ishmaelite traders were carrying gum, balm and laudanum. These plant resins, including balsam, were used for a range of medical disorders, such as fevers, stomach disorders and excessive sweating. When Jacob sent his sons for the second time to Egypt to buy food they were to take some of the produce of Canaan, including balm, honey, gum, laudanum, nuts and almonds as a gift to Joseph. The *Book of Exodus* records details of the special ointment used to consecrate the vessels of the Temple and anoint the *kohenim*. This ointment contained cassia, cinnamon, myrrh, calamus and olive oil. Calamus remains an essential ingredient in the manufacture of perfumes while it is also a psychoactive product, being hallucinogenic at high doses. Cassia is closely related to cinnamon and was prised for its aroma whereas myrrh has analgesic properties and can stimulate the appetite. Hyssop, which has mild purgative properties, is mentioned in the *Book of Psalms* (51:9) as a cleanser from sin (Figure 11.1).

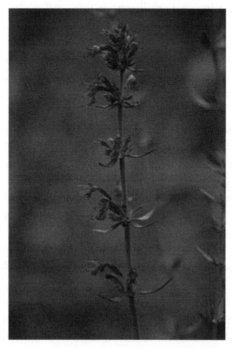

Figure 11.1 Hyssop (*Hyssopus officinalis*): purgative and 'cleanser from sin'.

We have seen the reference to the healing of King Hezekiah. However, one of Hezekiah's acts, for which he was praised by the rabbis, was to conceal the legendary *Book of Remedies* which was said to have contained the cures for all diseases and the authorship of which was attributed to King Solomon by the great mediaeval rabbi–physician Nachmanides, Ramban, (1194–c.1270). The Biblical commentator Rashi (1040–1105) believed that people were being healed so quickly by these remedies that they did not develop the humility that their illness should have produced, and so they failed to see God as the true Healer.[5] Maimonides, however, commented that the *Book of Remedies* contained treatments based on astrological phenomena and magical incantations, which might lead people to use them for idolatrous purposes. Further, it contained details of the formulae for poisons and antidotes, and this might have led unscrupulous people to use the poisons to kill their enemies.

Medicine in the Talmud

The nature of the Talmud, with its encyclopaedic view of the Jewish world spanning many centuries of Jewish life in both the land of Israel and the Babylonian diaspora, lent itself to coverage of a wide variety of traditional medical themes, including folk remedies and health beliefs. The Talmud builds on the range of medicinal products and hygienic procedures in the Bible supplemented by oral traditions, some said to have been preserved from the time of Moses. In addition, the Talmud contains a large number of medical references dealing with the rights and duties of the physician. From Talmudic times it was recommended that no wise person should live in a town that did not have a doctor. It was required for a patient to seek help for healing even on the Sabbath when religious restrictions might be set aside if there is any possible danger to health.

Some of the popular medicine traditions recorded in the Talmud will naturally seem strange, even outlandish, to the modern mind but we should remember that in mediaeval Europe as late as the sixteenth century the apothecary was legally required to keep woodlice, ants, vipers, scorpions, crabs, sparrow brains and fox lungs in stock.[6] Leading rabbis of the Talmudic period, such as Abbaye and Raba, did have concerns about the use of magic and charms but, mindful of contemporary sentiment, accepted that whatever is done for therapeutic purposes is not to be regarded as superstitious.[7] Further, given the strictness of Jewish dietary laws and their proscription of certain animals and birds for food, they record cases of permitted and forbidden treatments.[8] The use of forbidden animal products for medication remained a problem for observant Jews. Although the theoretical lists of available Jewish traditional remedies and materia medica contain many products from such animals as the eagle, lion, frog, hyena and crocodile, they feature much less in lists of Jewish practical pharmacy. This is thought to be less due to commercial availability than to halachic considerations.[9]

The medication mentioned in the Talmud is derived mainly from plants and trees. Often the trees are used in their entirety, while sometimes just the leaves and rarely the bark are used. Plant oils were popular and olive oil might be used as a gargle for sore throat. The most important animal product is honey: 'with sweet a person heals the bitter.'[10] Drugs might be prepared in different ways. Mostly the drugs were cooked individually or together – a liquid remedy called *shikyana*. Sometimes drugs were pulverised and taken internally either as dry powder or suspended in water. *Samma de naftza,* an abortifacient remedy, was imbibed in this way.[11] Wax and base tallow were used as the base for salves. One such, *collyria,* was used for eye disease. Salves could also form the basis of poultices and plasters. Plaster, *retiya,* may be applied to a wound, or if the whole body is injured as in a fall then the whole body is covered with a plaster, one of the ingredients of which is wheat. Theriac, a great compound medication with a variety of often potent ingredients, such as snake flesh, was widely employed in Talmudic times. The rabbis counsel against the use of theriac from heathen sources because of the risk of adulteration with poisons.[12]

Other products used for treatment include many common foodstuffs. Bread soaked in wine is recommended as an eye compress and green leaves may be applied to inflamed eyes.[13] Ripe or unripe gourds can be placed on the forehead to relieve fever.[14] Mar Samuel (*c.*165–*c.*257), a leading scholar and physician of the Talmudic period, considered that cool water for eye compresses is the best collyrium in the world and children were bathed in wine for healing purposes[15] (Tosefta Shabbat 12:13). The use of natural springs and waters was also well known – and the springs of Tiberias, on the shore of the Sea of Galilee, were particularly prized for their healing properties. Rabbi Yochanan explains that the absence of *tzaraat,* leprosy, in Babylon was because of their bathing in the Euphrates.[16]

In addition to the use of specific medications the Talmudic records, additional details would seem to add a magical dimension to the treatment. The use of garland, or knotted plants, is said to be especially efficacious – three knots arrest the illness, five heal it and seven help even against magic.[17] A particularly efficacious medication was said to be *samtar.* If this is placed on a wound caused by an arrow or spear it would help the victim survive.[18] If someone is bitten by a rabid dog they would be given liver from that animal to eat.[19]

There is little in the way of so-called *filth pharmacy* in the Talmud, which appears extensively in Greek and Roman sources. In the Talmud Rabbi Chanina records the use of a measure of 40-day-old urine for a wasp sting or scorpion bite – presumably this was to be applied externally.[20] In the

Jerusalem Talmud, a shorter and less complete compendium produced in the land of Israel rather than in Babylonia, Rabbi Yochanan records that he learned from a Roman woman that children's faeces were a cure for scurvy.[21]

Many non-medicinal remedies are also recorded in the Talmud. These include the application of heat, e.g. by the use of warm cloths on the abdomen and hot cups on the navel.[22] The beneficial effects of sunshine on health were also known from Biblical times and recommended by the rabbis.[23] Dietary considerations relative to health were also recorded in detail in the rabbinic literature. The rabbis took care that, although patients might be given advice about diet, for incurable patients some are of the opinion that such patients be allowed to eat what they want.[24] Physicians were advised that they should handle such situations with delicacy – not giving specific difficult orders but saying the same: 'don't sleep in a damp place or drink anything cold', adding 'lest you die like so and so' – as this will make a better impression.[25] Sick people were advised to avoid eating gourds but could eat the more delicate food known as *hatriyot*. A physician came to heal Rav Yirmiyahu and saw gourds present and exclaimed, 'How can I heal him – the Angel of Death is in this house!'[26] Eating beef, fat meat, poultry, roasted eggs, cress, milk and cheese could make illness worse while beneficial foods, which could heal sickness, included: cabbage, mangold, camomile and small fish.[27] Specific foods for the sick would include the gruel-like tisane or *arsan*, which is made from old peeled barley from the bottom of the sieve, or fine barley flour. *Schathitha*, dried baked corn flour mixed with honey, was prepared in thick and thin forms. The thick version was used as nourishing food and the thin form as medication. A similar product, made from lentil flour mixed with vinegar, was used as a remedy for fever.[28]

The most common forms of surgical treatments to be considered within the framework of traditional medicine include bleeding and cupping. Bleeding, by performing phlebotomy, is often mentioned in the Talmud, sometimes accompanied by a special blessing, and was widely performed as a medical treatment until as late as the nineteenth century. Sanhedrin 129b gives directions for cupping and bleeding. Mar Samuel, the greatest of Talmudic physicians, advised that a patient should fast before bloodletting and take their time before resuming normal activities after the procedure.[29] The rabbis were concerned about the risks of bleeding and constructed a calendar of propitious days for the procedure.

There is a voluminous literature in the Talmud and in the New Testament (*Matthew* 10:1) about demons and their role in the causation of illness and the rabbis believed that magic and the evil eye operated through them. The demon aetiology is even susceptible to a theory of contagion. One should not drink liquid left by another or the spirit that comes out of the other, if he has a disease, can pose a mortal danger. Demons inhabit marshy places, damp and deserted houses, latrines, squalid lanes and foetid atmospheres, which obviously became associated with disease and ill-health.[30]

Mediaeval Jewish medicine

In the Middle Ages there was often a narrow line delineating the role of traditional healers and practising physicians. The physician was often seen as a powerful exponent of science and religion while the rationale of superstition and magic in medicine had become part and parcel of the Jewish cultural heritage.[31,32] Magical cure and incantations were occasionally permitted by the rabbis – not because of their likely efficacy but to set at ease the mind of the superstitious. Thus, it was not really necessary for the patient to resort to the magician for treatment as the ordinary remedies used by doctor and layman used the full range of magical devices. Many of these treatments follow theories of aetiology and pathology, which we can readily see today as being wrong but from mediaeval beliefs about cause and effect the treatments follow a logical pattern.[33-35] The traditional Jewish healer required knowledge of the Jewish lore surrounding his practice besides an expertise in medicinal plants and an ability to exorcise the evil eye.[36]

Jews and Christians shared much of this popular medicine. Rabbi Menahem of Speyer was quoted as saying that, as sound effects a cure so a Christian may be permitted to heal a Jew by incantation, even if he invokes the aid of Jesus and the saints in his spell.[37] However, religious views differed on the attitude to healing. Important rabbinic authorities, such as Nachmanides, considered that righteous people should be protected by God's blessing while Moses Maimonides, Rambam (1138–1204), the greatest of Jewish mediaeval rabbis and himself a physician, believed that the divine mandate to heal derives from the Torah (Figures 11.2 and 11.3). In short, true healing is a gift from God who has given the doctor what is required to heal by natural means.

Mediaeval medicine had inherited from late antiquity the conviction that there was a close correlation between the universe, the macrocosm, and humans, the microcosm. Both were said to be formed of the four elements – air, fire, earth and water – and

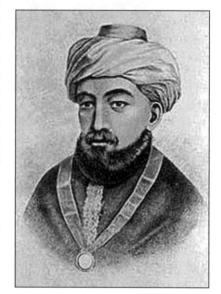

Figure 11.2 Moses Maimonides (1138–1204): rabbi and physician.

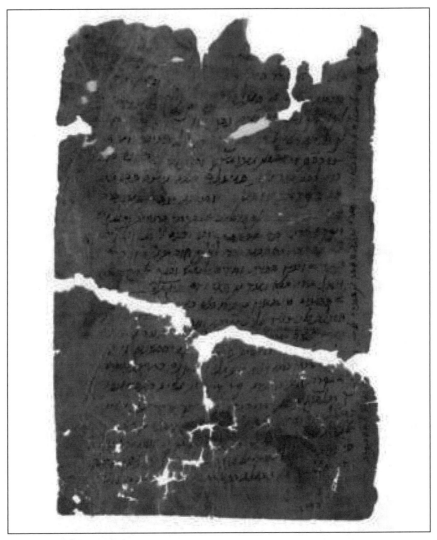

Figure 11.3 Fragments of a letter written by Maimonides. (*Taylor-Schecter Geniza Newsletter* 2005.)

endowed with the same four qualities – heat, cold, dryness and humidity. The four humours – blood, yellow and black bile, and phlegm – had to be kept in balance by, for example, bloodletting, and doctors had special zodiacal calendars to identify the best times for bleeding.[38] The Talmud gives clear evidence of the widespread practice of bloodletting and although Maimonides himself counselled against it as a reliable treatment it retained its popularity down to modern times.

The rabbinic *Responsa* literature of the Middle Ages, where the mediaeval rabbis respond to questions by their followers, contains much of medical interest. Here, we see the attitudes of people, distressed by illness, to healing practices and what they had recourse to in the hope of returning to full health. Some treatments seem benign. There was an association between sanctified wine for the ceremonies of *kiddush* and *havdalah* and the strengthening of weak eyes because mediaeval Jews saw the drinking of the wine or merely bathing the eyes with it as a remedy in itself.[39] Other treatments posed religious problems. Patients would ask the rabbi for permission to undergo procedures that might be in conflict with the laws of Shabbat and many of the medications would have required the taking of foodstuffs forbidden by a kosher diet. In general permission seems to have been given for the consumption of the most outlandish products if it would benefit health, although some rabbis indicated that they would withhold consent 'to all remedies which are biblically forbidden'.[40]

Zimmels records what he calls medicines in their natural state such as goats' milk, fish oil, warm animal blood, human milk and urine. More commonly, medicines contained a number of ingredients. One celebrated ingredient was the Egyptian mummy, the embalmed flesh of which was taken internally or more often applied as a plaster. Given the scarcity of mummies from Egypt, eventually the bones and flesh of ordinary corpses were ground up and sold as mummies. Some rabbis had problems about using 'the flesh of corpses' which the mummy represented, but usually permitted it considering that the product no longer resembled its original matter. Using the principle of sympathy it was the upper half of the mummy, containing as it does the heart, lungs and stomach, that was considered most likely to be effective.

Some treatments were considered to have specific effects. A modest Jewish herbal of the fifteenth century copied and illustrated in Italy preserves a sense of plants and their properties. Here St John's wort (*Hypericum perforatum*) is considered to be a diuretic and expectorant.[41] Treatments included fish oil for coughs, and drinking urine for jaundice and ass milk for asthma and haemoptysis. People with epilepsy could be given such products as broth from a reptile or a mole whereas people with mental illness could be given the flesh of a fowl that had died a natural death. Topical treatments, including ointments, bathing and the application of plasters and poultices, such as oats or barley, were also used. One plaster that was 'proved by experience' had sheep fat, butter, olive oil, wax, egg yolk, almonds, alum and herbs all fried together.[42]

Mediaeval herbal therapy

Herbs often have natural healing properties that have been accepted by medical science and the search for active ingredients in traditional medicines has intensified in modern times. Substances of medicinal plants played a major part in the lives of mediaeval Jews. They served as foodstuffs, herbs, cosmetics, condiments and incense as well as in home industries such as tanning, dyeing and ink production.[43] The mediaeval mind often associated the healing herbs with magical qualities, and it is usually impossible to divorce the purely therapeutic from the magical and superstitious in such prescriptions. Thus, herbs gathered in a cemetery were considered of high medicinal value because of their association with the spirits and their occult potency.[44]

In the Roman period medicine sellers had their own professional and social organisation and, in the Middle Ages, during periods of both Moslem and Christian rule, herbalists and purveyors of medication had proper supervision and were educated in medicine and pharmacy. In the Arab world many of these practitioners inherited their skills through numerous generations of the same family. It should not be thought that these medications were without effect. Indeed, the efficacy of many plant medicines has long been understood for simple symptom control and some products could be used for more specific conditions. To this day there are many plant-based remedies in official national pharmacopoeias that have stood the test of time and have met the criteria of randomised control trials.[45] The Jewish community in Cairo relied on the trade in medicinal remedies for much of its commercial success with Jewish traders in port cities around the extensive mediaeval diaspora.[46]

Hebrew sources record use of fennel for abdominal disorders and threatened miscarriage, celandine sap for cataracts and columbine taken internally for bad eyes (Figure 11.4).[47] A decoction of sage was employed as a cure for paralysis and to aid digestion. The mixture included saltpetre, sage, bay and cinnamon, which was beaten thoroughly with honey. After drinking the decoction the disturbance should leave and the patient is then recommended to drink some wine.

In the *Materia Medica* of Maimonides there are a number of plant medications with an identifiable psychoactive effect and, given his custom of tailoring his prescriptions to individual patients, we have a clear idea of his clinical practice. Maimonides, practising in Cairo and personal physician to the Sultan of Egypt, was well aware of psychosomatic factors in disease, considering that 'the skilled physician should place nothing ahead of rectifying the state of the psyche by removing these passions'. There has been considerable concern in recent years to understand the nature of the placebo response as it is conceded that one of the reasons for the popularity of alternative complementary medicine is the time, support and empathy provided by its practitioners. Indeed, it is concluded that a good doctor–patient relationship can tangibly improve patients' responses to treatment, placebo or otherwise.[48]

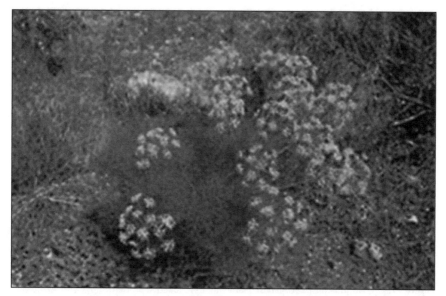

Figure 11.4 Fennel (*Foeniculum vulgare*): Hebrew sources recommend fennel as a purgative and to prevent miscarriage.

Paavilainen records more than 100 different drugs used by Maimonides for the treatment of melancholy with about 24 of them used most frequently.[49] Most commonly prescribed were *Rosa canina*, *Citrus*, oxtongue (*Helminthia echioides*) and pistacia (mastic and pistachio), along with the mineral jacinth and castoreum, a secretion from beaver glands used today in the manufacture of perfumes (Figure 11.5). She considers that almost two-thirds of Maimonides' treatments for melancholy would have had some level of efficacy either as a mood enhancer or as a tranquilliser. Basil is antidepressant and sedative whereas citrus may also be a mood enhancer, neuroprotective and anti-amnesiac. The pepper genus has numerous psychoactive properties while raisins and grapes are also neuro-protective, and wine, of course, can relieve stress and improve the mood if taken in appropriate quantities. Maimonides also liked to prescribe spike-nard (*Nardostachys jatamansi*), also called nard, which is a flowering plant of the valerian family with flowers and stems that can be crushed and distilled into an intensely aromatic, amber-colored, essential oil, which is used as a perfume, as well as a sedative and hypnotic.

Ibn Ezra (1092–1167) was a poet, astronomer and Bible commentator whose writings detail his own medical knowledge as well as that of contem-porary physicians, usually accompanied with the formula 'and this has been verified with testing'.[50] He divided active medications into those that purge the body whether by vomiting or by diarrhoea, those that are beneficial for diseased organs when hung on the arm or neck or by ablution or by drinking,

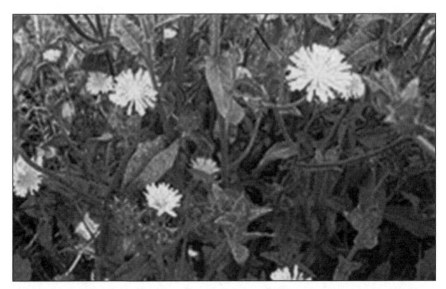

Figure 11.5 Oxtongue (*Picris echioides*): plant with psychoactive properties.

in a poultice or by fumigation, and others that counteract the poison of creeping animals or deadly poison of beverages.[51] He wrote that, when drugs are acting through their whole essence, it is impossible to define their action by logical judgement, but when people examine them by testing the truth of their efficacy will come to light.[52]

Among the hundreds of Ibn Ezra's treatments are extract of absinth together with ashes, commonly used in his time in place of soap. The patient wraps it tightly round the head in a bandage, then rinses the ashes from the head. This is done two or three times a week to cure headaches of every kind.[53] The juice of a sempervivum plant that has been buried for a year underground, if instilled into the ear, is said to cure any deafness even if it is from childhood.[54] A further treatment for a headache involves taking the peganum herb with marjoram and pennyroyal and putting them in a bag on the sufferer's head. The pain, throbbing and swelling of haemorrhoids will be relieved by finely ground leek, cooked with butter.[55] However, he also recorded that excrement of a bear when hung on the thigh of one who has colic pain makes him healthy and soothes his pain. Among his recordings of spells and incantations is that if you write the following three names on the patient's forehead – *kita*, *zvi* and *lekh* – while blood comes out of his nostrils it will stop immediately.[56]

Alternative therapies

Some traditional remedies did not require ingestion of medication but rather relied on *segulot*, which originally referred to charms but came to be attached to the concept of an 'occult virtue' which was inherent in a particular object. Nachmanides believed that King Solomon had gained all the appropriate knowledge in this area from the Torah – 'even the potency of herbs and their *segulot*'. Rabbi Bayha ben Asher (died 1340) believed that God had taught Moses the nature and occult virtue of plants and herbs that had the power to heal but could also 'sweeten the bitter and make the bitter sweet'.

The principles of 'sympathy', where the effect resembles the cause, and 'contact', where objects that have been in contact continue to act on each other after the contact has ended, can also be found in the Jewish sources. Accordingly, we find such remedies as rubbing a stillborn baby with its placenta or eating the liver of a mad dog as a cure for the dog's bite. Sympathy was even extended to looking at specific colours to influence the red or black humours or trying to destroy an enemy by destroying his image. As for contact, it was believed that anyone who got possession of someone's cut hair or nail clippings could assume power over them. The name given to a person gives them some of the character of its original owner. Rabbi Jacob Emden (1697–1776) referred to a drug that heals sword wounds when the drug is in contact with the blood on the sword, even if the wounded person is now some distance away. The noted physician Tobias Hacohen (1652–1729) reported cases of family illness where brothers, even those living in different countries, developed the same illness or died at the same time.

The principle of antipathy was the basis for the use of amulets. Thus the supposed antipathy between deer and snakes led to people wearing the tooth of a deer to keep snakes away. Maimonides was careful to avoid magical treatments unless there was evidence as to their efficacy and claims for their benefit could be proved, or if withholding them would cause psychological distress to the patient. Rabbi Samson Morpurgo (died 1740) noted the principle of sympathy as well as the working of specific remedies. He also noted that other 'remedies', whether of vegetable or animal origin, were hung on the neck or arm of the patient, who had fever, jaundice, epilepsy or dysentery, and these were to be considered *segulot* because doctors were aware that they were not conventional treatment. However, Morpurgo made a specific case for the use of snake products, found in the medication known as theriac, because doctors had indicated that it could be prescribed for disorders of the white humour and thus did not work by occult virtue alone. In general, however, the consumption of many of the noxious medicaments was not recommended for Jewish patients and there was a particular revulsion to the use of blood and products of vermin and reptiles.[57]

There is a wide variety of treatments recorded within the rabbinic *Responsa*. Among the popular prescriptions are many items that owe their place to tradition and long established associations such as cutting the beard as a cure for sore eyes or washing being harmful to aching teeth. As a treatment for toothache salt, pepper and a little garlic were mixed, and the mixture was left on the pulse overnight.

A couple of years ago the actress Gwyneth Paltrow made headlines when wearing a backless dress showing the marks from having cupping during an acupuncture treatment. Today cupping is most commonly used to treat coughs, asthma, and muscle aches and pain, especially back pain, but it has been used in cultures across the world for centuries and was especially popular in eastern European Jewish traditional medicine, where it was known as *bahnkes*. Cupping was especially popular as a treatment for weak and obese patients and pregnant women. Despite the enduring popularity of the procedure, the old Yiddish proverb, *Es vet helfen vi a toiten bahnkes,* 'it will help like applying cups to a dead person', indicates a more sceptical view of its efficacy. Cupping techniques vary but *bahnkes* involves the use of small cups containing a small amount of alcohol which is heated and a vacuum is produced by the absence of oxygen (Figure 11.6). The cup is then pressed tightly against the skin. This suction is thought to draw out noxious substances from the body, thus restoring the balances of bodily humors.

Numbers also played an important part in healing. The numbers 3, 7 and 9 were particularly efficacious and invocations used were similar for Jews and Christians with the wording adapted to the sensitivities of the patient. *Sefer Hasidim,* a book of mediaeval pietistic literature, records that a person who has been harmed by a demon needs to have the charm repeated nine

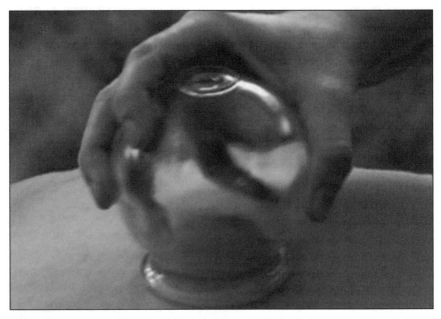

Figure 11.6 Cupping glass.

times, as they do in Germany, for a cure.[58] The principle of transference was also employed in treatment. For a severe headache a thread was wound three times around the patient's head and hung in a tree. When a bird flew through the loop it took the headache with it.[59] The placing of the patient's excrement on a growing plant to which the illness will be transferred is recorded by Tobias Hacohen, who indicates that its value is greatly exaggerated.[60] The principle could even be used to gauge the progress of the illness. The patient's belt was stretched over the length and width of his body and then hung on a nail with the appropriate incantation and measured: any change in length was interpreted as being prognostic of the course of the illness. Circling round the patient, initially seen as preventing the action of demons, could also be used as a remedy against various diseases.[61]

The mere repetition of a magic name may affect a cure, or the magic name may be written on the person or inscribed on an amulet. Having the name written on the forehead was said to be very effective in stopping bleeding. A magic name written on an apple and consumed on three separate occasions was used to heal fevers.[62] To ease a confinement Psalm 20 was to be recited nine times. This might be repeated or combined with a call on the angel Armisael, who governs the womb, to help the woman and baby to life and peace.[63] The variety of spells available for treatment was infinite and in many cases did not need to be accompanied by medication or bloodletting. Many German magical cures, which would otherwise have been lost, have been preserved in Hebrew manuscripts.

A person's name is considered to play a role in deciding his fate; it is given to him when he enters the Jewish world and has been described as serving as a social and cosmological identity card.[64] The Talmud records that a change of name can cause a change of fortune.[65] To confuse the Angel of Death it may be necessary, *in extremis*, to change the name and thus the fate of the patient. In the Middle Ages the name might be chosen by lot or by randomly finding a name in the Bible whereas in more modern times the change of name was usually to one associated with life, health or old age, such as Chaim or Alter.[66] Change of name was also used for childless couples wishing to have children and for those parents whose previous children had died. The ritual for such a name change can be found in many contemporary Jewish prayer books. The angelic name Rafael, shares the same Hebrew root as *refuah*, medicine, and is thus an auspicious name for health or for inscription on an amulet. Many of these amulets carry the numerical equivalents of holy words because of what is seen as the intrinsic holiness of the Hebrew letters.

There are passages in the Torah the recitation or inscription of which can be efficacious in treating illness. Particularly popular are talismans from the *Book of Psalms*. The entire *Book of Psalms* was considered as a potent protection against danger whereas Psalm 121 is used especially for protecting women after childbirth and Psalm 91, using either the first or last letters of each verse, is for general protection.[67] Charms and incantations remained popular in Jewish traditional medicine, especially for the treatment of eye disease, headache and epilepsy.[68]

The early modern period

The migration of Jewish physicians during the sixteenth to eighteenth centuries, many with an Iberian background and trained in Italian medical schools such as Padua and Pisa, brought modern medicine into the Ottoman Empire. These Jewish doctors filled an important gap in the numbers of physicians in the area and records indicate that they formed a larger proportion of the population than the number of Jewish inhabitants might have indicated.[69]

During this period there was a wide variety of medication available, whether of animal, vegetable or mineral material, mostly based on locally available products. One such, a potion made from almond milk, honey and roses, was popular among Jerusalem's Jews. Rabbi Rafael Mordekhai Malkhi, who arrived in Jerusalem from Italy in 1676, mentions many items in his writings.[70] He noted that the potion of almond milk, honey and roses could cause diarrhoea and suggested the use of sweet wine with sugar. However, he expressed his concern about the poor quality of medication on offer and noted that much of what was available to the Jewish population was based on superstition.[71] A poultice for the eyes was made from dried plums and seedless raisins cooked with some spices such as cinnamon, ginger or rose water. Malkhi's grandson, Rabbi David de Silva, describes some compounds in a chapter entitled *Pri Megaddim*, choice fruit, in his work *Pri Hadas*. De Silva includes about 200 items in his pharmacopoeia, which Amar notes shows similarities with works from Hippocrates and the early modern period, as well as contemporary popular medicines.[72] At the same time the baths and hot springs at Tiberias were restored during the sixteenth century and thousands of Jewish, Muslim and Christian pilgrims came to enjoy the curative power of the waters.[73]

While modern medicine developed rapidly, especially in western countries during the eighteenth and nineteenth centuries, much of the new knowledge remained out of the reach of most of the population usually because of cost. At the same time there was little popular understanding of the pathology or physiology of disease and many could easily be fooled by exaggerated claims of effectiveness. Consequently, a market grew from the seventeenth and eighteenth centuries in Britain and North America for commercial medications supplied by apothecaries, as well as by untrained and unlicensed providers of patent medicine.

Patent medicines were marketed effectively and their popularity can be gauged by the existence of over 1000 such products by 1830. British products dominated the international market until well into the nineteenth century. Many of the suppliers of these medicines were known as quacks, usually described as someone who pretends to have qualifications that they do not possess, and often called medical charlatans. In the late eighteenth century a couple of Jewish quack doctors in Britain tested the boundaries of orthodox medicine by providing both patent medicine and obtaining genuine medical qualifications.[74]

They were aware that a university degree could enhance the value of their practice and used the lax regulations of Marischal College at Aberdeen University to obtain medical degrees *in absentia,* with affidavits provided by *bona fide* medical practitioners, as at this time only the Scottish universities were open to Jews. The University was alarmed at the award of their medical qualifications to medical charlatans, but in an era where there was difficulty in drawing a clear line between the dispensing practice of a properly qualified practitioner and the sales practices of unregistered medicine traders there was little that they could do.

William Brodum, known also as the Empiric Brodum, had a stall at Covent Garden selling his Botanic Syrup. Brodum had courted official notoriety, and considerable financial success, with his book *A Guide to Old Age: A Cure for the Indiscretions of Youth*. His rival, Samuel Solomon, was born in Cork in 1745, the younger son of the minister to the Jewish community there. Solomon had also made a fortune from sales of his *Guide to Health* and his patent medicine Cordial Balm of Gilead. The Cordial Balm cost the enormous sum for the period of 33/– (£1.65) and was essentially a mixture of brandy and a concoction of various herbs, and was claimed to cure virtually every disease but was especially valuable for sexual disorders. Solomon's financial success was recognised in Liverpool where a number of streets were named after him and his medication.

The boundaries were to be tested further by the practices of the Jewish Levenston family who were active in Glasgow, but also other British centres, during much of the nineteenth century.[75-77] Michael Jacob Levenston and his sons were already involved in medical herbalism by the 1840s. Claiming to be medical qualified they were forced to drop pretensions to medical degrees once the General Medical Council began licensing procedures in 1859. They had an extensive pharmacopoeia of British and American remedies of the type that were much in demand at the time. While Michael and his sons continued to trade in herbal medicine, one son, Samuel, entered Glasgow University obtaining the MD degree in 1859, though he had previously practised as a medical botanist claiming a non-existent medical qualification. Though medically qualified Samuel was struck off the Medical Register in 1877 by the General Medical Council regulations for advertising and selling patent medicines and, despite appealing in 1881, he was never reinstated.

Contemporary Jewish popular medicine

Judaism's approach to healing is illuminated in the traditional centuries old *MiSheberach* prayer for healing which is said when someone is ill. The prayer calls for a 'complete healing' (*refuah shleimah*) which includes a 'healing of body' (*refuat ha-guf*) and a 'healing of spirit' (*refuat ha-nefesh*). It is understood that this is no guarantee of a cure but gives patient, family and community voice to their belief that the course of the illness will reach a favourable outcome. Prayer is naturally a familiar source for achieving a cure and, even in modern times, despite studies of prayer effectiveness producing negative results, it retains its popularity as evidenced by the existence of websites such as www.jewishinghealing.com. Many believe that prayer can aid in recovery, due not just to divine influence but also to the psychological and physical benefits to a person who knows that he or she is being prayed for. The increase in morale may thus aid recovery. Many studies have suggested that prayer can reduce physical stress and that 'the psychological benefits of prayer may help reduce stress and anxiety, promote a more positive outlook, and strengthen the will to live'. The rise of the pietistic Hasidic movement in eastern Europe in the eighteenth century, with its veneration of leaders, known as *Zaddikim*, led to a belief in the power of the *Zaddik* to cure the sick.

It should not be thought that traditional Jewish medicine has disappeared in the modern period with its emphasis on scientific progress and evidence-based procedures. Customs common in eastern Europe a century ago, such as placing pigeons on the abdomen of a jaundiced patient, have become common practice in Israel among all sectors of the population.[78] Popular adherence to the use of amulets and charms has persisted even among contemporary Jews. These amulets are often made of stone or metal to be worn by the patient and, over the past few years, it has been observed that there has been an increasing tendency for the use of amulets in Israeli hospitals. A study of parents of children admitted to a paediatric intensive care unit in Zerifin (Sarafand), Israel showed that around a third of Jewish families used such amulets, claiming that it reduced parental anxiety and warned medical staff to respect the emotional and psychological value that they represent.[79] Such people find the contact with the healer to be of value even if he fails to bring a cure. Moslem patients in Israel also made use of healing charms, many of Jewish origin with Hebrew lettering, reflecting a tradition dating back to mediaeval times. Amulets have persisted despite almost universal opposition through the ages by rabbis and Jewish physicians who consistently described their use as irrational and superstitious.

Of course, religious Jews have long regarded positively the value of prayer, whether by the reciting of Psalms or the direct blessing of the patient, and as we have seen there remained a strand within the rabbinic leadership that preferred to see healing in divine hands without negating the value of medical interventions. In extreme cases, which I have witnessed myself on a couple of occasions, the name of a seriously sick person was changed in an attempt to thwart the evil designs of the Angel of Death.

Given the survival of these customs, and an increasingly pervasive concern about the direction of modern medicine, it is not surprising to record the continuing use of traditional practices. In recent years studies have indicated the use of medicinal plants among the rural population of Israel and within the country's ethnic groups, especially those from such countries as Iraq, Iran and Yemen. These substances, usually obtained from local rather than imported products, are considered to be based on the Galenic tradition and adapted to an Arabic and Moslem form during the Middle Ages. The contemporary emphasis on modern therapeutics has modified this tradition but not eliminated it.

Lev and Amar have identified animal, mineral and especially plant products used in the modern Israeli popular medicine market.[80] They found well over 200 plant products in common usage. While enumeration of all the products is beyond the scope of this article many will be familiar to those who would keep a supply of simple herbal home remedies for minor ailments not thought sufficiently important to call on the services of a physician. Thus, there are such common vegetables as onion, cauliflower and garlic, cereals such as oats, and herbs and spices such as tarragon, wormwood, cumin, cloves and dill. Hyssop oil is used for backache, clove oil for toothache and rosemary remains a popular remedy for kidney stones, while the use of the seed of the emetic nut *Strychnos nux vomica*, substantially having the properties of the poison strychnine, is used for its stimulant action on the gastrointestinal tract, for itch and for inflammations of the external ear. In chronic constipation it is often combined with cascara and other laxatives to good effect. The list of products includes only cultivated plants. Wild plants are still gathered by healers and patients but they are not commonly sold in the traditional shops.

The 20 animal products include such substances as beeswax and honey used for burns, eye inflammation and coughs, but also deer horn employed as a general tonic and for drug addiction. Musk oil and grain is used for high blood sugar while snail operculum, from the shell lid, deals with the evil eye. There were fewer than 20 mineral products available, many, such as clay, earth, sulphur and ferrous citrate, known also as green vitriol, used to treat skin problems. Galena, otherwise known as lead sulphide but often containing silver admixtures, antimony and zinc products, is used for eye problems. Apart from sulphur the most frequent mineral prescribed was alum, long known to have antibacterial properties and used in modern deodorants, is not only used as a disinfectant but also to reduce liver size and as a general tonic. Nevertheless, Lev and Amar relate that the commercial field for the sale of traditional medicines in Israel is declining and businesses have closed and the inventory of medicines has diminished.[80] Their work in documenting the decline of this sector is a window into the mediaeval world, using philology, comparisons across Levantine cultures and comparisons with Biblical and Talmudic medicine.

If commercial popular medicine is fighting for survival against the current fads for modern alternative medicines, one Jewish folk remedy still seems to hold sway. From Talmudic times rabbis such as Rabbi Abba used chicken soup as a remedy (Figure 11.7).[81] Maimonides stated that chicken soup is an excellent food suitable for those convalescing from illness and fattening those who have lost weight due to illness, finding it beneficial for those with asthma while noting that it helps the chronic fevers that develop from white bile.[82-84] Chicken soup is not without its risks: hypernatraemia and anaphylaxis have been recorded and one child has been recorded as choking on a chicken bone that lodged in his bronchus while drinking unstrained chicken soup.[85,86] Nevertheless, Ohry and Tsafrir,[85] Rosner[86] and Lieberman[87] all conclude that the medical uses of chicken soup are part of the armamentarium of successful traditional remedies.

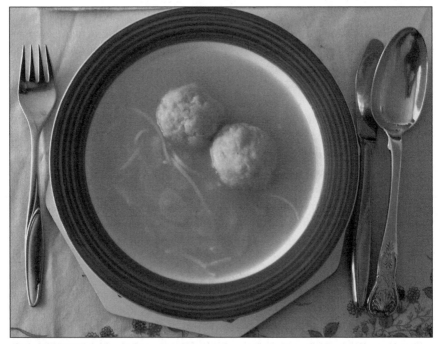

Figure 11.7 A bowl of chicken soup – sometimes called 'Jewish penicillin' – is traditionally served with *lokshen* (noodles) and *kneidlach* (matzoh balls). (Courtesy of Marion Woolf.)

Conclusion

The subject of Jewish medicine has a long history described in literature stretching back to the Biblical period. The practice reflects the Biblical and Talmudic period with additions reflecting the encounter between Jews and their Christian and Moslem neighbours over 1500 years of the diaspora. The resurgence of interest in medical botany and herbalism in recent years has encouraged further study of the content and practice of popular medicine in its widest context and has emphasised its cross-cultural nature. Even the spells, charms and incantations of an earlier era still find their echo today and might claim a place in the search for cure as long as patients are given recourse to the evidence-based medicine that they require for recovery.

References

1. Bermant C. *The Jews*. London: Sphere Books, 1978: 138.
2. Matras H. *Jewish Folk Medicine in the 19th and 20th Centuries*. Tel Aviv: Beit Hatfutsot, 1995: 113–135.
3. Matras H. *Jewish Folk Medicine in the 19th and 20th Centuries*. Tel Aviv: Beit Hatfutsot, 1995: 122.
4. II *Kings*, 3:15; I *Samuel* 16:16.
5. Epstein I (ed., trans.). *The Talmud. Commentary on Tractate Pesachim, Babylonian Talmud*. London: Soncino Press, 1981: 56a.
6. Rosner F (ed., trans.). *Julius Preuss' Biblical and Talmudic Medicine*. New York: Sanhedrin Press, 1978: 433.
7. Epstein I (ed., trans.). *The Talmud. Shabbat 67a and Hullin 77b, Babylonian Talmud*. London: Soncino Press, 1981.
8. *Tosefta Shabbat*, VII, VIII (Hebrew).
9. Lev E, Amar Z. *Practical Materia Medica of the Eastern Mediterranean According to the Cairo Genizah*. Leiden: Brill, 2008: 511.
10. Rosner F (ed., trans.). *Julius Preuss' Biblical and Talmudic Medicine*. New York: Sanhedrin Press, 1978: 435.
11. Epstein I (ed., trans.). *The Talmud: Niddah 30b, Babylonian Talmud*. London: Soncino Press, 1981.
12. Epstein I (ed., trans.). *The Talmud: Shabbat 109b, Babylonian Talmud*. London: Soncino Press, 1981.
13. Epstein I (ed., trans.). *The Talmud: Shabbat 108b, Babylonian Talmud*. London: Soncino Press, 1981.
14. Epstein I (ed., trans.). *The Talmud: Yoma 78a, Babylonian Talmud*. London: Soncino Press, 1981.
15. *Tosefta Shabbat* 12:13 (Hebrew).
16. Epstein I (ed., trans.). *The Talmud: Ketubot 77b, Babylonian Talmud*. London: Soncino Press, 1981.
17. Epstein I (ed., trans.). *The Talmud: Shabbat 66b, Babylonian Talmud*. London: Soncino Press, 1981.
18. Epstein I (ed., trans.). *The Talmud: Baba Batra 74b, Babylonian Talmud*. London: Soncino Press, 1981.
19. Epstein I (ed., trans.). *The Talmud: Yoma 8b, Babylonian Talmud*. London: Soncino Press, 1981.
20. Epstein I (ed., trans.). *The Talmud: Shabbat 109b, Babylonian Talmud*. London: Soncino Press, 1981.

21. Shabbat 14:14d, *Jerusalem Talmud* (Hebrew).

22. Epstein I (ed., trans.). *The Talmud: Shabbat 40b, Babylonian Talmud*. London: Soncino Press, 1981.

23. Epstein I (ed., trans.). *The Talmud: Malachi 3:20. Nedarim 108b, Babylonian Talmud*. London: Soncino Press, 1981.

24. Freedman H, Simon M (eds, trans.). *The Midrash*. London: Soncino Press, 1977. See Exodus *Rabbah* 30:22; *Ecclesiastes Rabbah* 5:6.

25. Sifra on Leviticus 16:1 (Hebrew).

26. Epstein I (ed., trans.). *The Talmud: Nedarim 49a, Babylonian Talmud*. London: Soncino Press, 1981.

27. Rosner F (ed., trans.). *Julius Preuss' Biblical and Talmudic Medicine*. New York: Sanhedrin Press, 1978: 441.

28. Epstein I (ed., trans.). *The Talmud: Avodah Zarah 38b and Gittin 70a, Babylonian Talmud*. London: Soncino Press, 1981.

29. Epstein I (ed., trans.). *The Talmud: Shabbat 128a/b, Babylonian Talmud*. London: Soncino Press, 1981.

30. Trachtenberg J. *Jewish Magic and Superstition: A study in folk religion*. New York: Atheneum Press, 1970: 198.

31. *Jewish Encyclopaedia*, Vol 8. New York: Funk & Wagnalls, 1925: 417. Available at: www.jewishencyclopedia.com (accessed 30 April 2009).

32. Zimmels HJ. Magicians, *Theologians and Doctors: Studies in folk-medicine and folk-lore as reflected in the rabbinic Responsa (12th to 19th Centuries)*. London: Edward Goldston & Son, 1952: 193–4.

33. Rivers WHR. *Medicine, Magic and Religion*. Fitzpatrick Lectures. London: Royal College of Physicians, 1924: 1915–16. (*London International Library of Psychology, Philosophy and Scientific Method* 1924;7:51.)

34. *Jewish Encyclopaedia*, Vol 5. New York: Funk & Wagnalls, 1925: 426–7. Available at: www.jewishencyclopedia.com (accessed 30 April 2009).

35. Trachtenberg J. *Jewish Magic and Superstition: A study in folk religion*. New York: Atheneum Press, 1970: 197.

36. Matras H. *Jewish Folk Medicine in the 19th and 20th Centuries*. Tel Aviv: Beit Hatfutsot. 1995, 123.

37. Trachtenberg J. *Jewish Magic and Superstition: A study in folk religion*. New York: Atheneum Press, 1970: 200.

38. Metzger T, Metzger M. *Jewish Life in the Middle Ages: Illuminated Hebrew manuscripts of the thirteenth to sixteenth centuries*. Fribourg, Switzerland: Chartwell Books, 1982: 174.

39. Metzger T, Metzger M. *Jewish Life in the Middle Ages: Illuminated Hebrew manuscripts of the thirteenth to sixteenth centuries*. Fribourg, Switzerland: Chartwell Books, 1982: 195.

40. Zimmels HJ. *Magicians, Theologians and Doctors: Studies in folk-medicine and folk-lore as reflected in the Rabbinic Responsa (12th to 19th centuries)*. London: Edward Goldston & Son, 1952: 124.

41. Metzger T, Metzger M. *Jewish Life in the Middle Ages: Illuminated Hebrew manuscripts of the thirteenth to sixteenth centuries*. Fribourg, Switzerland: Chartwell Books, 1982: 173.

42. Zimmels HJ. *Magicians, Theologians and Doctors: Studies in folk-medicine and folk-lore as reflected in the Rabbinic Responsa (12th to 19th centuries)*. London: Edward Goldston & Son, 1952: 132.

43. Lev E, Amar Z. *Practical Materia Medica of the Eastern Mediterranean According to the Cairo Genizah*. Leiden: Brill, 2008: 511.

44. Trachtenberg J. *Jewish Magic and Superstition: A study in folk religion*. New York: Atheneum Press, 1970: 207.

45. Lansky EP, Paavilainen, HM, Pawlus AD, Newman RA. *Ficus* spp. (fig): Ethnobotany and potential as anticancer and anti-inflammatory agents. *J Ethnopharmacol* 2008: 119:195–213.

46. Lev E, Amar Z. *Practical Materia Medica of the Eastern Mediterranean According to the Cairo Genizah*. Leiden: Brill, 2008: 510.

47. Lev E, Amar Z. *Practical Materia Medica of the Eastern Mediterranean According to the Cairo Genizah*. Leiden: Brill, 2008: 207.

48. Spiegel D, Harrington A. What is the placebo worth? *BMJ* 2008;**336**:967–8.

49. Paavilainen H. Psychoactive plants in Maimonides' Regimen Sanitatis and de Causis Accidentium, Korot. *Israel J Hist Med Sci* 2007;**18**:25–54.

50. Leibowitz JO, Marcus S (eds, trans.). *Sefer Hanisyonot: The Book of Medical Experiences*. Attributed to Ibn Ezra, *Medical Theory, Rational and Magical Therapy: A Study in Medievalism*. Jerusalem: Magnes Press, 1984.

51. Leibowitz JO, Marcus S (eds, trans.). *Sefer Hanisyonot: The Book of Medical Experiences*. Attributed to Ibn Ezra, *Medical Theory, Rational and Magical Therapy: A Study in Medievalism*. Jerusalem: Magnes Press, 1984: 137.

52. Leibowitz JO, Marcus S (eds, trans.). *Sefer Hanisyonot: The Book of Medical Experiences*. Attributed to Ibn Ezra, *Medical Theory, Rational and Magical Therapy: A Study in Medievalism*. Jerusalem: Magnes Press, 1984: 147.

53. Leibowitz JO, Marcus S (eds, trans.). *Sefer Hanisyonot: The Book of Medical Experiences*. Attributed to Ibn Ezra, *Medical Theory, Rational and Magical Therapy: A Study in Medievalism*. Jerusalem: Magnes Press, 1984: 171.

54. Leibowitz JO, Marcus S (eds, trans.). *Sefer Hanisyonot: The Book of Medical Experiences*. Attributed to Ibn Ezra, *Medical Theory, Rational and Magical Therapy: A Study in Medievalism*. Jerusalem: Magnes Press, 1984: 181.

55. Leibowitz JO, Marcus S (eds, trans.). *Sefer Hanisyonot: The Book of Medical Experiences*. Attributed to Ibn Ezra, *Medical Theory, Rational and Magical Therapy: A Study in Medievalism*. Jerusalem: Magnes Press, 1984: 213.

56. Leibowitz JO, Marcus S (eds, trans.). *Sefer Hanisyonot: The Book of Medical Experiences*. Attributed to Ibn Ezra, *Medical Theory, Rational and Magical Therapy: A Study in Medievalism*. Jerusalem: Magnes Press, 1984: 148, 183.

57. Trachtenberg J. *Jewish Magic and Superstition: A study in folk religion*. New York: Atheneum Press, 1970: 204.

58. Trachtenberg J. *Jewish Magic and Superstition: A study in folk religion*. New York: Atheneum Press, 1970: 201.

59. Trachtenberg J. *Jewish Magic and Superstition: A study in folk religion*. New York: Atheneum Press, 1970: 204.

60. Zimmels HJ. *Magicians, Theologians and Doctors: Studies in folk-medicine and folk-lore as reflected in the Rabbinic Responsa (12th to 19th centuries)*. London: Edward Goldston & Son, 1952: 141.

61. Zimmels HJ. *Magicians, Theologians and Doctors: Studies in folk-medicine and folk-lore as reflected in the Rabbinic Responsa (12th to 19th centuries)*. London: Edward Goldston & Son, 1952: 147.

62. Trachtenberg J. *Jewish Magic and Superstition: A study in folk religion*. New York: Atheneum Press, 1970: 201.

63. Trachtenberg J. *Jewish Magic and Superstition: A study in folk religion*. New York: Atheneum Press, 1970: 202.

64. Matras H. *Jewish Folk Medicine in the 19th and 20th Centuries*. Tel Aviv: Beit Ha-tfutsot, 1995: 118–119.

65. Epstein I (ed., trans.). *The Talmud: Rosh Hashanah 16b, Babylonian Talmud*. London: Soncino Press, 1981.

66. Trachtenberg J. *Jewish Magic and Superstition: A study in folk religion*. New York: Atheneum Press, 1970: 205.

67. Matras H. *Jewish Folk Medicine in the 19th and 20th Centuries*. Tel Aviv: Beit Ha-tfutsot, 1995: 120.

68. Zimmels HJ. *Magicians, Theologians and Doctors: Studies in folk-medicine and folk-lore as reflected in the Rabbinic Responsa (12th to 19th centuries)*. London: Edward Goldston & Son, 1952: 140 .

69. Amar Z. *The History of Medicine in Jerusalem*. BAR International Series 1032. Oxford: Archaeopress, 2002: 116–19.

70. Benayahu M. *Medical Works of Rabbi Rafael Mordekhai Malkhi*. Jerusalem: AI Weinberg Ltd, 1985 (Hebrew).

71. Singer A. Ottoman Palestine 1516–1800: Health, disease and historical sources. In: Wasserman M, Kottek SS (eds), *Health and Disease in the Holy Land: Studies in the history and sociology of medicine from ancient times to the present*. Lampeter: Edward Mellen Press, 1996: 200.

72. Amar Z. *The History of Medicine in Jerusalem*. BAR International Series 1032. Oxford: Archaeopress, 2002: 117.

73. Singer A. Ottoman Palestine 1516–1800: Health, disease and historical sources. In: Wasserman M, Kottek SS (eds), *Health and Disease in the Holy Land: Studies in the history and sociology of medicine from ancient times to the present*. Lampeter: Edward Mellen Press, 1996: 202.

74. Collins K. *Go and Learn: the international story of Jews and medicine in Scotland 1739–1945*. Aberdeen: Aberdeen University Press, 1987: 37–41.

75. Collins K. *Be Well! Jewish immigrant health and welfare in Glasgow 1860–1920*. East Linton: Tuckwell Press, 2001: 141–6.

76. General Council of Medical Education and Registration of the United Kingdom. Minutes. London: WJ Goldbourn, 1877: 37, 106, 231.

77. *Medical Times and Gazette*. London: J&A Churchill, 1881: II: 478–80.

78. Matras H. *The History of Medicine in Jerusalem*. BAR International Series 1032. Oxford: Archaeopress, 2002: 129.

79. Barr J, Berkovitch M, Matras H, Greenberg R, Eshel G. Talismans and amulets in the pediatric intensive care unit: Legendary powers in contemporary medicine. *Israel Med Assoc J* 2000;**2**:278–81.

80. Lev E, Amar Z. Ethnopharmacological survey of traditional drugs sold in Israel at the end of the 20th century. *J Ethnopharmacol* 2000;**72**:191–205 .

81. Epstein I (ed., trans.). *The Talmud: Shabbat 145b, Babylonian Talmud*. London: Soncino Press, 1981.

82. Rosner F (trans.). *The Medical Aphorisms of Moses Maimonides*. Haifa: Maimonides Research Unit, 1989: 293–312.

83. Rosner F (trans.). *Moses Maimonides Treatise on Asthma*. Haifa: Maimonides Research Unit, 1994: 176.

84. Rosner F. *Encyclopaedia of Medicine in the Bible and Talmud*. Northvale, NJ: Jason Aronson, 2000: 74–5.

85. Ohry A, Tsafrir J. Is chicken soup an essential drug? *Can Med Assoc J* 1999;**161**:1532–3.

86. Leiberman A, Bar-Ziv J. Unstrained chicken soup [letter]. *Chest* 1980;**77**:128.

87. Rosner F. Therapeutic efficacy of chicken soup. *Chest* 1980;**78**:672–4.

88. Rosner F. Its uncanny (letter). *Can Med Assoc J* 1980;**162**:973.

Index